Artificial Intelligence Platform for Molecular Targeted Therapy

A Translational Science Approach

Artificial Intelligence Platform for Molecular Targeted Therapy

A Translational Science Approach

Ariel Fernández

Former Karl F. Hasselmann Endowed Chair Professor of Bioengineering,
Rice University, USA

Daruma Institute for Artificial Intelligence in Pharmaceutical Research,
AF Innovation Pharma Consultancy, North Carolina, USA

INQUISUR/CONICET/UNS, Argentina

CONICET, The Argentine National Research Council, Buenos Aires, Argentina

World Scientific

NEW JERSEY • LONDON • SINGAPORE • BEIJING • SHANGHAI • HONG KONG • TAIPEI • CHENNAI • TOKYO

Published by

World Scientific Publishing Co. Pte. Ltd.
5 Toh Tuck Link, Singapore 596224
USA office: 27 Warren Street, Suite 401-402, Hackensack, NJ 07601
UK office: 57 Shelton Street, Covent Garden, London WC2H 9HE

Library of Congress Cataloging-in-Publication Data
Names: Fernández, Ariel, 1957– author.
Title: Artificial intelligence platform for molecular targeted therapy :
a translational science approach / Ariel Fernández, Daruma Institute, Argentina &
AF Innovation, USA & CONICET-National Research Council, Argentina.
Description: First edition. | New Jersey : World Scientific, [2021] |
Includes bibliographical references and index.
Identifiers: LCCN 2020057455 | ISBN 9789811232305 (hardcover) |
ISBN 9789811232312 (ebook) | ISBN 9789811232329 (ebook other)
Subjects: LCSH: Drugs--Design. | Drug development. | Artificial intelligence. | Molecular dynamics.
Classification: LCC RS420 .F47 2021 | DDC 615.1/9--dc23
LC record available at https://lccn.loc.gov/2020057455

British Library Cataloguing-in-Publication Data
A catalogue record for this book is available from the British Library.

For any available supplementary material, please visit
https://www.worldscientific.com/worldscibooks/10.1142/12160#t=suppl

Typeset by Stallion Press
Email: enquiries@stallionpress.com

In loving memory of Haydée Stigliano, my mother.

We are lucky to live in a time when revolutions based on physical, chemical, and biological methods enabled us to isolate, make, visualize and begin to understand the function of biological molecules and to explore opportunities emerging from these discoveries for medicine and pharmacology. The century of visualization of molecules began in the year 1912 with von Laue's X-ray diffraction experiments of crystals at the Universität München, followed by structure determinations of simple inorganic crystals by the Braggs, father and son, at the University of Cambridge, UK. The method was developed further by Max Perutz and others for the analysis of the three-dimensional atomic structures of biological molecules and has, with the help of new instruments and methods, revolutionized natural sciences and medicine.

With amazement we experienced in the past few decades the advent of a second revolution in the vision of molecules by utilizing the wide spectrum of radiation beyond X-rays, radiowaves and visible light and by employing particle diffraction, including electrons and neutrons. With the recent advance in understanding the rules which govern macromolecular structures guided by the dizzying mass of experimental data and the growing computer power we may approach the holy grail of biology: the reliable prediction of structures of biological molecules from sequence. I hope to see it happening. Meanwhile, I strive as I assist pharmacology with drug design and modeling of ligand-target interfaces, being aware that targets may rearrange upon ligand binding, that receptors may have floppy binding sites and that targets may attain activity only within the assembly of a multi-component complex. Another fascinating problem is the role of non-matching symmetry and frustration in chaperonin function as a folding catalyst.

These problems reach beyond the classical sequence-structure conundrum but are essential for structure-based drug development. This book addresses these imperatives and opens avenues of research and discovery for structural biologists who may find it very rewarding and of assistance in solving their problems.

Robert Huber
Nobel Laureate

Foreword

AI is taking the world by storm, and this book will help to pave the way for serious applications of AI in drug design. Ariel Fernández has extensive experience in the field including multiple patents based on his work on wrapping technology. He integrates this experience with leading AI software platforms to show how they can be used in drug design. The book will be essential reading for anyone involved in drug design and in biochemistry more broadly.

AI research began in the mid-1950's with a focus on some of the most daunting questions regarding humans, machines, and their interactions. One example is the question of how children learn a language. Thus "learning theory" emerged as a significant discipline in computer science. Techniques developed in subsequent research now allow machines to learn how to read license plates and addresses on letters, to understand your voice on phone calls, to recognize faces on the street, and much, much more.

A natural evolution in AI is thus to try to learn how to do drug design, despite the fact that humans have not yet broken the code. This is therefore a significant reach. It took AI years to do mundane tasks like character recognition that humans regularly do. But the advent of the big data era has raised expectations of AI, and it is natural to hope that AI can begin to do things better than humans. Many claims in this direction have been made.

One example of an AI challenge in drug design is to determine the three-dimensional structure of a protein from its one-dimensional amino acid residue sequence. This is still a work in progress, but the progress made so far is remarkable. Thus it is natural to look for further ways in which AI can aid in drug design.

But there is a need, especially in drug design, not just to solve a problem but to understand how it is solved. Knowing how is an essential first step to avoiding side effects. This requirement connects with an important theme in AI. For some, AI provides a way to understand how humans do what they do, e.g., in language acquisition. This book will help in this direction, since it links AI techniques with clear physical principles, sometimes lacking in protein folding methodology. One challenge addressed here is to use AI to include a more accurate physical context.

There is significant pressure in all fields to see what benefits AI can bring to improve conventional thinking. This book initiates a discussion of AI in drug design that will help a broad range of people assess what AI can do for the field.

Ridgway Scott
Professor Emeritus
University of Chicago

About the Author

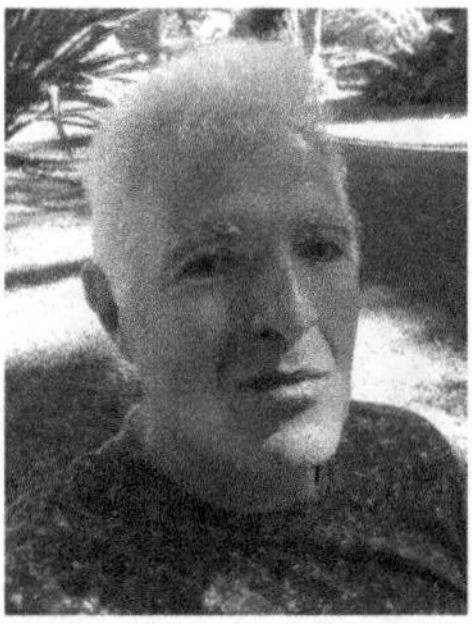

Ariel Fernández (born Ariel Fernández Stigliano) is an Argentine-American physical chemist and mathematician. He obtained a Ph.D. degree in Chemical Physics from Yale University and held the Hasselmann Endowed Chair Professorship in Bioengineering at Rice University until his retirement. He also held a faculty appointment at The University of Chicago, in the Computer Science Department. To date, he has published over 400 scientific papers in professional journals including *PNAS*, *Physical Review Letters*, *Nature*, *Nature Biotechnology*, *Genome Research* and *Genome Biology*. Fernández has also authored five books in biophysics and molecular medicine and holds several patents on biotechnological innovations. He is currently involved in research and entrepreneurial activities. Since 2018 Fernández heads the Daruma Institute, the research arm of AF Innovation, a Pharma Consultancy based in Argentina and the USA.

Preface

"To a man with a hammer everything looks like a nail."

Mark Twain

"To be is to be encoded."

Ariel Fernández

This book approaches drug design and, more broadly, molecular targeted therapy, through the translation of fundamental advances in biophysics and physical chemistry. The translation is enabled and leveraged by artificial intelligence (AI), which becomes instrumental as complex biological contexts need to be modeled or recreated.

Chapter 1 introduces AI in a heuristic fashion, delineating the basic architectures, operative work flows and free open-source software libraries for deep learning systems and their underlying convolutional neural networks (CNNs).

Chapter 2 introduces interfacial physics as required to provide a representational framework to be integrated in the software library of a CNN. The chapter lays the groundwork for AI-leveraged engineering of drug-target interfaces.

Chapter 3 presents a first illustration of the power of AI to handle biological complexity at molecular scales: Through AI, an *in vivo* context capable of expediting the protein folding process is recreated. Thus, *in vivo* folding pathways are generated and validated vis-à-vis experimental evidence on the converging state of the chain.

Chapter 4 explores functional genomics databases from the vantage point of epistructural biology, the conceptual framework introduced in Chapter 2 to enable the implementation of AI methods. Equipped with the conceptual and representational arsenal described, the chapter delineates an AI platform to infer amyloidogenic propensity at a genome-wide level.

Chapter 5 introduces an evolutionary axis to epistructural biology, needed to develop drug selectivity filters capable of telling apart paralogous proteins and avoiding off-target paralogs. The chapter emphasizes that the protein-water interface constitutes a unique marker for molecular evolution. This fact endows epistructural biology with a vantage point to explore the evolutionary axis, which is essential to understand and manipulate biological phenomena.

Chapter 6 delineates biological function from the perspective of epistructural biology and assesses the functional impact of molecular targeted therapy guided by AI-empowered epistructural design.

Chapter 7 illustrates the power of epistructure-based selectivity filters in AI-assisted drug design.

Chapter 8 introduces molecular targeted therapies that get redesigned to effectively synergize with cancer immunotherapies. The empowerment of the latter is guided by epistructural AI-leveraged design.

Chapter 9 deals with choreographed synergies between targeted therapy and immunotherapy guided by AI. The goal is to leverage cancer evolution as it evades the elicited immune response, thereby steering the tumor towards its annihilation with the aid of AI. In this chapter, a symbolic regression is carried out by AI, exploiting the scaling symmetry of the time-dependent data.

Chapter 10 deals with the possibility of leveraging AI to empower molecular dynamics (MD), whose true potential remains largely untested because relevant timescales are often beyond reach and infrequent events of direct relevance to biophysical processes are missed. We apply deep learning to a) encode the dynamics into a simplified embodiment that retains only essential topological features of the vector field that steers MD integration, b) propagate the simplified trajectory beyond the timescales accessible to atomistic MD, and c) reconstruct the coarse grained trajectory back at the atomistic level. Thus, AI constructs a generative model that provides hierarchical understanding of MD simulation while enabling access to realistic timescales and the capture of physically meaningful rare events.

Chapter 11 deals with rational drug design in the absence of reported structure for the therapeutic target and information on its regulation. This chapter delineates the leveraging of AI to steer the engineering of molecular targeted therapy in such challenging situations. The chapter focuses specifically on protein associations, where drug-based disruption of dysfunctional complexes poses a major challenge to targeted therapy. The problem becomes daunting when the structure and regulated modulation of the complex are unknown. To address the challenge, we leverage an AI platform that learns from epistructural information and infers regulation-susceptible regions that also generate interfacial tension between protein and water, thereby promoting contextually tuned protein associations. The AI-empowered discovery platform is benchmarked against a PDB-derived testing set and validated against experimental data.

Chapter 12 implements a deep learning (DL) platform that teaches drugs to target proteins. This is accomplished by introducing modifications in chemical scaffolds guided by *a priori* predictions of drug-induced binding-competent conformations of the intended target. In this way, we deal with the fact that target proteins are usually not fixed targets fitting a lock-key paradigm: they structurally adapt to ligands in ways that need to be predicted to empower drug discovery. In contrast with protein folding predictors that do not include disorder propensities as input, the neural network presented solves a "drug-induced folding problem" by incorporating as input sequence-derived signals for structural disorder. The DL system thus predicts conformations in floppy regions of the target protein that rely on associations with a conformation-selecting purposely designed drug to acquire and maintain their structural integrity. This is tantamount to generate within an AI-empowered drug discovery platform the *a-priori* drug-induced folding ensemble without committing to a specific ligand and then steer the modification of a lead compound to select a specific drug-induced conformation from within the ensemble.

Finally, based on the knowledge accrued from the 12 chapters, the Epilogue assesses the plausibility of a futuristic scenario where AI develops its own pattern-based physics.

As Ray Kurzweil would have it, computer technologies are entering a dramatic phase in their exponential development. In the next two decades, a revolution like no other will tear apart the fabric of civilization, prompting us to enquire whether our own future will be entirely human. This book is squarely placed at the inception of this revolution. This unique juncture makes the book necessarily transitional, even provisional, but also hopefully prescient in its scope. It is meant to reach out to what is perhaps the last generation of humans endowed solely with a "wet" intelligence. The future has never been so inscrutable, and yet we are confident that this book will be part of it.

I would like to express my heartfelt thanks to the marvelous people who inspired me, helping me in many different — often unfathomable — ways to pursue this line of thought and bring it to fruition: Ridgway Scott, Oktay Sinanoglu (d), Manfred Eigen (d), Kent Wilson (d), María Ines Platzek, Robert Huber, Herschel Rabitz, Steve Berry (d), Stuart Rice, Joshua Jortner, Jianping Chen, Xi Zhang, Keith Dunker, Ya-Yue Van, Jianpeng Ma, Michael Deem, Sangtae Kim, Andrés Colubri ... I am sure I am leaving out important people, and for that, I apologize.

Last but not least, I would like to thank Joy Quek, senior editor at World Scientific, and her excellent team in Singapore, who made possible the production of this book, working with great diligence, skill and care.

Ariel Fernández
Winston-Salem, North Carolina, USA

Contents

Chapter 1

Propaedeutic to artificial intelligence

"The reasonable man adapts himself to the world, the unreasonable one persists in trying to adapt the world to himself. Therefore all progress depends on the unreasonable man."

George Bernard Shaw

We introduce AI at a fairly elementary level adopting a heuristic perspective. The presentation focuses mostly on machine learning and specifically on deep learning. The narrative is tailored to drug designers and developers seeking to accelerate the discovery cycle. Basic knowledge of linear algebra and some familiarity with Python programming is all that is required for the pharma researcher to follow the presentation in detail. A crucial distinction is delineated between standard well-established cheminformatics and pharmacoinformatics applications and AI deployed to empower the design of dynamic drug/target interfaces, the focus of the book. Thus, the chapter sets the tone for the remainder of the book which advocates the deployment of AI to tackle dynamic problems in drug design, including the incorporation, mimicking and simulation of *in vivo* settings. In so doing, the book introduces the arsenal of epistructural biology to provide the proper representational/conceptual framework that enables inference through the tensor flow of convolutional neural networks.

1.1 Primer on artificial intelligence and deep learning

Artificial intelligence (AI) refers to machines endowed with traits that humans perceive as intelligent, such as learning and problem solving [1]. Within this vast protean field, machine learning (ML) refers to the ability to learn without being explicitly programmed to do so, while deep learning (DL) refers to an automated extraction of features and patterns from arrayed data that gets sequentially represented through a hierarchy of abstractions organized in a multi-layered neural network (NN) [2–4]. Deep learning will be the aspect of AI that this book mostly deals with.

DL is supremely efficient at unraveling underlying features directly from data [2,5]. As in face recognition, features are hierarchically organized, so that large-scale patterns (eyes, noses, face shapes) emerge after several layers of abstraction from more rudimentary patterns (lines, curves, shades). The beauty and power of DL lies in the fact that the feature extraction process is unsupervised: the features emerge from the training of the system without any human input or bias, and represent the optimal performance of the network in regards to its ability to make accurate inferences. Time is ripe to plunge into DL and master the field. This is because

- we have vast amounts of biomedical data that require interpretation are easily and inexpensively stored,
- we have the right hardware, i.e. graphics processing units (GPUs) that are massively parallelizable, and
- we have adequate software such as TensorFlow (TF) that enables suitable modular coding if the data can be pixelized or voxelized into a tensorial array, be it a vector, a matrix or a tensor proper [3, 4].

The building block of NNs is obviously the neuron, referred to as *perceptron*, in computer science [5]. The perceptron enables forward propagation of information encoded in an array of inputs $x_1, x_2, \ldots, x_n$ weighted by parameters $w_1, w_2, \ldots, w_n$ to generate an output of the form $y = f(\sum_{i=1}^{n} x_i w_i + w_0)$ where w_0 may be regarded as a bias term and f is a nonlinear activation function, often a sigmoid

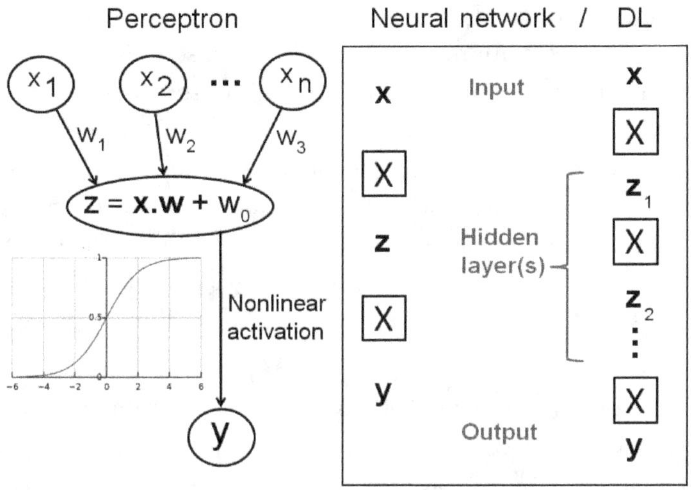

Figure 1.1. Scheme of the perceptron or neuron activation by linear transformation of input stimulus ($\boldsymbol{x}$) followed by nonlinear signal transmission as output y. The panels on the right show the organization of NNs with one and multiple hidden layers. The "boxed X" indicates full (dense) node connectivity between consecutive layers.

or sigmoid shaped, as shown in Fig. 1.1. The bias term enables to shift the activation function. In vector representation, we often write $y = f(z), z = \boldsymbol{x}.\boldsymbol{w} + w_0$, where $\boldsymbol{x}, \boldsymbol{w}$ are respectively input and weight vector. One can subsequently build a fully connected (dense) layer of perceptrons indexed by j, whereby $z_j = \boldsymbol{x}.\boldsymbol{w_j} + w_{0,j}$. The dense layer can be readily implemented in TF code, by simply specifying number of outputs/perceptrons [3, 4]. We usually refer to the vector of linearly transformed inputs z as "hidden layer", as it does not explicitly describe observables [5].

Hidden layers may be stacked as in DL architectures. Thus, for the *j-th* perceptron in the k-th hidden layer, we get $z_j^{(k)} = \sum_{i=1}^{n_{k-1}} y_i^{(k-1)} w_{ij}^{(k)} + w_{oj}^{(k)} = \sum_{i=1}^{n_{k-1}} f(z_i^{(k-1)}) w_{ij}^{(k)} + w_{oj}^{(k)}$. The sequential composition of the network by stacking hidden layers has a standardized script in TF that generates the propagation of information as specified by the equation above [3,4]. In a NN with K hidden layers, we may regard the output $y_j^{(K)} = f(\sum_{i=1}^{n_{K-1}} y_i^{(K-1)} w_{ij}^{(K)} + w_{oj}^{(K)})$ as an inference made by the DL system.

The accuracy of the DL inference represents the level of optimization of network performance and may be assessed vis-à-vis a training set of input/output paired data points. This assessment is often referred to as the *loss* of the network [2,5]. The loss is parametrically dependent on the full weight tensor $\boldsymbol{W} = [w^{(k)}_{i_{k-1}j_k}]_{k=1,\dots,K}$ which may contain a huge number of weights, in the thousands if not millions, depending on the size of the network. Thus, for DL NN with K hidden layers the loss function or empirical risk $J(\boldsymbol{W})$ becomes $J(\boldsymbol{W}) = |\Im|^{-1}\sum_{\xi\in\Im}\mathcal{L}(\boldsymbol{y}^{(K)}_{\xi}(\boldsymbol{W}),\boldsymbol{y}_{\boldsymbol{\xi}})$, where $\Im$ is the training set with number of elements $|\Im|$, $\boldsymbol{y}^{(K)}_{\xi}(\boldsymbol{W})$ is the predicted output vector for input vector $\boldsymbol{x}_{\boldsymbol{\xi}}$, $\xi \in \Im$, $\boldsymbol{y}_{\boldsymbol{\xi}}$ is the actual output vector and $\mathcal{L}(\boldsymbol{y}^{(K)}_{\xi}(\boldsymbol{W}),\boldsymbol{y}_{\boldsymbol{\xi}})$ measures the discrepancy between actual and predicted output. In regression problems, where the output is a numerical vector, it is often convenient to adopt $\mathcal{L}(\boldsymbol{y}^{(K)}_{\xi},\boldsymbol{y}_{\boldsymbol{\xi}}) = \|\boldsymbol{y}^{(K)}_{\xi}(\boldsymbol{W}) - \boldsymbol{y}_{\boldsymbol{\xi}}\|^2$. In such cases the optimization of the NN through training becomes a problem of least squares. To optimize the NN is tantamount to minimize the loss $J(\boldsymbol{W})$, which requires a careful fine tuning of the size of the training set vis-à-vis the size of the weight parametrization. In principle, the optimal network is defined as $\boldsymbol{W} = \boldsymbol{W}^* = Arg\min J(\boldsymbol{W})$.

An insufficient number of training input/output pairs relative to the size of the weight tensor would give rise to *overfitting*, requiring special techniques, generically known as *regularization*, in order to trim the network, i.e. randomly remove connections, without compromising predicting efficacy [2,5].

Optimizing the network is no trivial task, as it involves the laborious and costly computation of the minus gradient $-\frac{\partial J(\boldsymbol{W})}{\partial \boldsymbol{W}}$, which locally indicates the direction of steepest descent in the multidimensional surface $J = J(\boldsymbol{W})$. An iterative gradient descent computation generating a fine tuned weight updating $\boldsymbol{W} \to \boldsymbol{W} - h\frac{\partial J(\boldsymbol{W})}{\partial \boldsymbol{W}}$ should eventually lead to convergence to a local minimum of $J = J(\boldsymbol{W})$ when adopting a suitable learning step h. This parameter should be tuned to effectively escape local minima while avoiding overshooting in trying to reach the global mimimum. Most gradient descent algorithms use an adaptive learning step during training, in accord with the constraints indicated. In practice the gradient problem is approached by what is called the *stochastic gradient descent* method, whereby not all datapoints (input/output pairs) in the training set are used in each minimization step but the gradient is approximated by an average over randomly chosen batches of datapoints in a tradeoff between accuracy and computational efficiency. Obviously batch size and learning rate are correlated, so the more accurate the gradient estimation, the larger the learning step may be (a token of computational confidence). To achieve significant speed, the stochastic gradient descent computation may be massively parallelized by splitting up batches into multiple GPUs.

1.2 Early applications of AI in drug discovery

Vast amounts of biomedical and biostructural data have become the hallmark of the post-genomic era and the sheer size of chemical combination possibilities makes it forbiddingly difficult to parse chemical space in search for suitable leads for targeted therapy [6]. In this scenario it is only natural that pharma researchers have turned to DL for guidance in the drug discovery and development process [7–10]. Thus, areas like cheminformatics or pharmacoinformatics have benefited immensely from the advent of DL systems trained by pairing chemical compounds with molecular attributes that are relevant to targeted therapy. These computational and informational techniques enable the evaluation of chemical compounds for specific properties, including target affinity, affinity screening profiles, structural features of drug-target docking and ADMET (absorption, distribution, metabolism, excretion and toxicity) profiling [8].

A major challenge in implementing DL models for pharmacoinformatics in accord with the generic scheme outlined previously stems from the need to represent the chemical structure as a tensor array (vector, matrix or tensor proper) of pixelated or voxelated inputs that may be subsequently interrogated geometrically across the hidden layers of NN in search for features that are indicative of the molecular properties indicated. There are a number of representations of chemical space amenable to TF encoding. The most obvious one is to order the atoms in the compound on a 1D-array (following, for example the IUPAC numerical labeling convention) and represent the chemical structure of the molecule as a covalent bond matrix pairing atoms in row and column in accord with their covalent linkages, including single, multiple and resonant (aromatic) bonds. The matrix is subsequently transformed into a topological descriptor that describes the invariants arising from different atom ordering. The input describing chemical structure is paired within a training set against the molecular attributes of therapeutic relevance that the network is meant to infer. Then, compounds that need to be evaluated/profiled are inputted as the array of pixels/voxels, transformed into a topological representation, and feature extraction is achieved through the sequential activation of hidden layers at increasing levels of abstraction, eventually leading to the profile inference which is subsumed in the output layer.

1.3 Convolutional neural networks to predict drug-target associations and affinities

Feature extraction through the NN often requires particular architectures known as convolutional NNs (CNNs) [2–5]. The idea is to pixelize or voxelize the input data in a matrix or 3D tensor array and then scan (convolve) the array with a filter associated with a specific pattern to generate feature map. For the sake of the argument, let us consider a 2D-array input $\boldsymbol{M}$. The filter $\boldsymbol{F} = (w_{ij})$ is an mxm matrix actually representing a convolutional kernel, so that a neuron in the F-associated hidden layer $\boldsymbol{M_F}$ only senses the pixels in an mxm patch (receptive field), and the layer becomes the feature map $\boldsymbol{M_F} = \boldsymbol{M} * \boldsymbol{F} = (\sum_{j=1}^{m}\sum_{i=1}^{m} w_{ij}x_{i+ap\,j+bp} + w_0)_{ab}$, where p, usually set at p = 2, is the stride adopted as the filter slides along the input matrix array, with dummy integers a, b indicating the patch location. Essentially, the CNN is a NN where the set of weights in each mxm patch of inputs are always the same as the filter slides along the input array to generate the hidden layer that constitutes the feature map. The convolution operation becomes the entry-by-entry (Frobenius) matrix inner product as the filter slides along the input matrix with a given stride. Successive filters may be applied

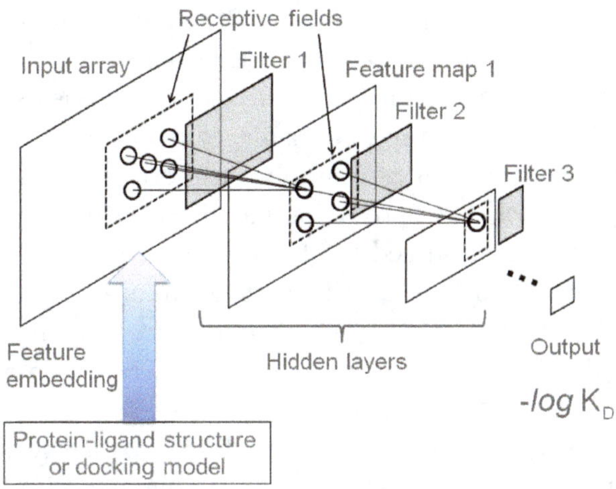

Figure 1.2. Scheme of a CNN used for inference of drug-target affinity through sequential application of filters that become optimized through minimization of the network loss.

reducing progressively the size of the feature maps as higher and higher levels of abstraction are achieved in the representation of the data (Fig. 1.2). Thus, the parametrization required for feature extraction in CNNs is relatively small, as all the neurons in a hidden layer partake the same connectivity parameters that define the filter that generated that layer.

The "beauty and magic" of CNN lies in the fact that the filters are not specified *a priori*, i.e. their weights are not fixed through human intervention. The filter parametrization is automatically determined by the training/optimization process without introducing any assumption, other than the size of the receptive fields for each convolution operation and the overall number of filters to be applied. Thus, feature extraction in a CNN is carried out in an unsupervised manner and only requires that we script (in TF coding) the number of hidden layers or feature maps and the size of the filters to be applied to generate each hidden layer. The features themselves emerge as the network is trained.

Thus, CNNs often constitute AI-empowered platforms for drug discovery, where the structure of a protein-ligand interface that serves as precursor for a predicted drug-target interaction is pixelated in a feature embedding process as a 3D spatial array of protein-drug atom pairs deemed to be interacting across the interface [11]. The inference of target affinity for a given drug is assessed through a sequence of feature extractions using convolution filters until the output feature map becomes a number directly associated with the affinity $pK_D = -log K_D$, where K_D is the dissociation constant for the drug-target complex inputted via feature embedding (Fig. 1.2). The training of the network is carried out by minimizing the network loss or empirical risk over a set of drug-target complexes whose structure and affinity are both known (preferably, experimentally determined). The proteins in the complexes of the training set are typically homologs of the one whose affinity for a specific drug we seek to infer, so that the features that enable the affinity inference may emerge from structural alignment.

As shown in the subsequent chapters, in more complex applications of CNNs, where the output is not simply a numerical parameter but rather a numerical array, it is often convenient to adopt a variation of the CNN architecture in which the patches that yield the pixels with the highest weights in the feature map are reconstituted into features perfectly stenciled by the filter, while other patches that do not yield discernible features are left invariant in non-overlapping regions. Thus, with the application of each filter, a feature-enriched reconstitution of the input layer is carried out prior to the application of the next filter (Fig. 1.3).

1.4 The cutting edge: AI-empowered engineering of dynamic drug-target interfaces

As previously highlighted [7–11], forays in ADMET and PK/PD (pharmacokinetics and pharmacodynamics) profiling, structural/ affinity predictions on drug-target associations, virtual screening and other cheminformatics or pharmacoinformatics applications are all successfully exploiting AI, and in particular DL, to develop useful predictors. In these studies, drug and target protein are represented as rigid entities not influencing each other's conformation, so the dynamics of the induced folding or structural adaptation of the

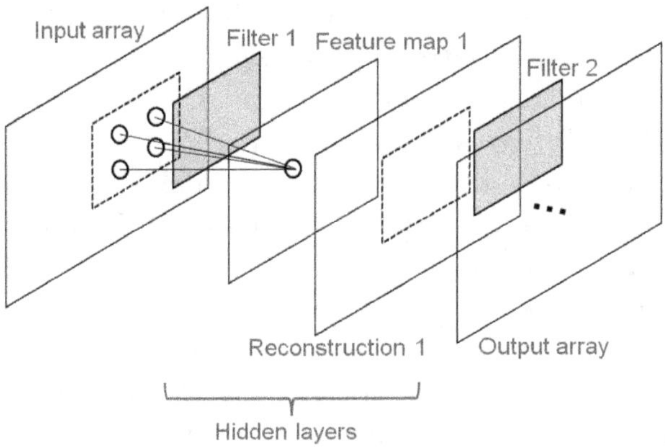

Figure 1.3. Scheme of a CNN with a particular type of architecture in which the patches that yield the pixels with the highest weights in the feature map are recreated as filter-stenciled "perfect" features. Thus, a feature-enriched reconstitution of each layer is carried out prior to the application of the next filter.

target protein to create an optimal drug-target interface [6] is absent altogether from the data analysis.

Therapeutic agents target dysfunctional or deregulated proteins in order to disable them, but the target itself is often a moving target, as protein regions prone to structural adaptation are typically the ones that bind to the drug [12]. Furthermore, the DL-compatible pixelated representation of the drug-target interface typically assumes pairwise interactions [11], but we now know that protein associations involve many-body energy terms: water exclusion from around pre-formed hydrogen bonds in one of the binding partners upon drug-target association plays a key role in driving the interaction [6]. Thus, AI-driven forays to investigate drug-target associations require a new discipline named epistructural biology [6]. As currently defined and understood, structural biology falls short of the proper conceptual/representational background to enable AI-driven forays into the design of drug-target interfaces [12]. Thus, a detailed representation of the dynamic drug-target interface incorporating many-body terms arising from water exclusion needs to be streamlined into the tensor flow of DL systems to bring drug design to the next level, i.e. mastering the engineering of drug-target interfaces and the dynamic problems arising thereof.

Last but not least, drugs target dysfunctional proteins in an *in vivo* setting, not an *in vitro* setting, while proteins are selected to fold efficiently *in vivo*, not *in vitro*, and the drug-induced folding upon binding occurs *in vivo*, not *in vitro*. Thus, the *in vivo* context needs to be factored into the dynamic analysis used to engineer the drug/target interface. At this juncture, AI and only AI can steer intuition and provide guidance to design therapeutic drugs and engineer drug-target interfaces in vivo by mimicking or simulating the cellular setting where such interfaces occur.

This book advocates the deployment of AI to tackle dynamic problems in drug design, including the incorporation, mimicking and simulation of *in vivo* settings. In so doing, it introduces the arsenal of epistructural biology to provide the proper representational and conceptual framework to enable inference through the tensor flow of CNNs.

1.5 DeepMind has solved a grand challenge of biology

As the final touches are being placed on this book on November 30, 2020, DeepMind, a Google company, announced that their AI system AlphaFold2 has solved the "protein folding problem" [13,14]. That is, by adopting a deep learning CNN trained on structural data and correlating it with evolutionary input, AlphaFold2 is capable of predicting the 3D structure of a protein chain from its amino acid sequence. This constitutes a towering achievement because the protein folding problem is the biggest challenge in biology or biophysics, has remained an open problem for over 50 years and has been deemed by most scientists as almost intractable. Perhaps the most astonishing and paradoxical aspect of this achievement is that the expertise profile of the team that developed AlphaFold does not resemble even remotely that of the researchers that have worked (almost fruitlessly) on the problem for the last 50 years. Thus, molecular biophysics is the most underrepresented field in the team's expertise and yet the problem they have solved is one of the paramount problems in molecular biophysics.

To solve the paradox, we need a better grasp on what DeepMind has truly done. They have not tried to predict protein folding pathways that converge to the native fold as the protein chain explores conformation space governed by physical principles. That effort, that has distracted biophysicists for decades, is in all likelihood completely misplaced and misleading. Natural proteins are selected to fold *in vivo*, not *in vitro*, and current computational technologies are completely at a loss in terms of modeling the complexities of an *in vivo* environment. This situation is likely to change with the advent of AI, as clearly demonstrated in Chapter 3.

By contrast, DeepMind has trained the AlphaFold CNN with plenty of structural information on native structures from PDB (protein data bank) entries, hence subsuming in those patterns all the physics and complexity of the *in vivo* environments. In other words, the relevant information is enshrined in the training set without requiring anyone developing the CNN to know about it. Then, through sequence alignment, the test sequence is evolutionarily related with sequences associated with structures in the training set, and the result of the alignment is inputted into the CNN along with the test sequence itself. The beauty and magic of the AI system is that it is able to infer the structure without explicitly learning the physics that governed the formation of the structure. In fact, it is most likely that the feature extraction in the CNN would reveal a completely novel, and hopefully perfectly equivalent!, set of physical principles tailored to the different levels of representational abstraction in the hidden layers. The features extracted in the hidden layers probably enshrine a novel and fascinating set of physical principles optimally tuned to the biology they govern. They are just waiting to be discovered.

1.6 AI encoding for hierarchical dynamical systems: adiabatic regimes, center manifolds and quotient spaces

Encoding is a necessary category in AI. The type of AI we are mostly concerned with involves deep learning, which requires an encoding of the raw information that needs to be acquired and processed. Just like with human intelligence, the encoding problem stems from the core question: what is essential and what it superfluous? The encoding problem becomes solvable when the system under scrutiny is hierarchical and the hierarchical structure is fairly obvious or at least discoverable. In the cases treated in this book, the structure of the data is always hierarchical, implying that the learning process admits and profits from a reductive approach enshrined in the encoding.

We shall deal mostly with time-dependent data, where detailed fast motions may be systematically averaged out, so the relevant information may be stored in a coarse grained representation. Rigorous mathematical constructs will be introduced to implement the hierarchical encoding. Some examples are:

- Chapter 5 deals with very long timescales associated with the evolutionary fate of proteins with common ancestry. We know that protein structure, being typically conserved across homologs, is not the relevant encoding representation to serve as evolutionary marker. This role is played by the *epistructure*, i. e. the way in which the structure relates to the surrounding solvent. Epistructure is a meta-category introduced and “tensorialized” in a voxelated form in chapter 2, and extensively exploited throughout the book. To be able to voxelate the epistructure, we need to subsume very complicated multiscale solvent-structure dynamics into simple structurally encoded features. Thus, the epistructure takes advantage of an intrinsic dynamic hierarchy in the protein-solvent relationship.
- Chapter 6 deals with the quantum mechanics for specific chemical processes that take place at the epistructure, where water is chemically functionalized. A rigorous treatment of this problem would require that we solve the time-dependent Schrödinger equation. In this context, an AI approach would need to be incorporated to learn to infer the nodal structure of molecular orbitals within a voxelated 3D grid. With current technologies, this AI approach is plausible only under the adiabatic regime of the Born-Oppenheimer approximation.

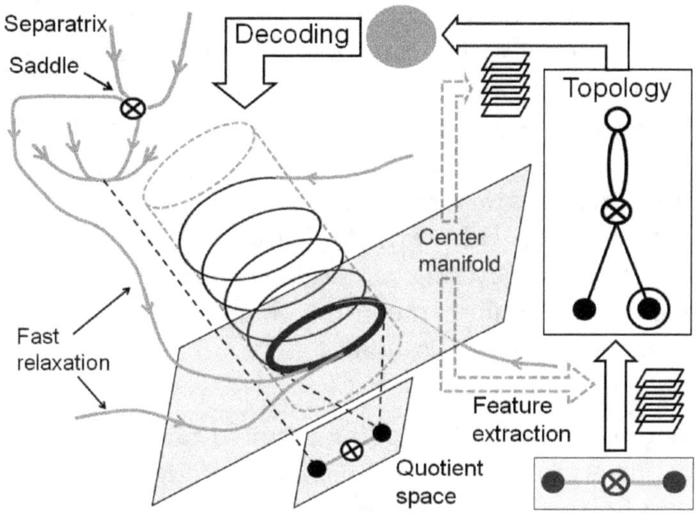

Figure 1.4. Schematics of two levels of encoding of dynamic data. The encoding processes are symbolized by dashed lines, and the enslaving center-manifold dynamics is highlighted by a thick dark circle. Both reductions become equivalent for dynamical systems that do not dissipate free energy.

- Chapter 9 deals with the clonal population dynamics of cancer phenotypes that become selected under therapeutic pressure. This dynamics is complex but hierarchical, and the mathematical procedure to "encode what is essential" in this context fortunately exists and is called center manifold reduction (Fig. 1.4). This reduction is actually a projection of the dynamical system onto a lower dimensional system that entrains it. In Chapter 9, AI simply discovers the center manifold by interrogating vast amounts of time-dependent data, as it seeks to meaningfully reduce dimensionality in such hierarchical systems. Thus, a symbolic regression is carried out by AI, taking advantage of the scaling symmetry introduced by the center-manifold entrainment of the dynamics.
- Chapter 10 introduces *quotient space*, a fundamental mathematical construct to take advantage of dynamic hierarchy in order to encode information as required to implement deep leaning systems. Quotient space requires an underlying dynamics and may be equated with orbit space, i.e. points in the same trajectory are

regarded as equivalent, and the quotient space is the set of equivalence classes with a topology inherited from the underlying space and its dynamics (Fig. 1.4). Thus, we simplify the space by lumping microstates into basins of attraction in the potential energy surface. The modulo-basin dynamics is far easier to encode as the system learns data generated by atomistic molecular dynamics simulations. In this way, AI learns to propagate dynamics in quotient space, covering physically realistic timescales usually inaccessible to detailed atomistic computations. The quotient space is obviously AI-discoverable.

While the center manifold encoding is suited for dissipative dynamics, where the attractor may be nontrivial (cf. Fig. 1.4), the quotient space simplification is better suited for Hamiltonian systems. Both levels of encoding converge as free-energy dissipation tends to zero. In fact, as the AI system encodes time-dependent raw data, it implicitly composes the two levels of encoding, with the center-manifold reduction averaging out of fast modes, followed by projection onto quotient space (Fig. 1.4).

In all cases dealt with in this book, the hierarchy of the data that makes it amenable to encoding is either AI-discoverable (Chapter 9), or it may be unraveled through a rigorous mathematical construct that needs to be incorporated to the deep learning code (Chapter 10). In the future, AI systems will likely be able to unravel such hierarchies without human intervention and engineer the multilayered CNN accordingly. Conceivable, in the future AI may also strive on systems that lack hierarchy, while it is doubtful that the human mind can ever handle such cases.

References

1. Russell S, Norvig P (2020) Artificial intelligence: A modern approach. Pearson, London, UK.
2. Kelleher JD (2019) Deep Learning. The MIT Press, Cambridge, Massachusetts.
3. Chollet F (2019) Deep learning with Python. Manning Press, Shelter Island, New York.

4. Atienza R (2020) Advanced deep learning with TensorFlow 2 and Keras, 2nd Edition. Packt Publishing, Birmingham, UK.
5. Schmidhuber J (2015) Deep learning in neural networks: An overview. *Neural Netw* 61:85–117.
6. Fernández A (2016) Physics at the biomolecular interface. Springer International Publishing, Switzerland.
7. Aliper A, Plis S, Artemov A, Ulloa A, Mamoshina P, Zhavoronkov A (2016) Deep learning applications for predicting pharmacological properties of drugs and drug repurposing using transcriptomic data. *Mol Pharm (ACS)* 13:2524–2530.
8. Lavecchia A (2019) Deep learning in drug discovery: Opportunities, challenges and future prospects. *Drug Disc Today* 24:2017–2032.
9. Jiménez J, Škalič M, Martínez-Rosell G, De Fabritiis, G (2018) Kdeep: Protein–ligand absolute binding affinity prediction via 3D-convolutional neural networks. *J Chem Inf Mod* 58:287–296.
10. Stepniewska-Dziubinska MM, Zielenkiewicz P, Siedlecki P (2018) Development and evaluation of a deep learning model for protein–ligand binding affinity prediction. *Bioinformatics* 34:3666–3674.
11. Hassan-Harrirou H, Zhang C, Lemmin T (2020) RosENet: Improving binding affinity prediction by leveraging molecular mechanics energies with an ensemble of 3D convolutional neural networks. *J Chem Inf Model* 60:2791–2802.
12. Fernández A (2020) Artificial intelligence teaches drugs to target proteins by tackling the induced folding problem. *Mol Pharm (ACS)* 17:2761–2767.
13. Callaway E (2020) 'It will change everything': DeepMind's AI makes gigantic leap in solving protein structures. Nature, published online Nov. 30, 2020. doi: https://doi.org/10.1038/d41586-020-03348-4.
14. Heaven WD (2020) DeepMind's protein-folding AI has solved a 50-year-old grand challenge of biology. MIT Tech Rev Nov 30, 2020 https://www.technologyreview.com/2020/11/30/1012712/deepmind-protein-folding-ai-solved-biology-science-drugs-disease/

Chapter 2

Epistructural biology: A conceptual and representational framework for AI-based drug design

Biological processes at molecular scales remain difficult to understand and control and the efficacy of AI approaches to design targeted therapeutic interventions would be limited unless such processes are properly represented in the data under scrutiny and in the features extracted thereof. First-principle approaches to the standing problems in molecular biophysics are still facing daunting challenges. Thus, the protein folding problem, the physical underpinnings of enzyme catalysis and protein associations, and the molecular etiology of aggregation-related disease remain almost as intractable now as when they were first posed decades ago. Not surprisingly, the molecular design of therapeutic agents remains more serendipitous than rational. This state of affairs takes us now to a cross-road of several disciplines wherein a new field, *epistructural biology,* is emerging as a scaffolding field to AI approaches to drug design. As shown in this chapter, this is so because the protein epistructure is actually encoded in the structure, with a single structural feature, the dehydron, encompassing the multiscale complexity of the structure-solvent relationship. This is a crucial step in order to leverage AI, as the dehydron pattern may be represented in tensor form, hence becoming tractable within an AI context.

The complex dynamical interaction between protein structure and its surrounding aqueous environment is central to the new discipline and attests to an overdue appreciation that biomolecular phenomena cannot be properly grasped without a firm understanding of the interfacial behavior. Thus, it becomes imperative that we provide a rigorous framework to deal with "epistructural" molecular processes. This chapter addresses this imperative and introduces the new discipline, paving the way for an AI-empowered feature extraction process that will ultimately be essential to implement molecular targeted therapies. Thus, this chapter provides the fundamentals for a meta-analysis of the information enshrined in the protein structure and dialectically related to the structure and dynamics of the surrounding aqueous solvent.

2.1 Epistructural biology and its supporting role in AI-driven drug design

Structural biology is traditionally regarded as a knowledge platform for the molecular understanding of life on earth, regarded in its broadest sense [1]. A combination of insights from structural biology, and other well established fields like biochemistry, physical chemistry, biophysics and even nanotechnology has been deemed essential to fully grasp most processes taking place in the cell, from mechanical delivery of cytosolic molecules to signal transduction, from metabolic pathways to developmental steps. Even the human interference with those processes, say, for therapeutic purposes, is typically guided by a blend of cross-disciplinary insights borrowing heavily from those fields [2].

Be as it may, scientists would be delusional if they believe that these interdisciplinary forays have been effective in addressing the grand challenges of molecular biophysics or translational medicine. Thus, protein-protein interfaces remain nearly as obscure and confusing today as they did decades ago, the physico-chemical underpinnings of enzymatic activity remain elusive, and the protein folding problem remains open, as we seek a solution based solely on first principles of physics. Furthermore, the therapeutic disruption of protein associations is still daunting, largely a hit-and-miss issue, and the rational design of therapeutic agents has not lived up to the expectations of the post-genomic era [2].

This baffling reality prompts the question: are we missing some fundamental science, or it is simply a matter of the overwhelming complexity of the issues at stake, a complexity that readily calls for the deployment of AI methods? At this point, we are almost confident we can rule out the latter possibility. The effective application of AI-based methods at this stage would be premature. AI requires that a conceptual and representational framework be developed first, in order to enable the fruitful extraction of relevant features that will lead to meaningful progress. This is precisely the thrust of this book.

From the perspective of structural biology, elucidation of the 3D structure of key machinery in the cell, from single-domain proteins to ribosome or DNA polymerase, has witness great progress. Furthermore, the dynamics subsumed in structural information is becoming accessible and empirical, semiempirical or ab initio methods can now handle canonical ensembles with a number of atoms ($\sim 10^8$) and timescales ($\sim 10\,\text{ms}$) probably sufficient to address some of the molecular complexities of cellular or physiological events. It is also worth emphasizing that the aqueous solvent can be incorporated explicitly into the molecular dynamics computations, and the empirical or semiempirical force fields governing interparticle interactions have reached a level of refinement probably sufficient to handle the physical complexities of polarizability or the electrostatic screening influence of the solvent [3]. Yet, all the problems or challenges mentioned above remain open, with only incremental progress reported and no fundamental advance been made that would instill confidence in their solution. In what pertains to the protein folding problem, vast empirical knowledge has been subsumed into the force fields, and even this extensive data fitting has only enabled researchers to obtain meaningful conducive folding trajectories for only a handful of small (in the order of 25–50 amino acids) single-domain proteins with explicit solvent [4]. As for protein-protein interfaces, standard pairwise potentials incorporated into docking algorithms can hardly make sense of a vast proportion of interactions across the interface typically regarded as mismatches. Perhaps an even worse state of affairs is found in the molecular underpinnings of enzyme activity, where seemingly anomalous ionizations or nucleophilic functionalization is magically attributed to a "special microenvironment" sculpted by the enzyme structure [2]. On the other hand, the therapeutic disruption of protein-protein interfaces with small drugs is regarded as a holy grail in molecular ingenuity, which is not surprising given the current perfunctory understanding of such interfaces [5]. Lastly, drug discovery remains by and large a serendipitous endeavor, where high throughput screening and combinatorial approaches have largely superseded rational design. This is due precisely to the dearth of fundamental concepts that may effectively guide design and lead optimization, as required to control specificity and dodge side effects. For these reasons, the cost of drug development is so forbiddingly high, as only a minuscule proportion of leads can be optimized into therapeutic agents with an impact confined to clinically relevant targets with few unpredicted off-target effects. Rather than being engineered based on selectivity filters, these drugs capable of withstanding the long-term attrition along the discovery pipeline are only identified during the later progressively more costly stages of clinical trials.

Given this state of affairs and the need to deploy AI-based methods, the "mantra" put forth in this book is that fundamental science is missing from the current approaches to the grand challenges and that the missing knowledge is essential to develop the proper representational and conceptual framework to enable AI-based approaches to drug design. One by one, the aforementioned problems will be addressed in the book as the missing fundamental science is developed. But, what is this lacking knowledge that precludes significant progress in the interrelated areas of molecular biophysics and drug design? How is the new knowledge articulated as a representational framework to enable AI-based feature extraction effectively guiding the design of drug-target interfaces?

To address these matters, we need to revisit accepted concepts that are not necessarily correct. In the interdisciplinary context discussed, the structure of a soluble protein (or the lack thereof, in the case of intrinsically disordered proteins) is perceived as an object in and of itself. This book upholds the view that there is information enshrined in the protein structure (or lack of structure) that can only be extracted when the structure is regarded in relation to the solvent. This assertion can be justified *a priori* since the solvent enables the folding process that led to the structure and mediates the intermolecular interactions that may stabilize or even induce the structure. This information, while dynamic in nature needs to be derived directly from structural information. To become of use to drug designers, it needs to be decoded in such a way that it does not require complicated molecular dynamics computations, often plagued with uncertainty.

This is precisely the purview of epistructural biology, a meta-reading of protein structure to incorporate the long-overdue understanding and codification of the interplay between structural and solvent dynamics. Because epistructural biology deals with the aqueous interface of a soluble protein, an object of nanoscale complication, it demands a nanoscale theory of water that would reproduce its dielectric response down to single molecules. Once equipped with this knowledge, we become acutely aware that folding process or protein associations cannot be grasped by using a potential that only includes pairwise contributions, as the local nanoscale solvent environment where the interactions occur is a crucial modulator of the screening effects. We also become aware that such a dielectric modulation, valid at nanoscale dimensions, cannot be obtained by upholding the Debye picture of water dielectrics, conjectured in 1929 for featureless condenser plaques and extrapolated without justification by Nobelist Arieh Warshel and others to the nanoscale complexities of the protein-water interface [2]. Indeed, a nanoscale theory of water is called for and derived in the first two chapters of this book. But what is truly the trademark of epistructural biology is not its ability to provide a physical understanding of the dynamic interplay between structure and solvent, but the possibility of digitally codifying this dynamic information in a useful handy manner, deriving it directly from a meta-analysis of the protein structure. As it turns out, this information proves to be immensely valuable to develop a selectivity filter in drug design, a concept with far-reaching impact in the pharmaceutical industry.

If it is ever intended to become rational, targeted drug design will require operational straightforward rules. Such rules should and will be cast in a manner akin to the simple combinatorial rules of synthetic organic chemistry, extracted from the underlying cumbersome quantum mechanical computations that lead to the principle of conservation of orbital symmetry. Evidently, a structural analysis of the drug target cannot provide such rules, as we have already witnessed the considerable degree of confusion and obscurity when it comes to rationalize and engineer protein-ligand interfaces. All along, this book argues that the biomolecular structure by itself, as obtained from X-ray diffraction or nuclear magnetic resonance (NMR), does not make complete physical sense unless it is considered in relation to the solvent (water for soluble proteins) and that the crucial information describing the dynamic interplay between structure and solvent is encoded in the protein structure itself and may be represented digitally upon the structural framework, yielding relatively simple combinatorial rules for protein associations and drug design.

To support this statement, a nanoscale theory of dielectric response suitable to study the protein-water interface needs to be put in place and the dynamics of the protein-water interface needs to be encoded in terms derived from structural information incorporating the insights provided precisely by the nanoscale theory of water behavior. Thus, the analysis leads to a meta-category, the epistructure, that subsumes the essential information on the solvent-structure interplay in a way that can be turned into an operational guiding principle for molecular design. Neither a structural analysis of the target, nor complicated molecular dynamics simulations incorporating the surrounding solvent can truly convey the sort of meaning that epistructure does. The latter requires a maturation of the dynamic analysis to identify specific structural features that only become apparent when the structure is regarded in relation to the solvent and can serve as blueprints for the drug designer.

At this point in the discussion it becomes natural to inquire what is the structure-derived feature that enshrines the main aspect of the structure-solvent interplay. The answer to the question depends of course on what goals the drug designer or drug developer seeking to create an optimal ligand has in mind as he/she analyzes the target structure. We can safely assume that the designer/developer main concern is the control of specificity and affinity as required to enhance clinical impact and minimize or mitigate side effects due to off-target associations. In such cases, we can anticipate that the structure-derived feature that defines the epistructure is the dehydron, defined as a backbone amide-carbonyl hydrogen bond that is partially exposed to the solvent [2]. Since by definition dehydrons signal sites prone to backbone hydration, which is always a disruptive factor in the protein structure, we are obviously dealing with a packing defect in the protein structure, a "hole" where the structure opens up to the solvent. The reasons why such defects are of keen interest to the designer of a ligand that "corrects" the packing defects upon target-ligand association are manifold: First, as demonstrated in this book, they constitute hot spots for the exclusion of interfacial water, secondly, the removal of specific water molecules enhances the underlying electrostatics of the backbone hydrogen bond, thereby strengthening and stabilizing the target structure upon association with the ligand, and thirdly, the dehydron is essentially sticky in the sense that it exerts a "wrapping" drag on the ligand, promoting the target-ligand association. These physical properties surely invite the formulation of a new paradigm for drug design in the context of targeted therapy: the drug as wrapper of dehydrons in the target structure. Complementing its central role as drug target, the dehydron is also a functional feature of the protein whose chemical role has not been yet appreciated: Dehydrons are enzymatic elements in so far as they induce hydrogen-bond frustration on solvating water molecules, thereby stabilizing adjacent hydroniums. The chemical role of dehydrons will be also explored in the book.

This emerging paradigm prompts the question: what is wrong with structure-based design? Or rather: why is structure-based design not the standard for drug design, especially if the goal is the control of specificity? The culprit needs to be sought in the elusive nature of protein-ligand interfaces. In standard approaches, the matching of opposite charges for polar groups on both sides of the interface is regarded as a major contributor to the free energy of the association, when in fact, it is a marginally contributor at best. This is so since paired charges across the interface must necessarily relinquish their hydration, which has an adverse thermodynamic cost typically commensurate with the electrostatic contribution associated with the pairing of the charges. More commonly, the matching of hydrophobic patches is regarded as a major contributor to ligand affinity, and sometimes it is, particularly when surface curvature issues are not prompting hydrophobic hydration. Yet, be as it may, hydrophobic patches do not constitute good targetable features. The problem in this case is different, and relates to the often overlooked evolutionary aspects of drug discovery. Hydrophobic patches on protein surfaces are highly conserved across proteins of common ancestry in humans (paralogs), thus inducing cross reactivities that are often undesirable as they may promote health-threatening or pernicious side effects, or interfere adversely with the on-target effect.

This critique brings up a major evolutionary issue advocating for dehydrons as the main targetable features in drug design: The dehydron pattern of a soluble protein is not conserved across its paralogs [2], hence a drug that wraps a dehydron in a specific target is certain to be fairly specific, with an impact confined only to the coterie of paralogs that share the same dehydron. We may safely assume paralogous structures are superimposable, as proteins with a common ancestry share the same fold. We may state that the main reason why epistructural drug design should and will supersede structural drug design resides then in the fact that dehydrons are biomarkers for protein evolution, enabling the designer to tell paralogs apart, while structural features do not constitute suitable evolutionary biomarkers.

Even if epistructure-based targeted therapy ends up being established as a paradigmatic design concept, as this book argues it will, targeted therapy has a major shortcoming when administered as monotherapy. This is especially true in cancer treatment, which provides the main therapeutic focus of the book. This relates again to evolutionary aspects, but this time at the level of somatic evolution: cancer evolution makes the disease a moving target whereby the selective pressure imposed by therapy on the cancer cell population leads to a prevailing drug-resistant phenotype. So even if specificity can be mastered in drug therapy, be it through epistructural design or by other means, the fact that targeted therapy selects for resistance in relatively short timespans (often in the order of months) creates a major hurdle and limits its clinical value.

This book squarely addresses this reality and emphasizes that the clinical impact of AI-enabled targeted therapy does not generally reside in its efficacy as monotherapy but rather in its complementary role in combination with immunotherapy. The latter, primarily represented by blockers of tumor-induced immunosuppression, has become the most promising modality for cancer treatment, with resistance patterns arising far later in treatment than what is usually expected for targeted therapy. Yet, eventually immunoediting arises, yielding immune-evading phenotypes selected by the surveillance imposed upon the tumor by the adaptive immune response. The book argues that at precisely this juncture, targeted therapy may admirably complement immunotherapy by annihilating the immune evading tumor. The timing and dosing regime can be tuned so that selection pressure is not maintained for too long, so the tumor never gets a chance to fully select for resistance. These hybrid treatments combining immune and drug targeted therapy will be extensively discussed in the book.

For targeted therapy to serve as a complement to immunotherapy, significant issues of compatibility arise, as the targeted therapy may adversely impinge on the pathways that are activated to trigger an adaptive immune response. Thus, the exquisite control of specificity developed in the first seven chapters becomes essential to resolve compatibility issues arising in combined therapies as described in the final four chapters. Combinations of targeted therapy and immunotherapy geared at launching an immune attack on the tumor, inducing an immune-evading phenotype and subsequently eliminating it require a fine tuned control of specificity in the targeted therapy, with the capacity to tell apart isoforms of a single target protein, as described in the book. To the best of our knowledge, the only technology so far capable of such level of control of specificity is the wrapping technology which uses epistructural biology as its knowledge platform and AI as the enabling tool.

On the practical side, this book offers an open source approach to epistructural drug design, introducing operational concepts that harness the latest advances in biophysics and molecular evolution to leverage AI-based methods. The epistructural drug designs may be exploited in targeted monotherapy or, alternatively, in companion treatment complementing immunotherapy, as shown in the book. The source code provided, its physical and evolutionary rationale and the instructions on how to use it to guide molecular engineering constitute the toolbox of epistructural drug design. The open-source platform enables a meta-analysis of the target protein structure or structural model, yielding the structurally encoded dehydron pattern, the main object in epistructural biology and the blueprint for the designer of the next-generation pharmaceuticals. Being open source and rooted in fundamental advances in molecular biosciences, epistructural drug design is not only inherently more accessible and transparent than other approaches to drug design but it also opens up the possibility of continued improvement through broad participation. This is precisely the spirit of this book and the view it strives to convey as it leverages novel AI-based methods of drug discovery and development.

2.2 What is epistructural biology?

In his book "*The Nature of the Chemical Bond*", Linus Pauling, a towering figure of modern chemistry, became probably the first to recognize the importance of the hydrogen bond as a primary determinant of biomolecular structure. In this way, Pauling laid the foundations of structural biology, and protein structure and dynamics became a central theme in the field for several prolific decades. Yet, a growing concern began to develop as long-standing related problems like the protein folding problem, the physical underpinnings of enzyme catalysis and protein associations, the rational design of targeted molecular therapies, and the molecular etiology of aggregation-related disease remained nearly intractable with the standard methods of structural biology. In all those cases, sorely missing from the analysis was the dynamic relation of the biomolecular structure and the surrounding aqueous solvent.

The subtleties of the dynamic coupling between structural protein motions and their aqueous environment beyond attested to the overdue recognition that biological phenomena would not be effectively understood without dealing with interfacial behavior. Thus, there arose a pressing need to grasp how biologically relevant behavior is shaped by the structuring of biomolecular interfaces and how protein-water interfacial tension affects the molecular events that take place in the cell. These imperatives gave rise to a new discipline that we are now aptly naming *epistructural biology*. This chapter introduces the subject adopting a heuristic approach to address the physical complexities of the protein-water interface. Considerable simplification of practical interest is achieved in the following chapters as the physical intuitions gained in this chapter will enable a meta-analysis of structural information, well beyond the horizon provided by structural biology.

2.3 Epistructural water

Water is of course a central player in biology, at least on the planet where this book is being composed, and yet its influence on biomolecular events is far from being understood. Let us begin with a nanoscale glance at the aqueous environment where biology unravels. The water molecule provides two proton donor and two proton acceptor hydrogen bonding coordinations in a near tetrahedral arrangement dictated by the hybridized sp^3 atomic orbitals of the oxygen atom. As water interfaces with a solute endowed with nanoscale or subnanoscale surface detail, such as a biomolecule, the tetrahedral lattice is perturbed in a complicated manner, and this perturbation carries a thermodynamic cost which is difficult to estimate. More specifically, certain hydrogen bond opportunities for interfacial water may not be fulfilled, leading to "*frustration*", a phenomenon of immense ramifications in interfacial physics, as we shall see throughout this book. Such frustration may occur, for example when a solvent-exposed backbone hydrogen bond in a soluble protein accommodates a water molecule that hydrogen bonds with the carbonyl oxygen, which has an unused lone electron pair (Fig. 2.1). The confinement of the water molecule in the subnanocavity often hinders the complete fulfillment of the water coordination possibilities. On the other hand, the cavity may be sealed

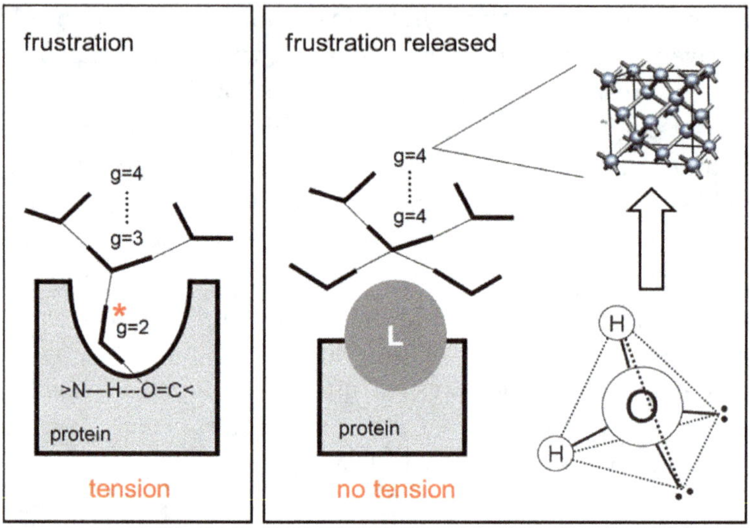

Figure 2.1. Disruption of water structure at the interface with a soluble protein. A structural defect exposing the protein backbone produces "frustration" in vicinal water molecules (thick angular segments) as its hydrogen-bonding coordination (g) is reduced when solvating the backbone. The frustrated molecule is marked by an asterisk. Thus, interfacial tension arises due to the disruption of the dynamic tetrahedral hydrogen-bond lattice characteristic of bulk water ($g = 4$). The electronic sp^3-structure of the water molecule with two lone electron pairs and two proton donors in tetrahedral arrangement dictates the arrangement of the supramolecular hydrogen-bond lattice. When ligand (L) seals the sub-nanoscale cavity, the disruption of water structure is reduced and frustration is released with concurrent decrease in interfacial tension.

by a ligand that has a good chance to stick if the water molecule in the cavity is too frustrated in the free nonbonded state, while the protein-ligand complex causes less of a distortion in the water lattice than the free subunits (Fig. 2.1). This picture, while intuitively appealing, needs rigorous support and has profound consequences for the understanding of biological events at the molecular scale. The book will revisit this picture over and over again from different complementary perspectives, beginning with a heuristic approach to "epistructural" interfacial tension and ending with a meta-analysis of protein structure in a dialectic relation to the solvent.

Water is known to be the matrix of life, and soluble proteins, like other solutes in the cytosol or intercellular space, perturb this matrix. A way of quantifying the magnitude of this perturbation is to compute the free energy change ΔG_{if} associated with spanning the aqueous interface that envelops the protein. If we normalize this extensive thermodynamic quantity by the surface area of the protein, we obtain the interfacial tension. Since the structure of the interface must be in principle determined by the structure of the protein, we may adopt the term "epistructural tension". It is evident that protein associations would tend to reduce ΔG_{if}, as such associations reduce the aqueous interface, so it is imperative that we find a way to compute epistructural tension and identify chemical and structural features in the protein that generate such tension. Thus, the first question we need to address in dealing with biomolecular interfaces is how are the structure and ultimately the thermodynamic properties of the interface determined by the structure of the soluble protein.

The multi-scale structure of water in the condensed phases of biological relevance remains a source of controversy [6, 7]. In bulk water, the controversy has been partly fuelled by the discovery of structural distortions in the fluctuating tetrahedral hydrogen-bond lattice due to asymmetric electron density [6]. On the other hand, the long-range tetrahedral hydrogen-bond network signatures are clearly present in the X-ray scattering intensity and structure factor data [7]. Thus, at nano-meter scales we may assume that the structure of water, with its resilient tetrahedral lattice of intermolecular hydrogen bonds, is largely responsible for its significant dielectric properties. As it is known, this resilience to the polarization induced by an external electrostatic field generated by a charge separation becomes apparent in the large permittivity coefficient of water.

Provided tetrahedral coordination possibilities are preserved as in bulk-like environments, polarization is believed to align with electrostatic fields determined by fixed charges, as first proposed by Peter Debye [8–12]. There are indications that this "Debye ansatz" may break down under confinement of water molecules in regions of nanoscale dimensions [9]. The breakdown is attributed to the fact that the bulk-like floppy tetrahedral lattice has been distorted to a point where water is effectively deprived of hydrogen-bond partnerships and tends to preserve its interfacial hydrogen-bond pattern in spite of the field-aligning torque imposed by the electrostatic field [9]. For instance, the complexities of dielectric properties at biological heterogeneous interfaces [13–15] bespeak of a spatial scale where the behavior of water dipoles cannot be accounted for through linear polarization relations [10, 16, 17]. The nanoscale structure of water must be inevitably incorporated into the electrostatic description of "*episteric*" fields at interfaces that confine the solvent to discrete levels [9, 10, 17]. By *episteric* we mean surrounding a solute particle with a defined interface and charge distribution, such as a soluble protein.

The laws of dielectric response are inherently continuous [12], at odds with the discrete structural distortions of water that promote anomalous polarization under nanoscale confinement. To exploit the mathematical apparatus of electrostatics, we face the conundrum of having to adopt continuous —actually differentiable-descriptors of water structure that are inadequate at scales where the discrete patterns of hydrogen-bond coordination becomes significant. To reconcile these conflictive aspects, we introduce a local indicator of time-averaged hydrogen-bonding patterns for water molecules at spatial locations. Specifically, we introduce a scalar field $g = g(\vec{r})$ indicating the expected number of hydrogen bonds of a water molecule computed while its oxygen atom is contained within a sphere of radius r = 4Å (∼van der Waals radius of carbon atom + thickness of one hydration layer) centered at position $\vec{r}$ and during a timespan $\tau = 10\,\text{ps}$ [9]. The (r,τ)-parametrization of this scalar field has been calibrated empirically, so that the choices guarantee second-order differentiability for g. This level of smoothness is required to introduce a nanoscale dielectric relation. The g-function indicates in a coarse grained way the number of interactions of a water molecule within a neighborhood of each point in space, remaining informative at ∼1 nm levels. By definition, $g = g(\vec{r})$ represents also an average over all water molecules visiting the sphere within the 10 ps-timespan. The hydrogen bonds in the counting involve neighboring water molecules and polar groups from the protein.

To examine the aqueous interface of a soluble protein we may embed and equilibrate the protein chain conformation in an explicit water bath. The chain conformation is determined by structural coordinates from the corresponding protein data bank (PDB) entry. Details of such computations will be provided subsequently and the robustness to different solvent models will be discussed in this and the four chapters that follow. The zest of this section is to simply delineate a relationship between protein structure and interfacial tension that will be operative to address core problems in molecular biophysics.

To obtain a description of the aqueous interface of a protein after equilibrated embedding of the protein structure, we have computed g-values at every atom on the surface of the protein, so that water molecules are present in the solvation shells of 4 Å-radius. It is entirely expected that g-values in the range $g \geq 3$ will occur on the interface, as $g = 3$ is the lower bound at the interface for an aqueous bulk phase. We are interested in "unusually low g-values, in the range $g < 3$, as those would entail the most significant perturbation of the water matrix. As an example, the surface g-values for *ubiquitin* are displayed in Fig. 2.2(a,b). Fig. 2.2(a) displays van der Waals radii of all surface atoms and in lighter color the 4 Å-radius solvation shells with $g < 3$. Fig. 2.2(b) shows the location of the hot $g < 3$-spots in relation to a ribbon rendering of the ubiquitin backbone in the native fold. Examination of the hot spots prompts us to ask: How does this interfacial pattern relate to the 3D native structure of ubiquitin? What are the structural features causative of such hot spots? The $g < 3$ values result from severe confinement of water molecules at the interface as it would be feasible at sub-nanoscale cavities. Such cavities would involve a special kind of packing defect involving unusual arrangements of the side chains of the protein. This is as far as intuition takes us, so we computed a strictly structure-based feature: The backbone hydrogen bonds that are incompletely shielded from the solvent, also known as *dehydrons*. The partial exposure of the backbone to water as represented by a dehydron clearly constitutes a packing defect since intramolecular backbone hydrogen bonds exposed to water are inherently weak and prone to cause a disruption of the protein structure as the amides and carbonyls become maximally hydrated. Thus, we contrasted the dehydron pattern for ubiquitin (Fig. 2.2(c), details on dehydron

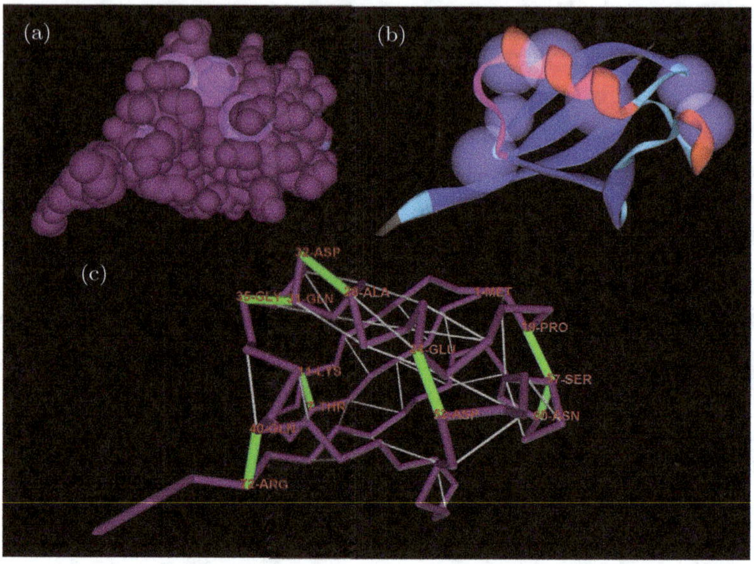

Figure 2.2. **(a)** The structure of *ubiquitin* (PDB entry 1UBI) with atoms represented by their van der Waals spheres (magenta) with semi-transparent blue spheres indicating 4 Å-solvation shells with g < 3 (hot spots). **(b)** Location of the solvation shells with g < 3 within a ribbon rendering of the ubiquitin backbone in the native structure. **(c)** Dehydron pattern for ubiquitin. The backbone is represented by virtual bonds (magenta) joining α-carbons of residues adjacent in the chain, dehydrons are represented by green sticks joining the α-carbons of hydrogen-bonded paired residues, while well-wrapped backbone hydrogen bonds are displayed as grey sticks joining paired residues.

computation will be revealed subsequently) with the $g < 3$ hot spots displayed in Fig. 2.2(a,b). A clear correlation emerged: *The $g < 3$ hot spots invariably corresponded to the solvation shells of the atoms closest to dehydrons.* This result can be carried over to all soluble proteins reported in PDB and clearly implies that protein *dehydrons play a decisive role in shaping the interface as they promote the most significant distortions in the water matrix.*

In fact, the solvation shells with the highest vacating probability $P(N = 0)$ (i.e. the probability of the solvation shell to be spontaneously deprived of water molecules, with $N =$ number of water molecules in solvation shell) are precisely those with the lowest g-values, in accord with the empirical relation $P(N = 0) = 1 - g/4$

hereby established and found across all soluble protein interfaces with reported structure [2]. Since $P(N = 0) = \exp[-< N >^2/2\sigma^2]$ with $\sigma^2 =< (N- < N >)^2 >$, we may assert that *dehydrons generate the largest fluctuations in interfacial water density and promote the most significant spontaneous local dehydration of the aqueous interface.* This result sets the agenda for the rest of the chapter, as it strongly suggest that dehydrons are crucial determinants of protein associations and therefore deserve to be studied closely from a physico-chemical perspective.

Thus, the heuristic physical arguments on epistructural interfacial tension presented in this chapter will invite the meta-analysis of protein structure unraveled in the remaining chapters, while laying the foundations of the new discipline named *epistructural biology*.

2.4 Epistructural interfacial tension

At the time when Debye's "molecular theory" of dielectric response emerged [12], the nanoscale structure of water, with its resilient tetrahedral lattice of intermolecular hydrogen bonds [6, 7, 9], was largely unknown and the importance of hydrogen bonds as determinants of water structure was not yet recognized. With virtually no information on the nanoscale structure of water and merely assuming the existence of a polarizable "sea of dipoles", Peter Debye derived a theory applicable in contexts where the dielectric response could be treated as a bulk attribute. The theory postulates an alignment of water polarization $\vec{P}$ with the internal electrostatic field $\vec{E}$. This ansatz enables the computation of the effective permittivity ε of the dielectric medium by assuming that the proportionality between the vector fields $\vec{P}$ and $\vec{E}$ can be expressed without loss of generality as $\vec{P} = (\varepsilon - \varepsilon_0)\vec{E}$, where ε_o is the vacuum permittivity. The ansatz yields a simplified Poisson electrostatic equation $\vec{\nabla}.(\varepsilon_0\vec{E} + \vec{P}) = \vec{\nabla}.(\varepsilon\vec{E}) = \rho$ (ρ = fixed charge distribution) that holds for an electrostatic condenser with planar featureless parallel plates and for virtually all aqueous dielectric media provided it lacks nanoscale detail.

The success of Debye's simplification encouraged researchers to extrapolate his linear polarization assumption to biophysical contexts such as protein-water interfaces [18, 19]. This extrapolation proves to be unwarranted and ultimately incorrect, as we shall presently demonstrate. The theoretical results obtained thereof proved to be nearly impossible to reconcile with experiment, as recent work suggests [13–16]. In the case of biological water, the supramolecular structure of the solvent and the nanoscale distortions relative to a bulk-like organization cannot be ignored. The crux of the problem is that confinement of water at the biological interface often creates dipole organizations that result from deprivation of hydrogen bonding opportunities, thereby creating uncompensated effective charges that are not a resultant of polarization along the direction of the internal field $\vec{E}$ of the protein [9].

In critically assessing the applicability of Debye's model to protein-water interfaces we first note that a single parameter, the effective permittivity coefficient ε, cannot possibly quantify the dielectric response of water. Recent computations reveal that there is a component of polarization generated by the nanoscale topography and chemical composition of the protein surface that offers resistance to the torque imposed by the field $\vec{E}$ on the water dipoles [20].

The biological interfaces confine water into patterns that cannot simultaneously minimize the disruption of the hydrogen-bond lattice and align the water dipoles with the electrostatic field. There are polarization components that do not align with the field and arise from tight local nanoscale organizations of water molecules deprived of hydrogen bonding opportunities [9]. This picture brings about a complex dielectric structure that cannot be subsumed into a single permittivity parameter. The nanoscale water structure must be incorporated into the electrostatic description of the resultant fields at interfaces that confine solvent to discrete levels.

We expect and hereby postulate that nanoscale local organization will introduce a significant component of polarization, $\overrightarrow{P^{\#}}$, orthogonal to the protein internal field $\vec{E}$. This "anomalous" polarization is a predictable resultant of the partial hindrance in the alignment of water dipoles with the field $\vec{E}$ due to nanoscale confinement. The departure from the "linear dielectrics" picture is described by writing the Poisson equation in its utmost generality as follows [9]:

$$\vec{\nabla}.(\varepsilon_0 \vec{E} + \overrightarrow{P^{\|}} + \overrightarrow{P^{\#}}) = \rho \tag{1}$$

where, without loss of generality, $\vec{P}$ has been decomposed into a field-aligned component $\overrightarrow{P^{\|}} = (\vec{P}.\vec{e})\vec{e}; \vec{e} = \vec{E}/\|\vec{E}\|$, and a component $\overrightarrow{P^{\#}}$, orthogonal to $\vec{E}$. Accordingly we obtain:

$$\vec{\nabla}.\left(\overrightarrow{P^{\#}}\right) = \rho - \vec{\nabla}.\left(\varepsilon_0 \vec{E} + \overrightarrow{P^{\|}}\right) \tag{2}$$

In (2) the term $\rho - \vec{\nabla}.(\varepsilon_0 \vec{E} + \overrightarrow{P^{\|}})$ measures the departure from the Debye dielectrics, with $\rho - \vec{\nabla}.(\varepsilon_0 \vec{E} + \overrightarrow{P^{\|}}) = 0$ when the Debye ansatz $\vec{P} = \overrightarrow{P^{\|}}$ is fulfilled, i.e. in the Debye limit conventionally adopted in molecular biophysics.

Defining the electrostatic potential φ through the relation: $-\vec{\nabla}\varphi = \vec{E} + \varepsilon_0^{-1}\vec{P}$, the total electrostatic energy becomes

$$U = -\frac{1}{2}\varepsilon_0 \int \varphi \Delta \varphi d\vec{r} = \frac{1}{2}\varepsilon_0 \int \left\|\vec{\nabla}\varphi\right\|^2 d\vec{r} = U_D + U^{\#} \tag{3}$$

where $\Delta = \boldsymbol{\nabla}^2$ is the Laplace operator, and

$$U_D = \frac{1}{2}\varepsilon_0 \int \left\|\vec{E} + \varepsilon_0^{-1}\overrightarrow{P^{\|}}\right\|^2 d\vec{r} \tag{4}$$

is the Debye contribution, and

$$U^{\#} = \frac{1}{2}\varepsilon_0^{-1} \int \left\|\overrightarrow{P^{\#}}\right\|^2 d\vec{r} = \frac{1}{2}\varepsilon_0^{-1} \int \|\vec{P} - (\vec{P}.\vec{e})\vec{e}\|^2 d\vec{r} \tag{5}$$

is the "orthogonal" polarization contribution to the electrostatic energy.

Since departures from bulk water structure (spatially measured by $\boldsymbol{\nabla} g \neq 0$) induce orthogonal polarization, we adopt the ansatz $\overrightarrow{P^{\#}} \propto \vec{\nabla} g$ or $\overrightarrow{P^{\#}} = \xi \vec{\nabla} g$ [9] where $\xi = (\lambda \varepsilon_o)^{1/2}$ and the parameter λ is obtained by estimation of the interfacial free energy of a nonpolar sphere with radius θ and contrasting in the macroscopic limit the result with the elastic integral $\int \frac{1}{2}\|\vec{\nabla} g\|^2 d\vec{r}$. The elastic integrand $\frac{1}{2}\|\vec{\nabla} g\|^2$ accounts for tension-generating reductions in water coordination and vanishes everywhere except at the solute-water interface. The comparison is valid since interfacial tension is related to the distortion of the tetrahedral coordination structure of bulk water. In the macroscopic limit, where $\theta \gg 1\,\text{nm}$, we get $\lambda = \frac{9.0mJ}{m} = limit\left\{\frac{\gamma(4\pi\theta^2)}{\int \frac{1}{2}\|\vec{\nabla} g\|^2 d\vec{r}}\right\}$ where $\gamma = 72\,\text{mJ/m}^2$ is the macroscopic surface tension of water at 298 K. From the ansatz $\overrightarrow{P\#} = \xi\vec{\nabla} g$, we obtain the relation:

$$U\# = \frac{1}{2}\varepsilon_0^{-1} \int \left\|\overrightarrow{P\#}\right\|^2 d\vec{r} = \int \frac{1}{2}\lambda \left\|\vec{\nabla} g\right\|^2 d\vec{r} \qquad (6)$$

This equation asserts that the interfacial tension has an electrostatic origin and may be characterized as the energy per unit of protein surface stored in the anomalous non-Debye polarization resulting from sub-nanoscale confinement at the interface (Fig. 2.3(a,b)). Since dehydrons create the biggest drops in g-value, we may intuitively assert that dehydrons cause the breakdown of the Debye electrostatic ansatz and at the same time, represent the culprit of interfacial tension. This in turn implies that dehydrons are the dominant features promoting protein associations (Fig. 2.1).

2.5 Perturbed water matrix in the epistructural interface

Cell functioning involves recruitment of biomolecular complexes, a process mediated by water that gets displaced as subunits bind. This process affects water frustration, that is, the number of unmet hydrogen-bonding opportunities at the protein-water interface (cf. Fig. 2.1). By searching for least-frustrated aqueous interfaces, this section delineates the role of frustration in steering molecular assemblage. The search entails a trajectory sampling using a functional measuring the gradient of frustration and computing the resulting non-Debye electrostatics within relaxation times for coupled protein-water systems. The minimal frustration principle

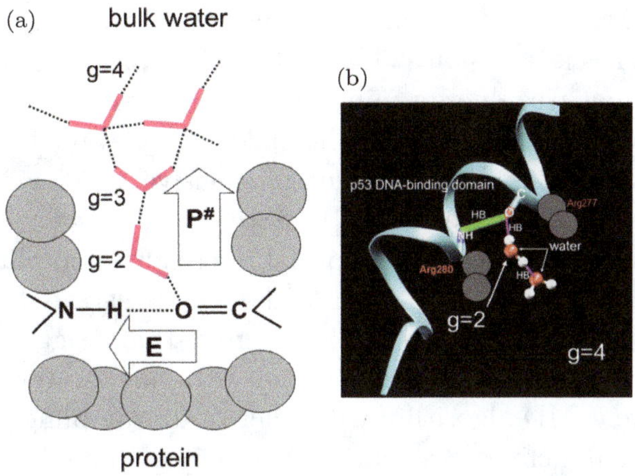

Figure 2.3. **(a)** Schematic representation of the non-Debye polarization of interfacial water constrained by the sub-nanoscale cavity created by a dehydron. The orthogonal polarization results from a deprivation in hydrogen-bonding opportunities for water molecules in the dehydron cavity. **(b)** Hydration pattern for dehydron Arg277–Arg280 in the DNA-binding domain of p53, displaying the paired backbone amide and carbonyl.

is validated against spectroscopic measurements of frustration-dependent dielectric relaxation, affinity scanning of protein-protein interfaces, and NMR-inferred association propensities of protein-complex intermediates. The methods are applied to drug design, revealing the targetable nature of the aqueous interface.

With the recognition that no cogent theory fully reconciles thermodynamic and structural characterization of protein associations, and that hydrophobicity is hardly operative at Angstrom-level curvatures, the forces that steer the formation of protein complexes remain under intense scrutiny [8,11,17,21–23]. This section addresses the problem, investigating protein complex formation from a solvent-centric perspective that takes into account the unusual properties of water near biomolecular surfaces. The approach requires a variational procedure to optimize the frustration state [24] of the aqueous interface. Frustration refers to unmet opportunities for hydrogen-bonding that cause interfacial tension [17]. It is at present unclear whether force fields and solvation models adopted in molecular dynamics (MD) computations can properly model frustration or capture interfacial tension [25–29]. It is also unclear -and unlikely- that the global free energy minimum would be a state of minimal interfacial frustration and, while the biological relevance of the former is still debated, the latter is clearly decisive in driving complex formation, as this section shows [13, 28].

As shown in this section, a special microstate sampling strategy steering MD computations towards the least-frustrated interface is essential to identify the molecular factors that trigger complexation. Accordingly, we implement and experimentally validate an explicit-solvent MD algorithm with microstate sampling guided by a functional that defines a variational principle to enable the search for minimally frustrated interfaces. The functional form of the variational principle hinges on the *ansatz* previously described that frustration creates a polarization component decoupled from the electrostatic field [17, 23]. The functional adopted exploits the link between frustration and electrostatics and computes the non-Debye electrostatic energy equivalently stored as the frustration-related interfacial tension [23]. Thus, the trajectories generated entail the computation of the gradient of frustration at each spatial location.

We demonstrate that frustration-related water polarization steers protein-protein (PP) associations with high specificity and drives the dynamics of complex formation. The validation of these assertions entails contrasting optimally frustrated states with affinity scanning of PP-interfaces [30] in complexes that assemble to mitigate frustrated hydration of free subunits, and with NMR information on the dynamics of complex formation [31]. Subsequently, we identify the optimal sequence of steps that maximize the mitigation of interfacial tension, funneling complex formation. Finally, we apply the solvent-centric approach to drug design in order to demonstrate the efficacy of the variational approach to engineer ultra-specificity, creating ligands that discriminate isoforms of target proteins.

To describe the local structural distortion of water, we introduce a "frustration scalar field" $\phi = \phi(\vec{r})$ that quantifies the expected number of unmet hydrogen bonds of a test water molecule placed at spatial location $(\vec{r})$ relative to the tetrahedral lattice representing bulk water structure. Thus we get $\phi(\vec{r}) = 4 - g(\vec{r})$, where $g(\vec{r}) \leq 4$ is the time-averaged number of hydrogen bonds (coordination number) that a water molecule sustains while it visits a sphere of radius r = 4 Å centered at position $\vec{r}$ for a minimum timespan 1 ps. The temporal averaging parameter is of the magnitude of the relaxation timescale for a decoupled water lattice [32], and the averaging is required to operate with a smooth scalar field [33]. A hydrogen bond is operationally defined by geometric constraints [21]: O-O distance <3.2 Å and O-H-O angle α_{HB} satisfying $120° \leq \alpha_{\text{HB}} \leq 180°$. Compared with bulk water, interfacial water may have reduced hydrogen-bonding opportunities, and may partly mitigate such losses by hydrogen bonding with polar groups on the protein surface.

A frustration functional $\Im(\phi) = \int \mathcal{L}(\phi) d\vec{r}$ is introduced to compute the free energy cost $\Delta G_{if}(\phi)$ of generating the water frustration field ϕ when spanning an aqueous interface with a solute molecule

$$\Delta G_{if}(\phi) = \Im(\phi) = \int \mathcal{L}(\phi) d\vec{r}$$
$$= \int \left[\frac{1}{2}\omega\|\vec{\nabla}\phi\|^2 - k_B T(\rho_0 - \rho)\ln\left(1 - \frac{\phi}{4}\right)\right] d\vec{r} \qquad (7)$$

where the elastic energy functional $\int \frac{1}{2}\omega\|\vec{\nabla}\phi\|^2 d\vec{r}$ penalizes distortions of the water structure, and the entropy differential $dS_{if}(\phi) = k_B ln[\frac{4-\phi}{4}]^{(\rho_0 - \rho)d\vec{r}} = [k_B(\rho_0 - \rho)\ln\left(1 - \frac{\phi}{4}\right)]d\vec{r}$ corresponds to the transference of a water molecule from bulk solvent with number density $\rho_0 = 0.033\,\text{Å}^{-3}$ to a differential volume region $d\vec{r}$ at position $\vec{r}$ with number density $\rho(\vec{r})$ and frustration $\phi(\vec{r})$. For small structural distortions $\phi \ll 4$, the linear approximation becomes valid, yielding: $dS_{if}(\phi) \approx -[k_B(\rho_0 - \rho)(\frac{\phi}{4})]d\vec{r}$.

The least-frustrated water interface is described by a frustration field $\phi = \phi(\vec{r})$ that satisfies the Euler-Lagrange equation [34]:

$$\nabla\partial\frac{\mathcal{L}(\phi)}{\partial\nabla\phi} = \partial\frac{\mathcal{L}(\phi)}{\partial\phi}, \qquad (8)$$

written explicitly as:

$$\Delta\phi = \left(\frac{k_B T}{4\omega}\right)(\rho_0 - \rho)\left(1 - \frac{\phi}{4}\right)^{-1}, \tag{9}$$

where $\Delta = \nabla^2$ is the Laplace operator, and hence $\Delta\phi$ gives the curvature of the frustration field. For small distortions $\phi \ll 4$, we get

$$\Delta\phi = \left(\frac{k_B T}{4\omega}\right)(\rho_0 - \rho). \tag{10}$$

To obtain ω, we use (9) applied to an equilibrating computation of ϕ obtained as a function of the distance X to a rigid nonpolar interface [30] consisting of a concave region of fixed curvature radius $\theta = 3.25$ Å, with X = 0 = center of curvature. An MD-equilibration of the NPT canonical ensemble is carried out for 1 ns (Fig. 2.4), a time incommensurably larger than the relaxation timescale for the decoupled water lattice dynamics (~1 ps) [32]. Thus, at T = 298 K, (9) yields $\frac{1}{9}\text{Å}^{-2} = \omega^{-1} \times 1.02 \times 10^{-20}\, mJ\text{Å}^{-3}$ or $\omega = 9.18 \times 10^{-20}\, mJ\text{Å}^{-1}$. To validate this estimation, we compute the interfacial tension $\Delta G_{if}(\phi(\theta))/4\pi\theta^2$ for a vapor spherical bubble equilibrated at radius $\theta = 2.48$ nm within a simulation timespan of 1 ns [33]. The bubble dimensions approximate a macroscopic limit at T = 298 K within an NVT canonical ensemble of 29,328 TIP3P water molecules [34] in a $10 \times 10 \times 10\,\text{nm}^3$ box with periodic boundaries. The equilibrated bubble is slightly larger than the original bubble at starting conditions, generated by water molecule removal from a spherical region with radius $\theta_0 = 2.00$ nm from an initial ensemble with density 958.5 kg/m^3. Thus, we obtain

$$\frac{\Delta G_{if}(\phi(\theta))}{4\pi\theta^2} = \int_{\partial B(\theta)}^{\infty} \frac{\mathcal{L}(\phi)d\vec{r}}{4\pi\theta^2} = \gamma = 53.8\, mJ/m^2. \tag{11}$$

This value is in good agreement with the Young-Laplace estimation: $\gamma_{YL} = -\frac{p_l\theta}{2} = 55.2\, mJ/m^2$, resulting from the virial computation of the bulk liquid water pressure $p_l = -46 \times 10^6\, N/m^2$, given a negligible vapor pressure in the bubble: $p_v \approx 0$, as no water molecule was

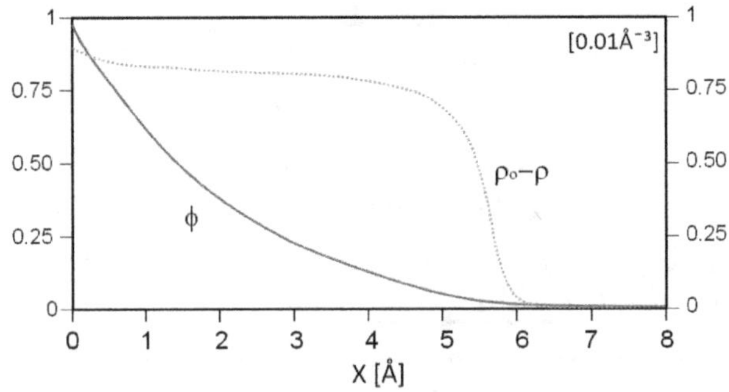

Figure 2.4. Computation of water frustration ϕ (ordinates, left axis) and number density ρ (ordinates, right axis, dimensions in Fig.) relative to the distance X to a rigid nonpolar interface consisting of a concave region of fixed curvature radius $\theta = 3.75$ Å, with X = 0 at center of curvature. We generated 10 lattice-equilibrating MD 1ns-trajectories for water dynamics within an isobaric/isothermal ensemble (1atm, 298 K) consisting of 10,190 water packed against a featureless concave layer of hydrogenated graphene (6×6 supercell, 72C, 72H) representing a nonpolar surface. The solvent bath provided at least four water layers of solvent envelope with water molecules extending 15 Å from the nonpolar surface.

detected escaping to the vapor phase at T = 298 K during the 1ns-computation.

The minimization of water frustration is now shown to translate into a major force steering protein associations, the elementary events in biology at the molecular scale. A major caveat holds as we incorporate water frustration into the canonical ensemble molecular dynamics of soluble proteins with explicit solvent: we cannot incorporate a frustration term directly into the potential energy since there is no explicit energetic penalty for missed interactions or unmet hydrogen-bonding possibilities. Yet, as shown in the microstate sampling scheme on Fig. 2.5, we can select at each stage of the simulation a representative from the set of *a-priori* equi-probable microstates to ensure a *probable* decrease in $\Delta G_{if}(\phi) = \Im(\phi)$ and, ultimately, an effective search for a state of minimal frustration. Let $[\mathbf{Q_n}, \mathbf{P^p_n} \bigoplus \mathbf{P^w_n}]$ denote the state of the system at stage n, specified by $\mathbf{Q_n}$ = atomic coordinates vector ($\mathbf{Q_n} = \mathbf{Q^p_n} \bigoplus \mathbf{Q^w_n}$), and $\mathbf{P_n} = \mathbf{P^p_n} \bigoplus \mathbf{P^w_n}$ = momentum vector, both decomposable as direct sums of protein (p) and water (w)

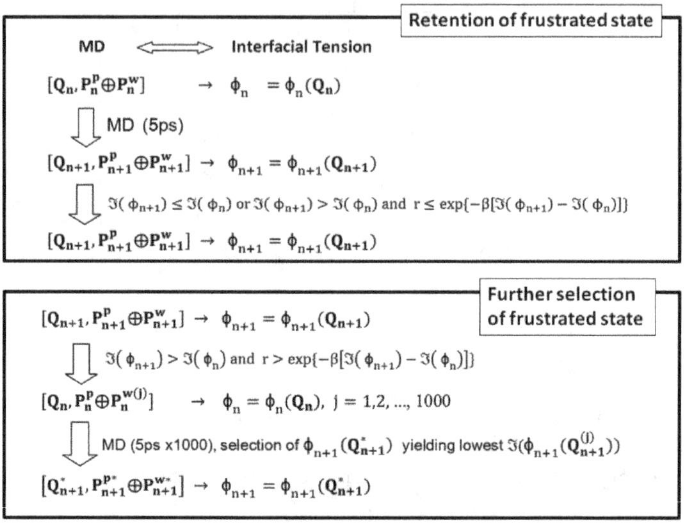

Figure 2.5. Microstate sampling scheme for a 5ps-MD iteration guided by interfacial frustration functional $\Im(\phi) = \int \mathcal{L}(\phi)d\vec{r}$. The upper box indicates flow under which the destiny microstate $[\mathbf{Q}_{n+1}, \mathbf{P}^{\mathbf{P}}_{n+1} \bigoplus \mathbf{P}^{\mathbf{w}}_{n+1}]$ is retained in the $n \rightarrow n+1$ iteration based on a comparison of scalar fields $\phi_n = \phi_n(\mathbf{Q}_n)$ and $\phi_{n+1} = \phi_{n+1}(\mathbf{Q}_{n+1})$. The lower box indicates the sampling procedure that takes place when the destiny state is not chosen to be retained. Reprinted from [Fernández A (2016) Non-Debye frustrated hydration steers biomolecular association: Interfacial tension for the drug designer. FEBS Letters 590:3481–3491] with permission from John Wiley & Sons.

contributions. The next state $[\mathbf{Q}_{n+1}, \mathbf{P}^{\mathbf{P}}_{n+1} \bigoplus \mathbf{P}^{\mathbf{w}}_{n+1}]$ resulting after 5 ps of MD simulation is retained depending on a comparison of the scalar fields $\phi_n = \phi_n(\mathbf{Q}_n)$ and $\phi_{n+1} = \phi_{n+1}(\mathbf{Q}_{n+1})$. Retention of the destiny state $[\mathbf{Q}_{n+1}, \mathbf{P}^{\mathbf{P}}_{n+1} \bigoplus \mathbf{P}^{\mathbf{w}}_{n+1}]$ occurs provided that either of the following inequalities holds:

$$\Im(\phi_{n+1}) \leq \Im(\phi_n) \text{ or } \Im(\phi_{n+1}) > \Im(\phi_n) \text{ and } \\ r \leq \exp\{-\beta[\Im(\phi_{n+1}) - \Im(\phi_n)]\},$$

with r = realization of random variable within the interval [0,1] and $\beta = [k_B T]^{-1}$. On the other hand, if $\Im(\phi_{n+1}) > \Im(\phi_n)$ and $r > exp\{-\beta[\Im(\phi_{n+1}) - \Im(\phi_n)]$, then we perform 5 ps MD runs on 1000 initial randomly selected *a-priori* equi-probable n-microstates $[\mathbf{Q}_n, \mathbf{P}^{\mathbf{P}}_n \bigoplus \mathbf{P}^{\mathbf{w(j)}}_n], j = 1, 2, \ldots, 1000$, with randomly chosen water momenta $\mathbf{P}_{\mathbf{n}}^{\mathbf{w(j)}}$ ($\mathbf{P}_{\mathbf{n}}^{\mathbf{w(1)}} = \mathbf{P}_{\mathbf{n}}^{\mathbf{w}}$) subject to the constraint of constant kinetic energy, and select the state $[\mathbf{Q}_{\mathbf{n+1}}^{*}, \mathbf{P}_{\mathbf{n+1}}^{\mathbf{p*}} \bigoplus \mathbf{P}_{\mathbf{n+1}}^{\mathbf{w*}}]$ as the (n + *1*)-destiny state that realizes the lowest $\Im(\phi_{\mathrm{n+1}}(\mathbf{Q}_{\mathbf{n+1}}^{(\mathbf{j})}))$ from within the set of 1000 destiny coordinate vectors.

2.5.1 *Epistructural interfacial tension drives specific protein-protein associations*

To assess the steering power of the water functional towards the minimally frustrated interfacial state, and illustrate the role of frustrated hydration as promoter of protein associations, we generated 500 ps-trajectories for soluble proteins known to engage in complexes with structures reported in the protein data bank (PDB). A TIP3P explicit solvent [35] within an AMBER package [36] and Coulombic interactions evaluated with the Ewald summation scheme [37] were adopted for MD simulation steered by the microstate sampling strategy described in the previous section (Fig. 2.5). An isothermal/isobaric ensemble at T = 298 K was adopted with initial structural coordinates for the protein chain obtained for the corresponding free subunit extracted *in silico* from the PDB-reported complex. The free (uncomplexed) protein subunits were solvated in a water box extending at least 10 Å beyond any protein atom and were thermalized for 5 ns. Following relaxation, positional restraints defined by force constant = 5 kcal/Å^2 were imposed on all protein nonhydrogen atoms.

In Fig. 2.6(a) we report the time evolution of $\Delta G_{if}(\phi) = \Im(\phi)$ for the free human growth hormone (hGH) receptor subunit hGHbp that forms the receptor/hGH complex, adopting the structural coordinates for the individual subunits provided in PDB entry 3HHR [30] with the structures thermalized as previously indicated. The thin solid line reports a single trajectory, the thick solid grey line, the average over 20 trajectories following the iterative scheme given previously, and the dashed line represents the control consisting of an average over 20 trajectories of 500ps-MD simulation without enforcing the microstate sampling strategy. The minimal $\Delta G_{if}(\phi)$-value is $\Delta G_{if}^{*}(\phi) = 121\ kJ/mol$, corresponding to interfacial tension

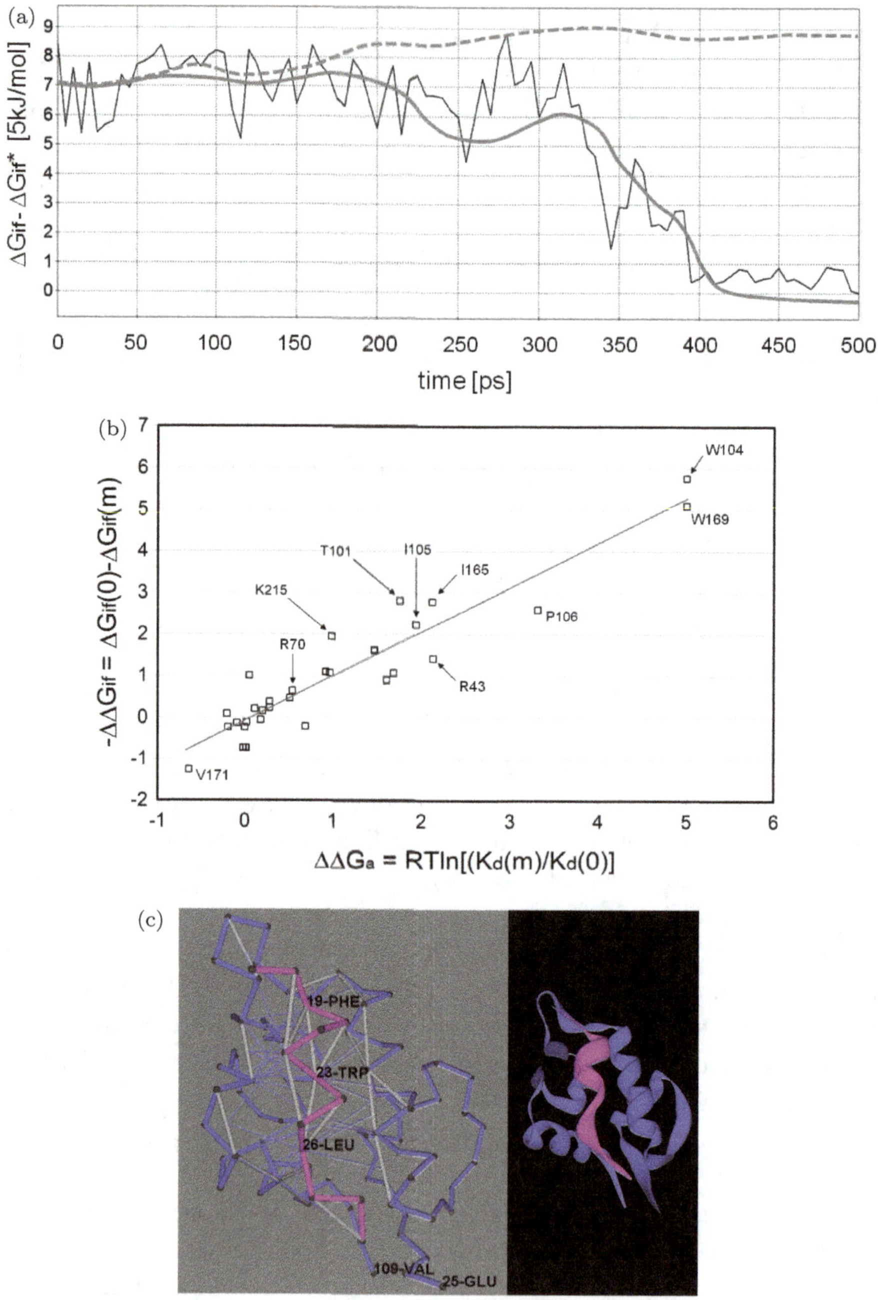

Figure 2.6. (*Continued*)

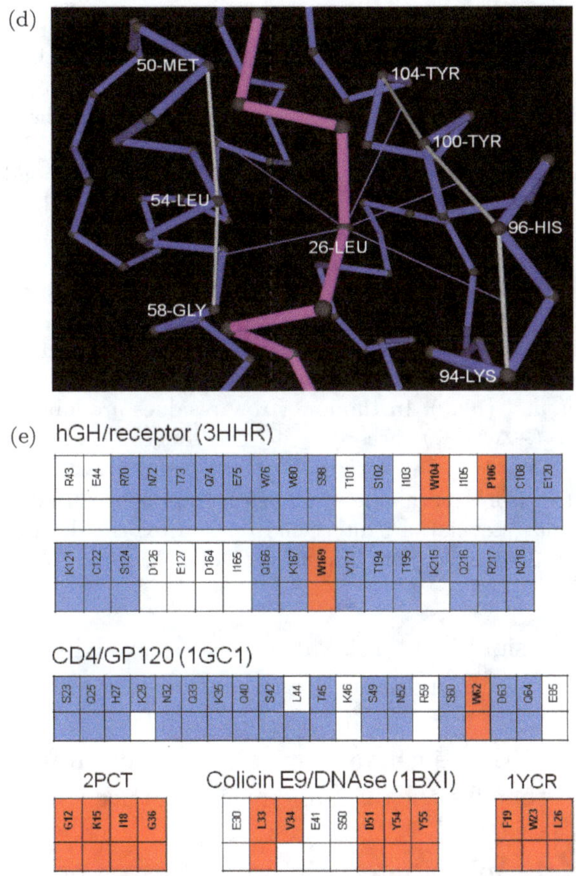

Figure 2.6. Water frustration as steer of protein associations probed by alanine scanning: **(a)** Steering power of microstate sampling. The search for the minimally frustrated interface state is evidenced by the time evolution of $\Delta G_{if}(\phi) = \Im(\phi)$ during 500ps-MD trajectories. The single trajectory is in solid thin line, the average over 20 trajectories in thick grey line, while the dashed grey line represents an average over 20 control 500ps-trajectories with no microstate sampling. Initial structural coordinates were obtained for the corresponding hGHbp receptor chain in the free state that forms a 1:1 complex with the human growth hormone (hGH) (PDB.3HHR). The minimal $\Delta G_{if}(\phi)$-value is reached within the 350–400 ps range. **(b)** Correlation ($R^2 = 0.88$) between $-\Delta\Delta G_{if}$ and $\Delta\Delta G_a$ for site-directed mutational substitution of interfacial residues in hGHbp, yielding the approximate relation $-\Delta\Delta G_{if} \approx \Delta\Delta G_a$. **(c)** Interfacial tension reduction in the MDM2-p53-transactivation domain complex (PDB.1YCR). Hot spots are identified as preformed backbone hydrogen bonds exposed to water (dehydrons) in the free p53 subunit, undergoing displacement of vicinal water upon association.

Figure 2.6. (*Continued*) The displacement results from the approach of a side chain of the binding partner and is marked by a thin line from the alpha-carbon of the displacing side chain to the center of the dehydron. The dehydrons from the MDM2 peptide are induced upon binding. Hydrogen bonds are represented as lines joining paired residues in a virtual-bond-alpha-carbon representation. The ribbon rendering on the right is an aid to the eye. **(d)** Displacement by MDM2 residue L26 of frustrated water around preformed hot-spot dehydrons in the p53-transactivation domain upon association. **(e)** Residue classification for PDB-reported protein complexes with available affinity scanning data according to $\Delta\Delta G_a$-values and $-\Delta\Delta G_{if}$-values. In the upper row for each PP interface, the classification is established according to the ranges $\Delta\Delta G_a \geq 3\,kcal/mol$ (red), $1\,kcal/mol \leq \Delta\Delta G_a < 3\,kcal/mol$ (white), and $\Delta\Delta G_a < 1\,kcal/mol$ (blue). In the lower row residues are labeled following the second classifier ($-\Delta\Delta G_{if}$), according to the ranges $-\Delta\Delta G_{if} \geq 3\,kcal/mol$ (red), $\frac{1\,kcal}{mol} \leq -\Delta\Delta G_{if} < 3\,kcal/mol$ (white), and $-\Delta\Delta G_{if} < 1\,kcal/mol$ (blue). Reprinted from [Fernández A (2016) Non-Debye frustrated hydration steers biomolecular association: Interfacial tension for the drug designer. FEBS Letters 590:3481–3491] with permission from John Wiley & Sons.

$2.13\,mJ/m^2$. A significant relaxation is observed in the 350–400 ps range (Fig. 2.6(a)), in agreement with experimental relaxation times for the coupling of protein motion and hydration pattern [38]. It should be noted that such values are incommensurably larger than the relaxation time for the decoupled water lattice (∼1 ps) previously incorporated [32].

To assert the role of interfacial water frustration as promoter of PP association, we determine the effect of site-directed mutations on the interfacial free energy increment $\Delta G_{if}(\phi)$, and compare the $\Delta\Delta G_{if}(\phi)$ values with the change in affinity quantified by the calorimetrically measured $\Delta\Delta G_a = RTln[\frac{K_d(m)}{K_d(0)}]$, where $\Delta\Delta G_a$ is the change in association free energy that results from a site-specific mutation [30], with $K_d(m)$, $K_d(0)$ indicating the equilibrium dissociation constants for mutant (m) and wild-type (0), respectively. Hot spots in PP associations were experimentally identified by alanine scanning of the PP interface [30]. This technique involves site-specific amino acid substitution for alanine (effectively, a side-chain truncation). The most comprehensively scanned interface corresponds to the 1:1 hGH-hGHbp complex [30]. Thus, the changes in affinity measured by $\Delta\Delta G_a$ and obtained from alanine scanning were contrasted with *in-silico* substitution effects computed as changes in interfacial free energy $\Delta\Delta G_{if} = \Delta G_{if}(m) - \Delta G_{if}(0)$. A tight correlation ($R^2 = 0.88$) between $-\Delta\Delta G_{if}$ and $\Delta\Delta G_a$ corresponding to the scanning of the receptor hGHbp (Fig. 2.6(b)), supports the relation $-\Delta\Delta G_{if} \approx \Delta\Delta G_a$, *and upholds the view that the complexes assemble to reduce the interfacial tension of the free subunits.*

To further support this assertion, other protein associations were considered where $\Delta\Delta G_a$-values were available [30, 39–42]. For example, the p53 trans-activation domain, that forms a complex with MDM2 (PDB.1YCR) [42], has been thermalized and equilibrated in free form following the protocol previously indicated to identify hot spots representing contributions $\geq$3 kcal/mol to ΔG_{if}. Such hot spots correspond to the frustrated water partially confined in the cavities formed by dehydrons in the protein structure (Fig. 2.6(c)). The backbone hydrogen bonds in the MDM2 fragment are induced upon binding and do not constitute hot spots, since no stable structure can be sustained by the MDM2 peptide in free form. Upon forming the complex, residues F19, W23 and L26 in MDM2 have been identified as removing frustrated water from the vicinity of the hot-spot p53 dehydrons shown in Fig. 2.6(c). For example, L26 displaces frustrated water from hot-spot dehydrons M50-L54, L54-G58, L94-H96, H96-Y100 and Y100-Y104, as shown in Fig. 2.6(d). These considerations lead us to identify MDM2 residues F19, W23 and L26 as the significant contributors, yielding $-\Delta\Delta G_{if} \geq 3\, kcal/mol$ upon *in silico* scanning of the PP interface. This result is in accord with the experimental alanine scanning yielding $\Delta\Delta G_a \geq 3\, kcal/mol$ solely for these three residues in MDM2 [42].

To extend and simplify the analysis, we classified residues according to $\Delta\Delta G_a$-ranges and independently according to $\Delta\Delta G_{if}$-ranges. Adopting the affinity classifier, hot-spot residues are labeled (upper row for each PP interface, Fig. 2.6(e)) according to the ranges $\Delta\Delta G_a \geq 3\, kcal/mol$ (red), $1\, kcal/mol \leq \Delta\Delta G_a < 3\, kcal/mol$ (white), and $\Delta\Delta G_a < 1\, kcal/mol$ (blue). Adopting the interfacial tension classifier (lower row for each PP interface), residues are labeled according to the ranges $-\Delta\Delta G_{if} \geq 3\, kcal/mol$ (red), $\frac{1 kcal}{mol} \leq -\Delta\Delta G_{if} <$

$3\,kcal/mol$ (white), and $-\Delta\Delta G_{if} < 1\,kcal/mol$ (blue). Using these two classifiers, the PP interfaces for five complexes with scanning data available were examined: hGH/hGHbp receptor (3HHR) [30], HIV-1-CD4/GP120 (1GC1) [39], trypsin inhibitor/beta-trypsin (2PTC) [40], colicin E9 immuno-protein/colicin E9 DNase domain (1BXI) [41] and p53/MDM2 (1YCR) [42]. *The significant correlation between the* $\Delta\Delta G_a$ *and* $-\Delta\Delta G_{if}$ *classifiers (Fig. 2.6(e), P-value* $< 10^{-5}$*) upholds the view that interfacial tension generated by frustrated hydration drives protein association.*

2.5.2 *Epistructural water frustration and association propensity in protein complexes*

To further validate the variational frustration principle we analyze the complex dissociation intermediates arising from progressive cold denaturation of homodimeric repressor protein CγIR2, a system for which the dynamic intermediates have been resolved at atomic resolution [31]. Thus, the frustration-related interfacial tension is given in Fig. 2.7(a) for PDB entries (absolute temperatures in brackets) 2LYJ (298K), 2LYK (270K), 2LYL (266K, dimer), 2LYP (266K, monomer), 2LYQ (262K), 2LYR (259K) and 2LYS (257K). The open disks correspond to the computation of interfacial tension $= \Delta G_{if}(\phi)/A$ for the free subunit with A = solvent-accessible surface area, while the filled disks represent the interfacial tension corresponding to one half of the $\Delta G_{if}(\phi)$-value for dimeric states, a valid estimation of the interfacial free-energy contribution for each subunit within a homodimer. It is clear that the inflexion point at 266 K represents a critically high interfacial tension beyond which the dimeric state prevails to mitigate the higher thermodynamic cost of spanning the interface as the temperature for complex renaturation is approached. A tight correlation ($R^2 = 0.921$, Fig. 2.7(b)) is obtained between dimer/monomer molar ratio X, a measure of association propensity obtained from average values of hydrodynamic radius [31], and the interfacial tension. This correlation validates the variational frustration principle and its dynamic steering role in complex formation. The protein surface regions causative of

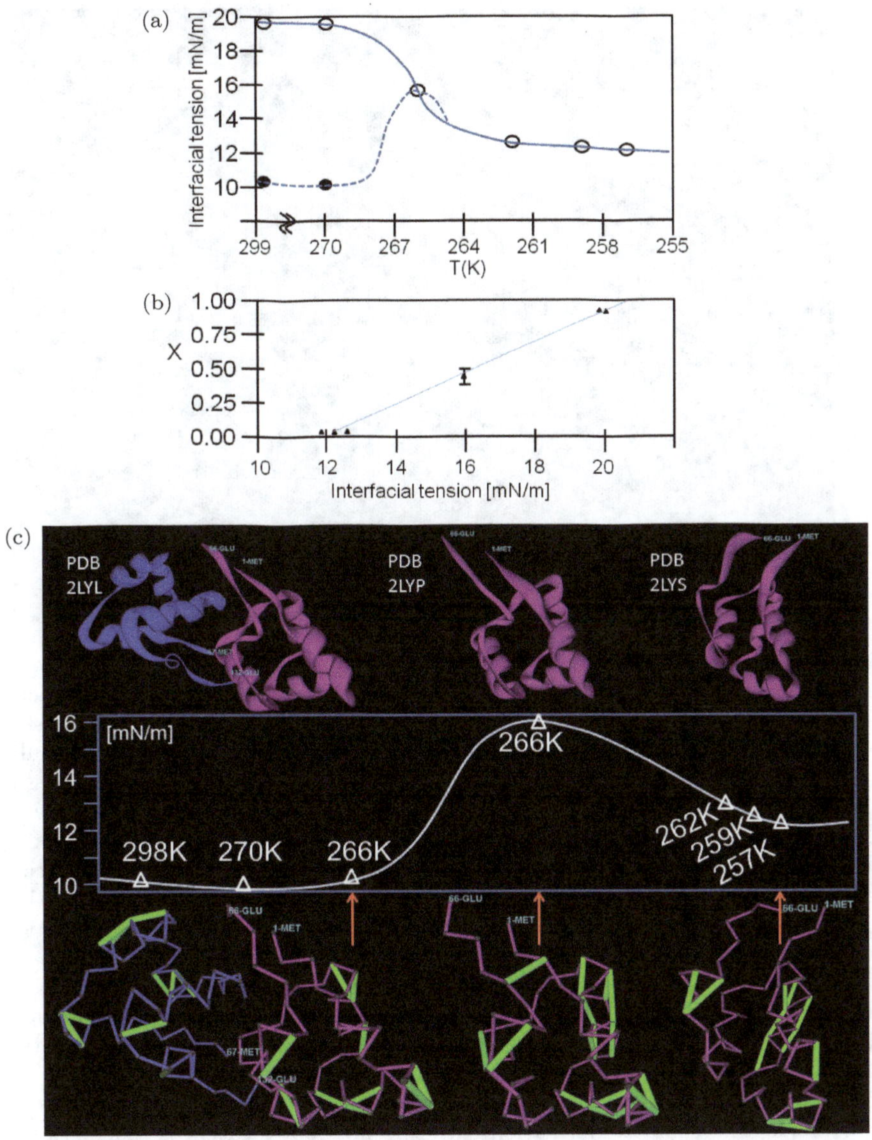

Figure 2.7. (*Continued*)

(d)

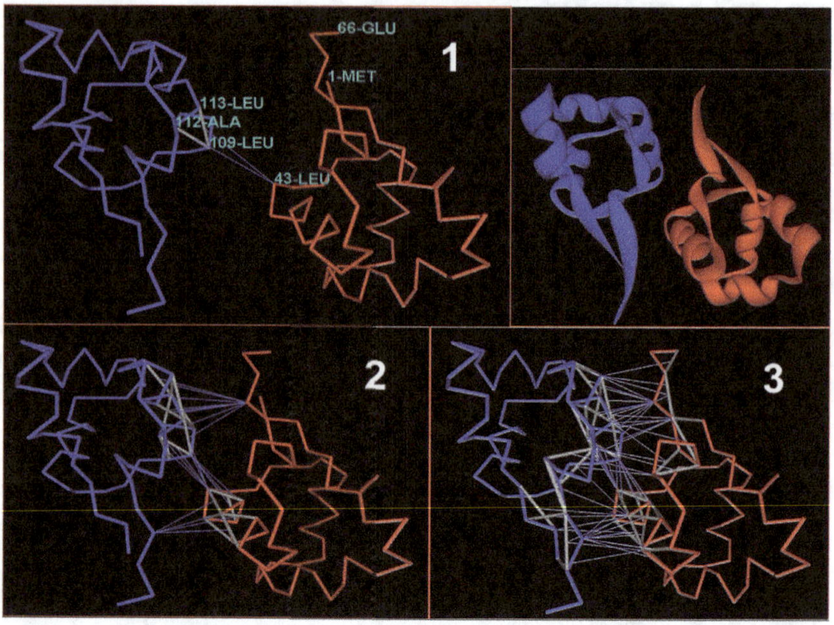

Figure 2.7. Interfacial frustration and dimerization propensity of cold denaturation intermediates of a protein complex: **(a)** Free-energy cost of interfacial frustration per unit surface area for the free monomeric subunit (open disks) and the subunit within the dimer (filled disks) for intermediate states resulting from progressive cold denaturation of the native homodimeric repressor protein CγIR2. The PDB files for the intermediates (absolute temperature in brackets) are 2LYJ (298K), 2LYK (270K), 2LYL (266K, dimer), 2LYP (266K, monomer), 2LYQ (262K), 2LYR (259K) and 2LYS (257K). **(b)** Correlation between molar dimer/monomer ratio and free energy cost of interfacial frustration per unit surface area for the free (uncomplexed) subunit in the cold-denaturation intermediates. **(c)** Hot spots of interfacial frustration (shown in green on the protein structure) for denaturation intermediate at 257K (PDB.2LYS), and the inflexion-point intermediate with monomeric state in PDB.2LYP and dimeric state in PDB.2LYL. The inflexion point intermediate is attributed two $\Delta G_{if}(\phi)$-values, one as free monomer and the other as subunit within the dimer. Hot spots are shown as solvent-exposed backbone hydrogen bonds or *dehydrons*. The chain conformation featuring hot-spot location is schematically represented by virtual bonds joining alpha-carbons. **(d)** Optimal frustration pathway leading to protein subunit association generated following the microstate sampling strategy (T = 298 K, computation time: 0.1 ms, number of iterations: 2–21 $\times$ 10^9). Initial conditions were provided by the structural coordinates of two dissociated CγIR2 subunits (PDB.2LYS). The chains are represented as virtual bonds joining alpha-carbons and intermolecular water exclusion from a

Figure 2.7. (*Continued*) PP interfacial dehydron is indicated by a line from the alpha-carbon of the approaching residue that promotes water removal to the center of the interfacial hydrogen bond. The latter are displayed as lines joining the alpha-carbons of the paired residues. Four runs reveal a unique nucleating configuration (**1**) at $\sim 1\,\mu s$. Other reproducible configurations (**2, 3**) occur at $\sim 19\,\mu s$ and $\sim 90\,\mu s$, with the latter (**3** and ribbon representation) presenting the fully dehydrated PP interface with RMSD < 0.80 Å relative to the homodimer crystal in PDB entry 2LYJ. Reprinted from [Fernández A (2016) Non-Debye frustrated hydration steers biomolecular association: Interfacial tension for the drug designer. FEBS Letters 590:3481–3491] with permission from John Wiley & Sons.

interfacial frustration [23] are shown in green on Fig. 2.7(c). Thus, hot spots in interfacial frustration are shown for the most denatured intermediate (PDB.2LYS, 257 K), and the inflexion-point intermediate whose critically high interfacial frustration promotes significant dimerization at 266K, with monomeric state in PDB.2LYP and dimeric state in PDB.2LYL. The inflexion-point intermediate is attributed two $\Delta G_{if}(\phi)$-values, one as free subunit (PDB.2YLP) and the other as subunit-within-dimer (PDB.2LYL).

Finally, the non-Debye frustration pathway leading to maximal reduction of interfacial tension conducive to protein subunit association is generated following the flow chart (Fig. 2.5) at renaturation T = 298 K. We computed the path to minimally frustrated hydration adopting the structural coordinates of two fully dissociated CgIR2 subunits (PDB.2LYS) as initial condition. Four runs reveal a unique nucleating step at $\sim$1 microsecond, ultimately leading to formation of the fully dehydrated PP interface. This step consists of intermolecular dehydration of dehydron Leu109-Ala112 and Leu109-Leu113 by Leu43 in the complementary binding subunit (Fig. 2.7(d)). The pathway leads to optimal mitigation of interfacial tension and ultimate formation of the dimer with RMSD < 0.80 Å relative to the homodimer crystal in PDB entry 2LYJ.

2.5.3 *Epistructural water for drug design*

The results presented so far reveal a protein "epistructure" defined by the frustration state of the aqueous interface. This concept impacts drug design geared at impairing protein function through target-drug association whereby the interfacial tension of the target is reduced. Such a design strategy explored throughout this book is expected to enable an ultra-selective control of the drug impact with discriminatory molecular recognition even at the level of isoforms of the target protein (>80% sequence identity). Homologous proteins typically possess high structural similarity but the differences in composition translate into differences at the epistructural level which may be harness to design selective drugs that can tell them apart.

For example, it has been recognized that the phosphoinositide 3-kinase (PI3K) family is implicated in human cancer through its role in the regulation of diverse cellular processes [43]. Yet, pan-PI3K inhibitors that bind indiscriminately with nanomolar (nM) affinity to isoforms PI3K alpha, beta, delta (class IA) are not desirable therapeutically due to off-target side effects [44]. It has become imperative to design drugs that can tell apart such isoforms. It would be desirable to re-engineering lead compounds to improve selectivity towards the beta–isoform recognized as a crucial target in PTEN (phosphatase and tensin homologue)-deficient cancers [45]. In this regard, the lead compound *2-[2-(2,3-dihydro-indol-1-yl)-2-oxo-ethyl]-6-morpholin-4-yl-3H-pyrimidin-4-one* (Fig. 2.8(a)) binds with nM affinity to PI3K beta and delta isoforms (IC_{50} = 4 and 28nM, respectively) [34]. The specificity towards the beta-isoform may be significantly enhanced by comparing the epistructures of both isoforms and modifying the lead compound to target epistructural differences (Figs. 2.8(b,c)). A first substitution (R-isomer, Fig. 2.8(a)) would in principle be suitable to selectively remove upon binding a pre-formed tension hot spot of interfacial tension present only in the beta-isoform (cf. Figs. 2.8(b,c)). Indeed, there is an interfacial tension hot spot in drug target PI3Kbeta corresponding to frustrated water partially hydrating dehydron Ala856-Leu859 (Fig. 2.8(b)). The crystal structure of the complex reveals that the methylation of the lead compound displayed in Fig. 2.8(a) targets dehydron Ala856-Leu859 upon drug-target association. However, the R-substitution *does not* endow the drug with higher discriminatory power towards the beta-isoform [43]. This is a-priori surprising because the

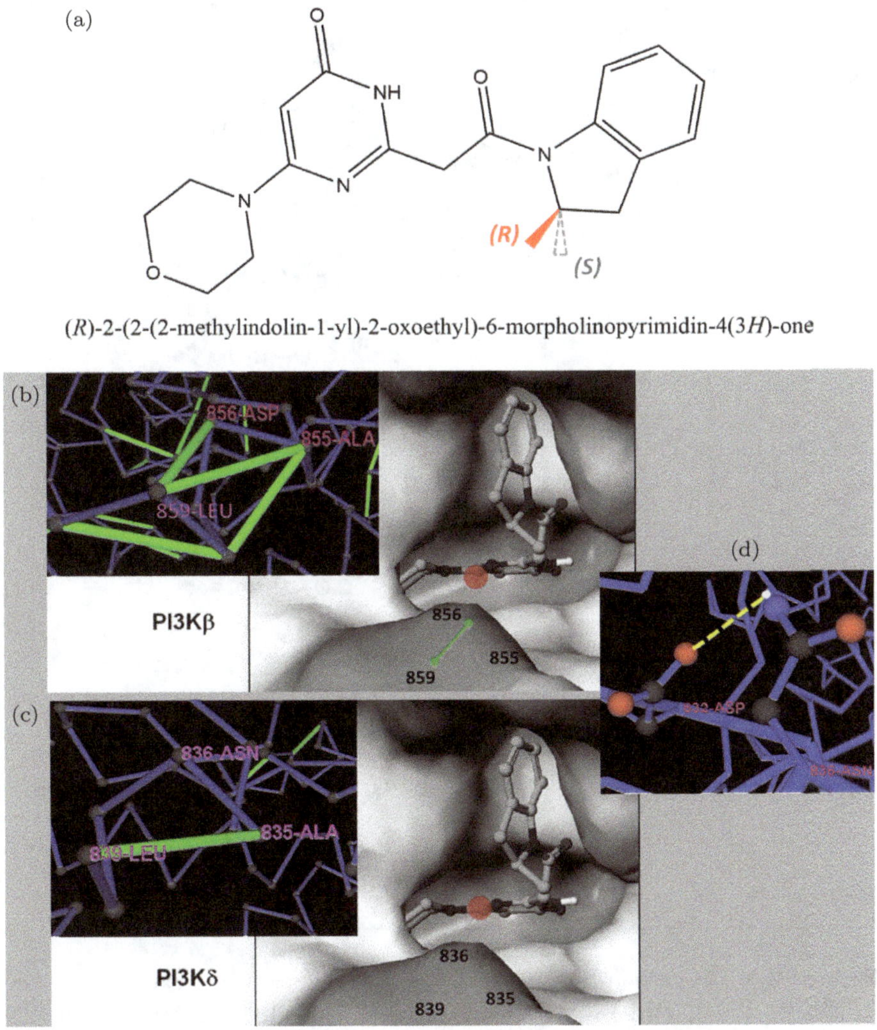

Figure 2.8. Drug design guided by the interfacial tension hot spots of the target protein: **(a)** Chemical structure of lead compound with nM affinity towards the beta and delta-isoforms of PI3K. Two methylation substitutions intended to improve selectivity are shown: R isomer in red, S-isomer in grey. The latter is predicted to endow the compound with discriminatory power, enhancing its selectivity towards the beta-isoform. The R-isomer is named using IUPAC convention. **(b)** Hot spot of interfacial tension in drug target PI3Kbeta corresponding to dehydron Ala856-Leu859 (inset, PDB.4BFR). Dehydrons are displayed as green segments joining the alpha-carbons of residues paired by

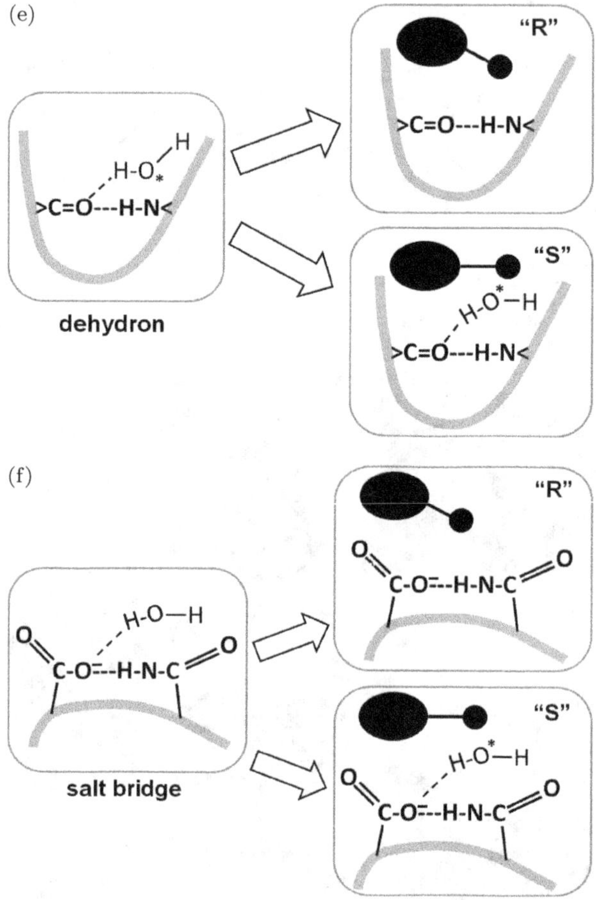

Figure 2.8. (*Continued*) solvent-exposed backbone hydrogen bonds. The structure of the complex (panel with space-filling atoms) reveals that the S-isomer methylation shown in (a) targets dehydron Ala856-Leu859 with retention of hydrating molecule (red circle). The ligand binding does not appreciably increase the frustration of the water molecule that was already frustrated due to sub-nanoscale confinement within the dehydron cavity and re-accommodates upon binding to the S-ligand. **(c)** Dehydron pattern for PI3Kdelta (PDB.4V0I). The Ala856-Leu859 dehydron in PI3Kbeta aligns with backbone hydrogen bond Ala836-Leu839 in PI3Kdelta which is not solvent-exposed and hence it does not cause significant water frustration. This local difference in interfacial tension between PI3Kbeta and PI3Kdelta suggests the modifications featured in (a) as a means to enhance drug selectivity towards the beta-isoform. **(d)** Salt

Figure 2.8. (*Continued*) bridge (dashed line) in PI3Kdelta absent in PI3Kbeta. **(e)** Scheme of frustration effects on dehydron-vicinal water upon binding the R- and S-isomer. Upon binding, the R-isomer excludes vicinal water, thus stabilizing the dehydron, while the S-isomer retains a water molecule but does not increase its frustration relative to the "apo" form. The frustrated loner pair on the oxygen is marked by an asterisk. **(f)** Scheme of frustration effects on water vicinal to a salt bridge upon binding the R- and S-isomer. Upon binding, the R-isomer excludes vicinal water, thus stabilizing the salt bridge, while the S-isomer retains a water molecule significantly increasing its frustration relative to the "apo" form. Reprinted from [Fernández A (2016) Non-Debye frustrated hydration steers biomolecular association: Interfacial tension for the drug designer. FEBS Letters 590:3481–3491] with permission from John Wiley & Sons.

Ala856-Leu859 dehydron in PI3Kbeta aligns with solvent-shielded backbone hydrogen bond Ala836-Leu839 in PI3Kdelta (Figs. 2.8(b,c)) which does not frustrate water nearby. The reason for the lack of specificity is that PI3Kdelta features *in lieu* of a dehydron the exposed salt bridge Asp832-Asn836 (Fig. 2.8(d)) which gets dehydrated upon binding with the R-ligand, thereby becoming stabilized to an extent comparable to the dehydron. The interfacial thermodynamics for ligand association reflect this observation, yielding $\Delta\Delta G_{if}(\beta, \delta, R) \approx 0 \pm \frac{0.22\,kcal}{mol}$ for the difference in the interfacial free energy change between the delta and beta isoforms upon binding to the R-ligand. To achieve specificity one may instead *retain* the frustrated interfacial water molecule upon ligand binding, adopting the methylated S-ligand to that effect (Figs. 2.8(b,c)). In the respective apo-states, water frustration is 1.7 for water around dehydron 856-859 in the beta-isoform and becomes 0.6 for the water molecule closest to Asn836 in the delta-isoform. The resulting local difference in interfacial tension between PI3Kbeta and PI3Kdelta suggests adopting the S-ligand with retention of interfacial water upon binding, as shown in Figs. 2.8(b,c) in order to enhance specificity towards the beta-isoform. Thus, the already frustrated water molecule around dehydron 856–859 simply rearranges to accommodate the S-ligand with frustration 1.7 turning 1.9 upon binding, whereas the 0.6 frustrated water hydrating salt bridge Asp832-Asn836, becomes severely frustrated, with frustration transitioning

$0.6 \to 1.8$, upon binding to the S-ligand (Fig. 2.8(e,f)). This trend is reflected in the thermodynamics: $\Delta\Delta G_{if}(\beta, \delta, S) \approx 2.8 \pm \frac{0.61\,kcal}{mol}$, indicative of a significantly higher affinity of the S-ligand towards the beta-isoform. Experimental results uphold this prediction [43]. With $IC_{50} = 23\,nM$ and $468\,nM$ for the beta and delta-isoforms, respectively, the S-ligand is three times more selective towards PI3Kbeta than the parental compound ($IC_{50} = 4\,nM$ and $28\,nM$, respectively).

This example illustrates the power of variational computations of frustrated hydration as a guide to design ultra-selective drugs that could not be rationally conceived adopting standard structure-based approaches.

To reconcile thermodynamics and structural data on protein complexation, this section focused on the steering role of frustrated hydration in biomolecular associations. To make frustration at the aqueous interface amenable to variational methods, we introduced a "frustration field" identifying locally unmet hydrogen-bonding opportunities due to sub-nanoscale confinement at each point in space. The frustration field was optimized variationally, and the dynamics resulting from the computational search were shown to drive protein associations with great specificity in order to mitigate frustration-related interfacial tension. Our computations entailed a microstate sampling method implemented to search for the state of minimal interfacial frustration within relaxation times for protein-water dynamic coupling. The crystallographic, affinity scanning and NMR record on protein assemblages attested to the validity of the minimal frustration principle.

The solvent-centric approach introduced in this section was shown to impact the design of ultra-selective drugs, as it highlighted the targetable nature of the aqueous interface enabling the discrimination of closely related protein isoforms that could not be operationally distinguished using structure-based designs. In this regard, the role of dehydrons as selectivity filters can be recognized, yet the physical underpinnings of the concept will be delineated further in the book.

2.6 Aqueous interfaces for structural biology

To complement and enrich the solvent-centric perspective on the epistructural interface provided in the previous sections, we now examine the features in the protein structure that most decisively contribute to determine the interfacial properties, i. e. the dehydrons, from a structure-centric perspective. Since we have identified the dehydron as the structural feature that contributes most decisively to the interfacial free energy, we may at this stage briefly switch from the solvent-centric perspective on biomolecular interfaces to a structure-centric perspective and examine dehydrons within the context of protein structure.

This approach naturally leads to the concept of cooperativity in the assembly of the protein structure, or rather, leads us to regard dehydrons as local indicators of failed cooperativity. Thus, dehydrons are viewed as structural defects that may be "corrected" upon association with protein binding partners or with man-made ligands such as therapeutic drugs. This conceptual framework becomes most efficacious to help improve drug design, as we shall see shortly.

While the biophysical principles governing the affinity of a drug for a target biomolecule are believed to be understood, the control of specificity, the safety, and the idiosyncratic efficacy of the therapeutic agents remain opaque subjects. Clinical uncertainty and unpredictable adverse effects often hamper drug development and this situation is unlikely to change unless a higher level of conceptual innovation is effectively incorporated in the discovery pipeline.

We shall narrow down our treatment of these vast problems to small-molecule drugs purposely engineered to target human proteins and thereby inhibit their biological function. Aiming at a paradigm shift in the field, we advocate a translational top-down approach that takes us back to the very fundamentals of protein associations as we introduce a foundational platform for a next generation of safer and more effective drugs.

In molecular therapy, we often deal with water-soluble proteins that are targeted by man-made ligands, therefore the efficacy and target-specificity of a molecular design depends pivotally on our understanding of protein-ligand associations. In this regard, there is a crucial property that seems have been missed altogether in rational drug design: *cooperativity*. We somewhat narrowly define this property as the concurrent participation of different regions of the biomolecule to promote and sustain intramolecular or intermolecular interactions. In plain terms, "cooperativity is the nonadditive contribution to protein interactions", a peculiar property often illustrated by the phrase "the whole is more than the sum of the parts". In our context of interest, the nonadditive nature of protein associations implies that *the rational drug designer faces a many-body problem*: the interactions between the protein target and the drug/ligand involve more than groups matched up in a pairwise fashion at the target-ligand interface. Because protein-ligand interactions take place in an aqueous medium, this many-body problem is a very special one. As we shall advocate throughout this book, matching groups with complementary biochemical properties across the target/ligand interface is only one aspect of what rational design is about and by no means the decisive one, as the evidence attests. The next generation of molecular designs must take into account modes of association or binding above and beyond pair-wise intermolecular interactions involving groups in the ligand and their purported matched groups in the target.

Be as it may, the current design paradigm is unlikely to change anytime soon unless a clear case can be made for cooperativity, and the right computational tools are brought to fruition to operationally incorporate this concept in drug design. As we deal with cooperativity, perhaps the first core question that needs to be dealt with is: *what sort of many-body problem is the drug designer facing and how can this knowledge play advantageously to address the major therapeutic imperatives of today and tomorrow?*

Protein structure in solution is assumed to arise and be sustained by forces that are essentially electrostatic [46–50]. Even the hydrophobic attraction between two nonpolar groups, an entropic effect arising from the minimization of unfavorable interfaces with water, includes a major electrostatic contribution as it increases the extent of hydrogen bonding among surrounding water molecules

[48]. The forces that drive protein folding and protein associations are actually modulated by an important factor often neglected: *the shaping of the solvent microenvironment wherein the forces become operational* [47]. Since the shaping of the microenvironment around a pair-wise intramolecular interaction requires the participation of other regions of the molecule, we may state that cooperativity is inherent to the folding of a protein chain [49–58].

To illustrate the importance of cooperativity, we may recall that an electrostatic interaction occurring in bulk water is 78 times weaker than the same interaction in an anhydrous medium [47,55]. Thus, the stability and strength of pairwise interactions between different parts of the peptide chain is determined not only by the atomic groups directly engaged in the interaction, but also by the groups involved in shaping their microenvironment by promoting the expulsion of surrounding water [55]. The latter contributors are just as important, as they determine either the persistence or the ephemeral nature of the interactions and, ultimately, the integrity of the protein structure [47]. In fact, low-permittivity microenvironments around the backbone hydrogen bonds of a self-interacting polypeptide chain are essential to promote and sustain its structure and have been the focus of much attention as we attempt to underpin the physical basis of cooperativity [47,49,56].

The backbone of a protein or peptide chain is highly polar, comprising an amide and carbonyl group per residue. This chemical feature introduces constraints on the nature of the hydrophobic collapse [54] and on the chain composition of foldable proteins, i. e. those capable of sustaining such a collapse [57, 58]. Thus, the hydrophobic collapse entails the dehydration of backbone amides and carbonyls and such a process would be thermodynamically unfavorable unless amides and carbonyls engage in hydrogen bonding with each other [54]. Only a hydrophobic collapse that ensures the formation and protection of backbone hydrogen bonds is likely to be conducive to sustainable folding [56].

The hydration of amides and carbonyls competes with the formation of the intramolecular hydrogen bonds. Thus, the structural integrity of proteins is compromised by a "deficiently wrapped" backbone [56, 59]. Wrapping refers to a cluster of nonpolar groups around a pre-formed coulombic interaction [58]. The need for protection of intramolecular hydrogen bonds from water attack is an important factor in determining the chain composition of a *foldable* protein, that is, of a chain capable of sustaining a soluble structure and folding expeditiously and reproducibly [56].

As noted above, the strength and stability of backbone hydrogen bonds clearly depend on the microenvironment where they occur: The proximity of nonpolar groups to a hydrogen bond enhances the electrostatic interaction by de-screening the partial charges or lowering the local environment permittivity [55, 57]. These nonpolar groups also stabilize the hydrogen bond by destabilizing the nonbonded state, i. e. by hindering the hydration of the polar groups in the nonbonded state [57, 58]. Thus, to guarantee the integrity of soluble protein structure, most intramolecular hydrogen bonds must be surrounded or "*wrapped*" by nonpolar groups fairly thoroughly as to become significantly dehydrated [56–59].

To make the wrapping concept more precise, we need a definition that enables a direct assessment of the extent of hydrogen bond protection from structure coordinates. This parameter, denoted ρ, is given by the number of side-chain carbonaceous nonpolar groups ($\mathrm{CH_n}, \mathrm{n} = 0, 1, 2, 3$) contained within a desolvation domain that represents the hydrogen-bond microenvironment. This domain is defined as the reunion of two intersecting spheres of fixed radius ($\sim$thickness of three water layers) centered at the α-carbons of the residues paired by the hydrogen bond. In structures of PDB-reported soluble proteins, backbone hydrogen bonds are protected on average by $\rho = 26.6 \pm 7.5$ side-chain nonpolar groups for a desolvation sphere of radius $\mathrm{r} = 6\,\text{Å}$. The desolvation domain adopted for a hydrogen bond is a residue-based feature, incorporating a descriptor of the local environment of each of the paired residues [58]. It fully subsumes the local environment of the hydrogen bond itself since the heavy atoms N and O are invariably within $6\,\text{Å}$ of the α-carbons of the paired residues and hence fully contained in the intersection of the desolvation spheres.

Accordingly, if we treat the solvent implicitly, we may identify a *wrapping interaction* as a three-body ijk-interaction, where nonpolar group k contributes to the removal of water from the microenvironment of an amide-carbonyl hydrogen bond that pairs groups i and j. In other words, the "wrapping" nonpolar group k lies within the desolvation domain of the ij-interaction. This type of three-body contribution is cooperative by definition and needed to maintain the structural integrity of the protein [57, 58]. An illustration of wrapping interactions in the native structure of human *ubiquitin* (PDB accession code PDB.1UBI) is given in Fig. 2.9. Thus, the wrapping of the Lys27-Gln31 backbone hydrogen bond by residues Ile36 and Lys29 is represented by thin blue lines. These residues contribute 4 and 3 nonpolar groups respectively to the desolvation domain (r = 6 Å) of the backbone hydrogen bond.

Taken together, the hydration propensity of amide and carbonyl and the dehydration-induced strengthening of their electrostatic association represent two conflictive tendencies, suggesting that there must be a crossover point in the dehydration propensity of a backbone hydrogen bond [60]. If the bond is poorly wrapped by a few nonpolar groups that cluster around it, then hydration of the paired amide and carbonyl is favored and prevails over a structured region, but as the hydrogen bond becomes better wrapped, the surrounding water loses too many hydrogen bonding partnerships and thus may be favorably removed [58]. This observation is essential to rationalize the cooperative two-state nature of the folding of single-domain proteins [61–63], as shown in Chapter 3: we may say that the state of hydration of a protein hydrogen bond is in a statistical sense a local reflection of the degree of progress of the folding process.

2.7 Dehydron pattern: The meta-analysis of protein structure

The structural integrity of a soluble protein is contingent on its ability to exclude water from its amide-carbonyl hydrogen bonds [56, 57]. Thus, dehydrons constitute structural weaknesses taking the particular form of wrapping deficiencies [57, 64, 65].

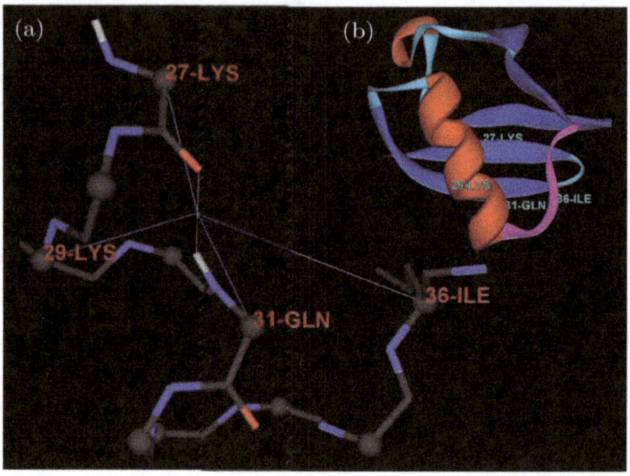

Figure 2.9. **(a)** Cooperative "wrapping" interactions involving residues Lys29 and Ile36 that contribute to stabilize and enhance the backbone hydrogen bond Lys27-Gln31 (thin white line) in human ubiquitin (PDB.1UBI). Each interaction generates a three-body energy term and a residue contributing with nonpolar side-chain groups to the desolvation domain of the hydrogen bond is represented by a thin blue line joining the α-carbon (grey sphere) of the residue with the center of the amide-carbonyl hydrogen bond. Conventional colors are used for atom representation and the protein backbone is represented schematically, except for the two residues paired by the backbone hydrogen bond that are displayed in full backbone detail. Only the side chains of the wrapping residues 29Lys and 36Ile are shown. **(b)** Location of the residues in a ribbon rendering of the native structure of human ubiquitin.

On the other hand, these defects favor the removal of surrounding water as a means to strengthen and stabilize the underlying electrostatic interaction [58, 65, 66], and thus are predictably implicated in protein associations [60], aberrant aggregation [61] and macromolecular recognition [62, 63]. By exogenously contributing to the wrapping of pre-formed hydrogen bonds, these associations in effect remove the wrapping defects, thereby stabilizing the structure.

Intramolecular hydrogen bonds that are not "wrapped" by a sufficient number of nonpolar groups in the protein itself may become stabilized and strengthened by the attachment of a ligand, i.e. a potential drug, or a binding partner that further contributes to their dehydration (Fig. 2.10) [64, 66]. Ample bioinformatics evidence on

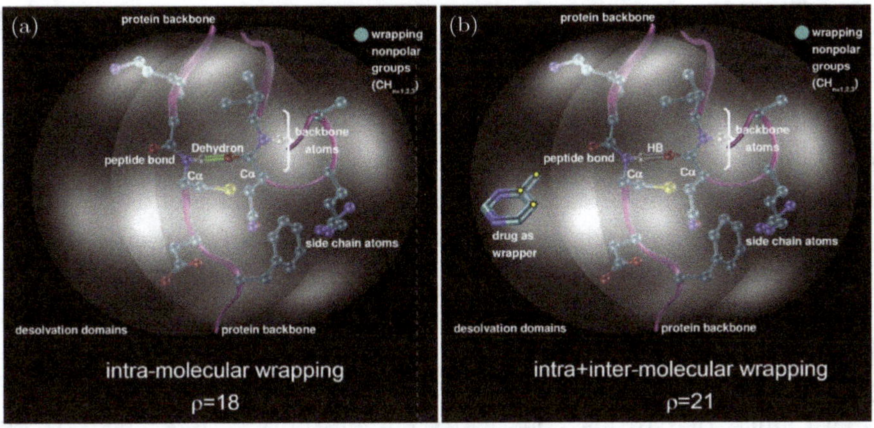

Figure 2.10. **(a)** Dehydron in a soluble protein. The dehydron ($\rho = 18$), marked in green, pairs two backbone groups (amide and carbonyl, conventional colors for atoms). The microenvironment is indicated by two intersecting grey spheres centred at the α-carbons of the paired residues. Wrapping side-chain groups are shown in light blue and only side chains contributing (fully or partially) to the dehydration of the hydrogen bond are indicated. **(b)** The drug depicted in the Fig. acts as an exogenous wrapper of the hydrogen bond (grey bond, $\rho = 21$) turning the dehydron into a well-protected bond (the 3 atoms marked with * complete the desolvation of the dehydron).

the distribution of dehydrons at the interface of protein complexes support this physical picture [58, 66]. Thus, dehydrons are decisive factors driving association in 38% of the PDB complexes and constitute significant factors (interfacial dehydron density larger than average on individual partners) in about 95% of all complexes reported in the PDB [58].

Dehydrons may be identified from atomic coordinates of proteins with reported structure, as illustrated in Fig. 2.10. Thus, we need to introduce an auxiliary quantity, the extent of hydrogen-bond wrapping, ρ, indicating the number of nonpolar groups contained within a "desolvation domain" around the bond. In structures of soluble proteins at least two thirds of the backbone hydrogen bonds are wrapped on average by $\rho = 26.6 \pm 7.5$ nonpolar groups for a desolvation ball radius 6 Å. Dehydrons lie in the tails of the distribution, i.e. their microenvironment contains 19 or fewer nonpolar groups, so their ρ-value is below the mean ($\rho = 26.6$) minus one standard deviation ($\sigma = 7.5$)[57, 58].

Thus, the overall under-wrapping of a protein may be assessed by determining the percentage of intramolecular hydrogen bonds satisfying the inequality $\rho \leq 19$, that is, the percentage of dehydrons in its structure. An example of the under-wrapping of a protein is given in Fig. 2.2(c), where the dehydron pattern of human ubiquitin is displayed.

Dehydron-rich regions in soluble proteins are typical hot spots for protein associations because of their propensity towards further dehydration [58, 66]. A functional perspective reinforces this view, since dehydrons constitute vulnerabilities that need to be "corrected" to maintain the integrity of the protein structure and its functional competence. Thus, specific residues of the binding partner contribute to the desolvation of dehydrons, as they penetrate the desolvation domain of intramolecular hydrogen bonds upon association. This intermolecular wrapping is illustrated in Fig. 2.11(a–c), displaying the functionally competent human HIV-1 protease dimer. The purported interfacial region of the homodimer contains 7 dehydrons when the monomeric domains are considered in isolation and separated from each other. Upon association, specific residues of the binding partner contribute to the desolvation of some of the dehydrons, as they enter the desolvation domain of the intramolecular hydrogen bonds. This inter-molecular wrapping reduces the vulnerability of the protease, which only has 3 dehydrons at the interface upon complexation, instead of the original 7 in the monomeric form. Similarly, the allosteric clam haemoglobin, a functionally competent homodimer utilizes 5 dehydrons of the monomeric state to accommodate its quaternary structure. These 5 dehydrons become well wrapped in the dimer (Fig. 2.11(d)).

Throughout the book, dehydrons will be referred to in different ways depending on the context. Thus, the terms *packing defect, wrapping defect, dehydron, structural deficiency, structural vulnerability*, will be used synonymously. Far from introducing a notational chaos, this name multiplicity bespeaks of the richness of the concept.

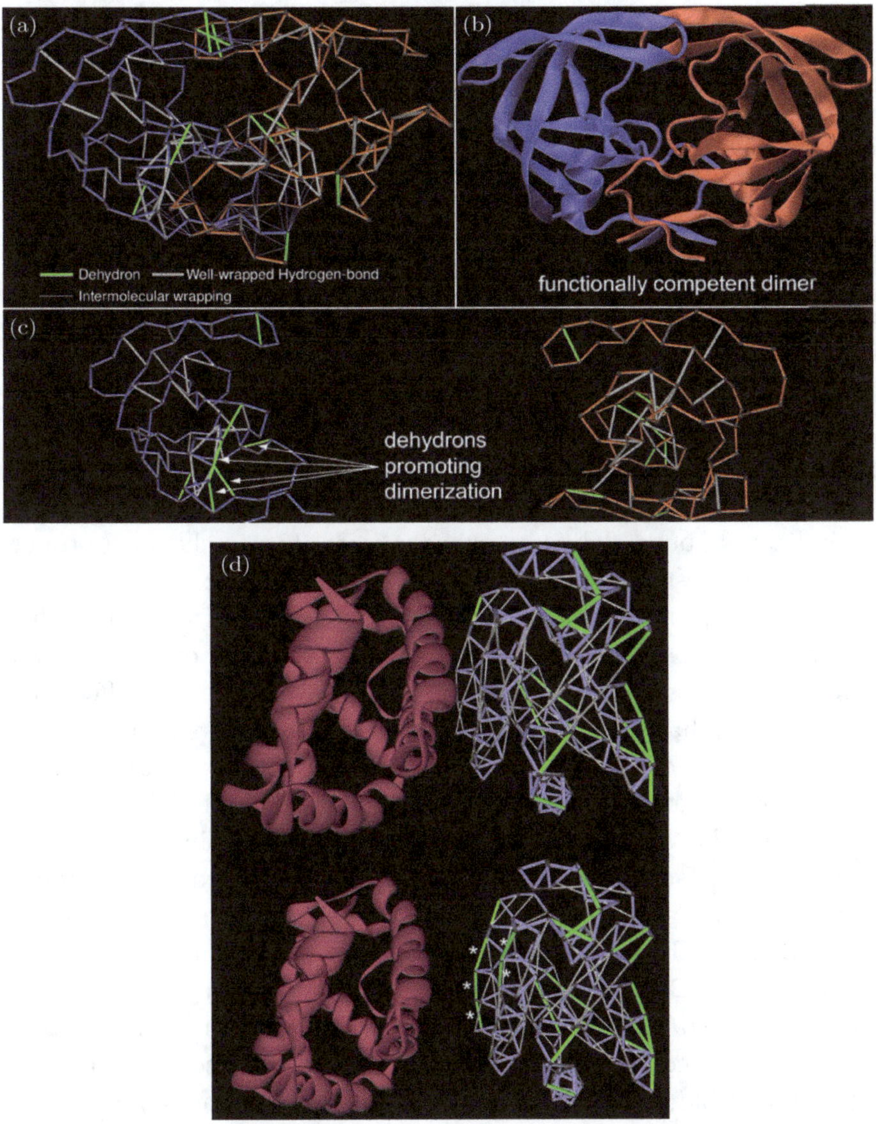

Figure 2.11. **(a)** Inter-molecular wrapping in the human HIV-1 protease dimer (PDB.1A30) as a means of protecting the enzyme structure from water attack. Dehydrons are indicated as green segments joining the alpha-carbons of the paired units, well-wrapped hydrogen bonds are shown in light grey, and the protein backbone is conventionally shown as virtual bonds joining the alpha-carbons of consecutive amino acid units. Complexation reduces the structural vulnerability

Figure 2.11. (*Continued*) of the protease by reducing the number of dehydrons at the interface from 7 to 3. Intermolecular wrapping is depicted by thin blue lines from the alpha-carbon of the wrapping residue to the middle of the hydrogen bond that is intermolecularly protected. Thus, an intermolecularly wrapping residue contributes with nonpolar groups to the dehydration of the preformed hydrogen bond from the binding partner. **(b)** Ribbon display of the dimer. **(c)** Wrapping of separate domains of the human HIV-1 protease. **(d)** Allosteric clam haemoglobin, a functionally competent homodimer that utilizes 5 dehydrons (marked by asterisks in lower panel) of the monomeric state to create a favorable interface for its quaternary structure. The 5 dehydrons become well wrapped in the dimeric state (upper panel). The wrapping pattern of one monomer is displayed while the other monomer is shown in ribbon representation.

2.8 Dehydron physics

As indicated above, dehydrons have unique physico-chemical properties: they represent structural vulnerabilities of the protein, but they also constitute sticky spots promoting the removal of surrounding water [56–59, 64, 66]. This latter property could only be established by addressing the following questions: How do we effectively demonstrate that a dehydron attracts nonpolar test groups? Can we measure the mechanical equivalent of its dehydration propensity?

Reported experimental work addressed these questions by measuring the adsorption of proteins with wrapping defects and equivalent surface hydrophobicity (area of solvent-exposed nonpolar surface) onto a "wrapping" layer [64]. This wrapping medium consists of a Langmuir-Blodgett phospholipid film coating a waveguide, as shown in Fig. 2.12. These high-precision experiments made use of evanescent-field spectroscopic interrogation of the wrapping medium enabling a direct measurement of the protein adsorption uptake. This observable is determined by detecting local changes in refractive index of the phase within which total reflection of the incident light occurred [64]. Thus, a beam from a He-Ne laser travels through a waveguide at an incidence angle suitable for total reflection within the medium. The adsorbed molecules alter the refractive properties of the hydrophobic layer and consequently alter the critical angle for total reflection. Thus, protein adsorption is commensurate

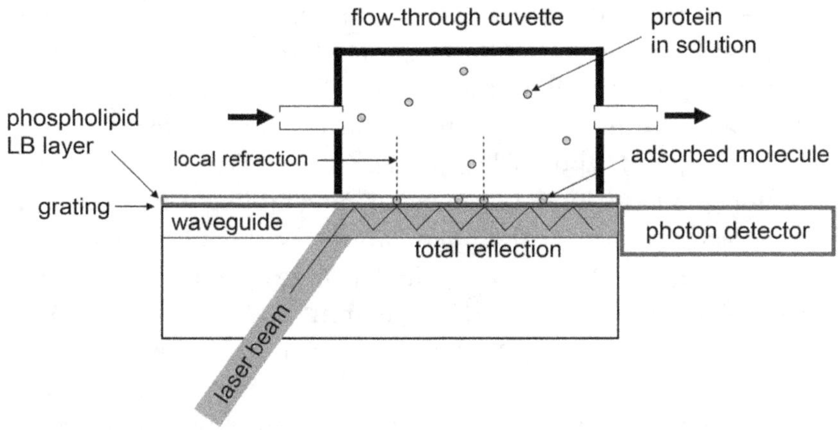

Figure 2.12. High-precision total reflection set-up to measure the adsorption uptake of proteins onto a hydrophobic surface under controlled hydrodynamic conditions. The adsorption uptake is proportional to the photon loss due to local alterations in the refractive index of a Langmuir-Blodget (LB) layer that constitutes the wrapping medium for the protein.

with photon loss resulting from the extent of local refraction or "evanescent field". Hence adsorption uptake can be determined by the loss of photons due to refractive photon leakage from the total reflection pattern.

For proteins with comparable surface hydrophobicity, the adsorption uptake correlates strongly with the extent of protein underwrapping [59]. As an adequate control, only proteins with the same extent of surface hydrophobicity or solvent-exposed nonpolar area were included in the comparative analysis. Hence, the attractive drag exerted by dehydrons on test hydrophobes became accessible. The net gain in Coulomb energy associated with wrapping a dehydron has been experimentally determined to be ~4 kJ/mol [64]. The adhesive force exerted by a dehydron on a hydrophobe at 6 Å distance is ~7.8 pN, a magnitude comparable to the hydrophobic attraction between two nonpolar moieties that frame unfavorable interfaces with water.

This study was motivated by the earlier observations that dehydrons play a pivotal role in driving protein associations, as such associations contribute intermolecularly to the wrapping of pre-formed structure, as discussed in the previous section. In consistency with current terminology, the force stemming from the dehydration propensity of the partially wrapped hydrogen bond is hithertofore termed *dehydronic.* The dehydronic force arises as a nonpolar group approaches a dehydron with a net effect of immobilizing and ultimately removing surrounding water molecules. This displacement lowers the polarizability of the microenvironment which, in turn, de-shields the paired charges [57, 64]. Thus, a net attractive force is exerted by the dehydron on a nonpolar group and this force represents the mechanical equivalent of the dehydration propensity of an unburied preformed hydrogen bond. Since the water molecules solvating an amide and carbonyl paired by a dehydron are necessarily depleted of some hydrogen-bonding partners, the work required for their ultimate removal from the bond surroundings is minimal [57,67]. The dehydronic field, denoted $\vec{\Phi}(\vec{R})$, is necessarily orthogonal to the Coulomb field generated by the polar (amide-carbonyl) pair, and may be described within a quasi-continuous treatment of the solvent by the equation:

$$\vec{\Phi}(\vec{R}) = -\vec{\nabla}_{\vec{R}}[4\pi\varepsilon(\vec{R})]^{-1}qq'/r \tag{12}$$

where $\vec{R}$ represents the position vector of the hydrophobe or nonpolar group with respect to the center of mass of the hydrogen-bonded polar pair, $\vec{\nabla}_{\vec{R}}$ is the gradient taken with respect to this vector, r is the distance between the charges of magnitude q and q' paired by the hydrogen bond (Fig. 2.13(a)), and the local permittivity coefficient $\varepsilon(\vec{R})$ subsumes the polarizability of the microenvironment, which is generically dependent on the position of the test hydrophobe [47, 59]. An appropriate expression for $\varepsilon(\vec{R})$, valid at nanoscales, is unavailable at present [70]. This is because of the discreteness of the dielectric medium and the need to include individual solvent dipole correlations [71]. Although a mean-field dielectric description is unsatisfactory, it is still possible to assert that $\vec{\Phi}(\vec{R})$ is an attractive force since a decrease in $\|\vec{R}\|$ entails a decrease in local polarization which, in turn, enhances the Coulomb attraction.

Building on this analysis, we may quantify the net hydrophobicity η of a hydrogen bond by taking into account the surface flux of the

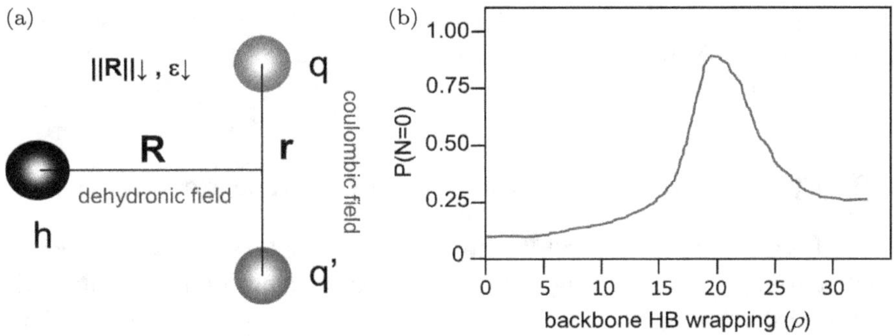

Figure 2.13. **(a)** Orthogonality between *dehydronic* field exerted on the test hydrophobe (h) along coordinate **R** and the coulomb field exerted along coordinate **r** between two spherical charges q, q'. **(b)** Water-vacating probability of nearest water-occupied solvation shell (P(N = 0)) versus wrapping (ρ) of backbone hydrogen bond for an ensemble of soluble proteins (main text), signaling the dehydron stickiness and the role of dehydrons as promoters of protein associations.

dehydronic field generated by the hydrogen bond. This field is given by $\omega^{-1}\vec{\Phi}(\vec{R})$ (ω = volume of test hydrophobe). Thus, in accord with Gauss theorem we obtain:

$$\eta = \oiint \vec{\Phi}(\vec{R}).d\vec{\sigma}(\vec{R}) \tag{13}$$

where integration extends over the closed surface of the dehydration domain of the hydrogen bond (cf. Fig. 2.10) and $d\vec{\sigma}(\vec{R})$ is the differential surface area vector.

To fully understand dehydron stickiness, it is useful at this stage to switch back to the solvent-centric view of the protein-water interface. The object we need to focus on is the 4 Å-radius solvation shell of the atom closest to the center of a backbone hydrogen bond and containing at least one water oxygen in the shell. The vacating probability P(N = 0) previously defined represents also a measure of the propensity for water exclusion from the protein surface, itself a local indicator of stickiness. The plot of P(N = 0) for the atom closest to a backbone hydrogen bond versus the wrapping of the backbone hydrogen bond (ρ) is displayed in Fig. 2.13(b) and obtained from 11,964 monomeric soluble proteins with PDB-reported structure.

The plot reveals that dehydrons are indeed the most significant promoters of water exclusion of all structured regions (i.e. with hydrogen-bonded backbone) in the soluble protein.

2.9 Epistructural biology for targeted drug design

The analysis of biomolecular interfaces presented so far suggests that, like in any protein-ligand complex, the wrapping intermolecular interactions between a drug and its target protein are expected to play an important role in determining the affinity. This paradigm will be thoroughly investigated and validated in Chapter 7. As previously indicated, such cooperative interactions between the drug and pre-formed hydrogen bonds in the target protein actually entail a net gain to the stability of the protein of $\sim$4 kJ/mol per wrapping interaction. Thus, the drug contributes with nonpolar groups to the desolvation of pre-existing dehydrons in the target and each wrapping contribution translates into a $\sim$4 kJ/mol decrease in the free energy change associated with drug binding. As an illustration, the wrapping contributions between the powerful anticancer drug imatinib (Gleevec®) and one of its primary therapeutic targets, the KIT kinase [72, 73], are depicted in Fig. 2.14. The wrapping interactions are promoted by the dehydronic fields generated by the deficiently wrapped hydrogen bonds 673Cys-676Gly, 595Leu-603Val, 640Glu-644Leu and 811Phe-814Ala.

The kinase inhibitor imatinib was not *purposely* designed as a wrapper of its purported protein targets, yet, as shown in Fig. 2.14, five wrapping interactions contribute to its affinity for the primary target KIT kinase. A crude estimate would indicate that this contribution to the association free energy is actually significant ($\sim 5 \times 4$ kJ/mol $= 20$ kJ/mol). Notice that while imatinib was selected for its pharmacological properties that conferred anticancer activity [72], it is unlikely to have emerged from a conventional structure-based design. Matching a nonpolar group in the drug against a carbonyl or amide in the target protein is hardly conceivable in conventional structure-based design as it would entail a hindrance to the hydration of the polar groups. Yet, as a three-body contribution, the proximity

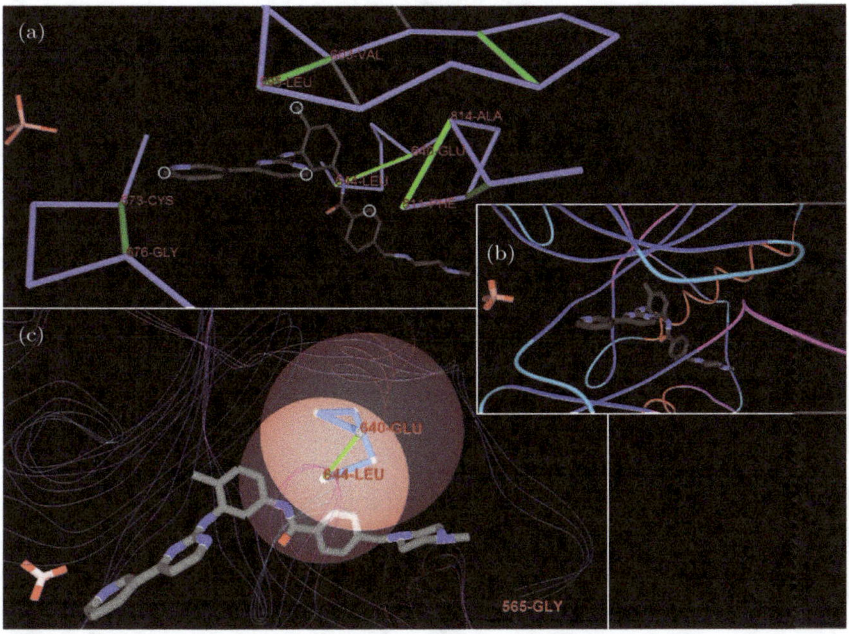

Figure 2.14. **(a)** Dehydrons in the KIT kinase wrapped intermolecularly by the kinase inhibitor imatinib in the crystallized drug/target complex (PDB.1T46). The drug nonpolar groups contributing to the wrapping upon association are marked by circles. The dehydrons (green) wrapped by the drug involve residue pairs 673Cys-676Gly, 595Leu-603Val, 640Glu-644Leu and 811Phe-814Ala. **(b)** Simplified tube rendering of the protein backbone provided as visual aid. **(c)** Detail of intermolecular wrapping interaction between imatinib and the KIT kinase. The drug penetrates the desolvation domain (intersecting pink spheres) of KIT dehydron 640Glu-644Leu upon binding, contributing with two nonpolar groups to the desolvation of the pre-formed hydrogen bond.

of a nonpolar group to an unburied polar pair is justified given the dehydronic field generated by the latter. Furthermore, given the extent to which wrapping interactions are likely to affect drug affinity, one wonders whether the wrapping concept can be fruitfully exploited to guide drug design.

This possibility naturally elicits some basic questions:

- Can we purposely design "cooperative drugs" that wrap dehydrons and thereby mitigate protein-water interfacial tension in the protein target?

- What is the potential impact of "epistructural design" on the technological base of drug discovery and what are the advantages it is likely to provide when compared with conventional structure-based design?
- Can this type of cooperativity-based design be integrated into an "epistructural bioinformatics platform", leading to a better exploitation of genomic information to develop safer and more efficacious therapeutic agents?
- Can we harness idiosyncratic differences in the wrapping patterns of gene products across patients to develop personalized treatments?

These are all crucial problems in molecular targeted therapy that will be addressed in the subsequent chapters as we assess the transformative power of the wrapping concept through a careful examination of biomolecular interfaces.

It is worth noting at this stage that our conceptual framework for drug design and the engineering of molecular interactions in general has evolved along this chapter. Thus, the drug-target dehydron-wrapping interaction (Fig. 2.14) is the counterpart of the displacement of specific frustrated water molecules at the epistructural interface upon drug-target association (Fig. 2.15). In this way, the interplay and mutual enrichment of two complementary views, a solvent-centric (Fig. 2.15) and a structure-centric (Fig. 2.15) actually shape the field of epistructural biology.

2.10 Epistructural biology for Covid-19: Molecular targeted therapy to defuse SARS-CoV-2

As this book gets written, the pressing need for targeted therapies against SARS-CoV-2, the culprit of Covid-19, has become all too apparent. Accordingly, an epistructural analysis of SARS-CoV-2 in its infection-promoting stage is hereby presented. Conformational changes in the virus spike protein are likely to occur at that stage, since the protein is enzymatically modified (cleaved). As shown in Chapter 12, AI is likely to play a key role to identify such chemically

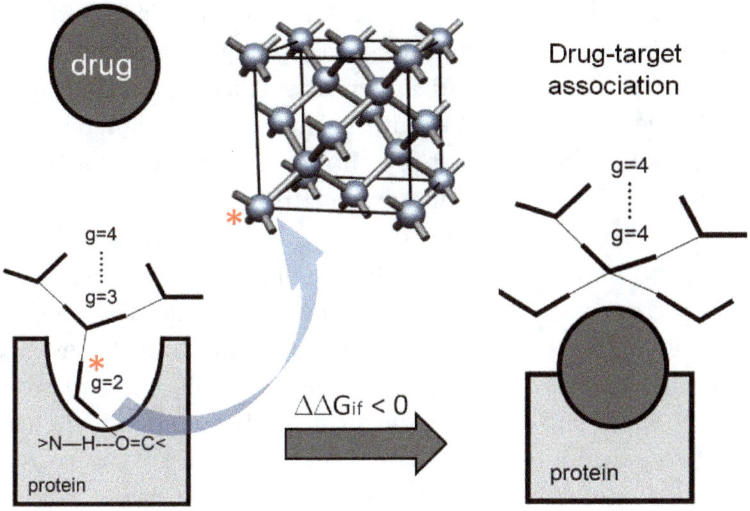

Figure 2.15. Interfacial physics counterpart of the intermolecular drug-target dehydron-wrapping interaction. The thermodynamic benefit associated with the wrapping interaction is complemented by the favorable decrease in interfacial free energy related to the displacement of a specific water molecule (marked by the asterisk) frustrated at the dehydron interface and turned a tetrahedral bulk-like coordinator upon drug-target association. Reprinted from [Fernández A (2016) Non-Debye frustrated hydration steers biomolecular association: Interfacial tension for the drug designer. FEBS Letters 590:3481–3491] with permission from John Wiley & Sons.

induced conformational changes that make the virus competent to penetrate the host cell.

The virus SARS-CoV-2 has propagated worldwide, causing the COVID-19 pandemic of 2020. With the awareness of this public health disaster, the evolutionary fate of the virus becomes a matter of the utmost concern [74–77]. Its evolutionary change is likely to impact transmission efficacy and severity, bearing directly on the course of the pandemic.

Korber *et al.* [74] provided epidemiological evidence that the amino acid substitution D614G in SARS-CoV-2 spike protein is becoming dominant, suggesting that the G614 mutant may entail a significant fitness advantage. Since the spike (S) protein mediates the viral recognition of the host receptor (angiotensin-converting enzyme 2, hACE2) as well as the fusion of viral and cellular membrane, it becomes imperative to find out how this mutation affects viral transmission and infectivity. Korber *et al.* argued that the rapid spread of the G614 mutant is related to higher infectivity. To support this hypothesis, they showed in that the G614 variant yields higher titers in pseudoviruses from *in vitro* experiments. These results appear to be corroborated by other groups [75, 76]. In infected individuals, the variant G614 is likely to cause higher upper respiratory tract viral loads, yet the severity of the disease does not appear to increase. These findings prompt a mechanistic assessment of the impact of the S-protein mutation on virus transmission as a guidance to steer the development of novel immunological cures.

The two competing phenotypes S^{D614} and S^{G614} were recently characterized and compared by Zhang and coworkers [78]. Their analysis revealed that retroviruses pseudotyped with S^{G614} infected hACE2-expressing cells significantly more efficiently than those with S^{D614}. To interpret the results, we first note that the S protein is organized as a trimer with each monomer containing two tethered and mutually interacting domains S1 and S2, the first involved in receptor binding (RB) through its RBD domain, while S2 mediates the fusion of viral and cellular membranes [74]. The greater transmission efficiency of the G614 mutant was proven not to correlate with higher epitope affinity or binding efficacy but with less S1 shedding and greater incorporation of the S protein into the pseudovirion, pointing to a higher stability of the S^{G614} phenotype [77]. Because S1 residue 614 is proximal to the S2 domain in the S-protein structure, Zhang *et al.* [77] first compared the ratio between the S1 and S2 domains in the virion that might signal altered release or shedding of the S1 domain after cleavage at the S1/S2 junction. The resulting S1:S2 ratio is markedly greater in $\mathrm{PV}^{\mathrm{G614}}$ compared to $\mathrm{PV}^{\mathrm{D614}}$, implying that G614 stabilizes the interaction between the S1 and S2 domains, which limits S1 shedding.

The epistructural analysis of the impact of the D614G substitution on the S1/S2 interface supports this picture, yet, as shown subsequently, the analysis needs to go beyond mere structural considerations and incorporate the relationship between structure and enveloping solvent. It has been postulated [74] that the carboxyl group in D614 forms a hydrogen bond with the hydroxyl group in T859 across the S1/S2 interface. The crystal structures of the complex do not support this picture, since the side-chain groups are not properly oriented for hydrogen bonding (Fig. 2.16(a)). Furthermore, this conjecture is completely at odds with the experimental results of Zhang et al. [77] because the substitution D614G would eliminate altogether the postulated hydrogen bond across the S1/S2 interface, hence the S^{G614} phenotype would be characterized by more S1 shedding compared with S^{D614}. The experimental evidence favors precisely the opposite conclusion [77].

A more thorough analysis of the impact of the D614G substitution takes into account the epistructure of the interacting S1 and S2 domains. The preformed D614-A647 backbone hydrogen bond (BHB) is partially exposed to the solvent (Fig. 2.16(b)), and hence it constitutes a dehydron in the S1 domain. As discussed, from a thermodynamic standpoint, the dehydron is an adhesive spot promoting removal of surrounding water for two mutually reinforcing reasons: a) the preformed BHB gets stabilized when a protein association (i.e. S1/S2 interaction) causes removal of surrounding water thereby hindering the structurally disruptive hydration of amide and carbonyl (destabilizing the unbound state is tantamount to stabilize the bound state); and b) the removal of backbone-solvating water molecules at the dehydron site is favorable because the partial confinement of such water molecules curtails their hydrogen bonding coordination possibilities, therefore their transference to the bulk becomes thermodynamically supported. The dehydron adhesiveness can be also justified from an energetic standpoint, as the screening of partial charges paired by the BHB is removed concurrently with the removal of surrounding water molecules, thus strengthening the BHB.

As previously argued, dehydrons compromise the integrity of protein structure, exposing it to disruptive backbone hydration, and promote protein associations as a means to exclude surrounding water. In this way, dehydrons become determinants for protein association because, by decreasing charge screening, exogenous removal of water

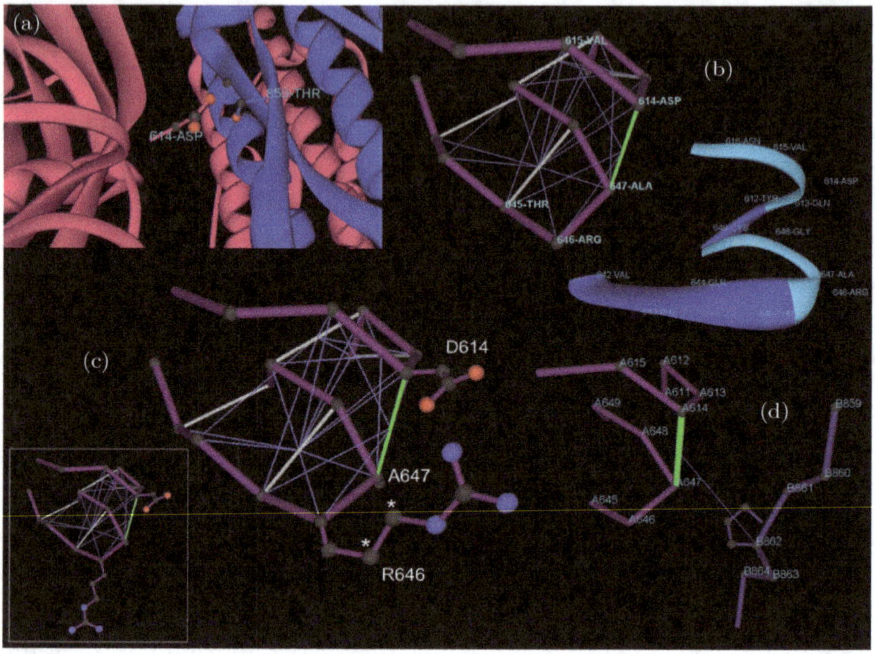

Figure 2.16. Structural and epistructural interactions at the S1/S2 interface in the spike protein of SARS-CoV-2. **(a)** Positioning of D614 in the S1 chain (magenta) relative to T859 in the S2 chain (blue) at the S1/S2 interface for the spike protein structure reported in PDB.6VXX. The protein backbone is rendered in ribbon representation. **(b)** Intramolecular wrapping of backbone hydrogen bonds (BHBs) around dehydron D614-A647 for the S1 chain. The protein backbone is represented as a polygonal (magenta) with lines joining the α-carbons of consecutive residues. Well wrapped BHBs are shown as grey lines joining α-carbons of paired residues, while the dehydron is shown in green. The wrapping of each BHB is indicated by thin blue lines from the center of the bond to the α-carbon of the residue that contributes side-chain nonpolar groups to the desolvation domain of the BHB. The ribbon rendering is an aid to the eye. **(c)** Improved intramolecular wrapping of dehydron D614-A647 achieved by forming the D614-R646 salt bridge. In this configuration, R646 contributes two extra side-chain methylene groups (asterisks) to the wrapping of the D614-A647 BHB when compared with the fully hydrated R646 side chain that occurs when S1 becomes part of the S1/S2 complex (inset). **(d)** The intermolecular wrapping of dehydron D614-A647 by P862 across the S1/S2 interface. The chains are labeled A, B, corresponding respectively to S1 and S2, as reported in PDB.6VXX.

from the dehydron microenvironment strengthens and stabilizes the electrostatic interaction that underlies the BHB. As discussed in this chapter, bioinformatics evidence on the distribution of dehydrons at interfaces of protein complexes supports this picture, pointing to dehydrons as important factors driving complex formation.

To identify dehydrons in protein structure, we have introduced a descriptor named *wrapping* that determines the reliance on binding partnerships to maintain local structural integrity. A dehydron is then an underwrapped BHB which possesses an insufficient number of side-chain nonpolar groups clustered around the BHB, so that the BHB is exposed to structure-disruptive hydration. Dehydrons and wrapping may be computed directly from structural coordinates (PyMol subroutine in Appendix 1).

In our case, the D614-A647 BHB in domain S1 is a dehydron wrapped intramolecularly by residues D614, A647, V615, T645 and R646 (Fig. 2.16b). It achieves maximum wrapping from R646 when this residue forms a salt bridge with D614 (Fig. 2.16(c)). In this way, the salt bridge D614-R646 contributes to stabilize BHB D614-A647 in the uncomplexed S1, while also blocking the S1/S2 association. As S1 gets associated with S2, the salt bridge gets dismantled (it is not present, as expected, in PDB structure 6VXX) and the dehydron D614-A647 completes its wrapping intermolecularly with a contribuition from P862 from the S2 domain (Fig. 2.16(d)). The substitution D614G has a major impact on the epistructure of S1, vis-à-vis the previous considerations. The effect results from two contributions: a) Mutation D614G eliminates the salt bridge that hampers the S1/S2 association as it improves the wrapping of the dehydron pairing residues at locations 614 and 647; and b) By reducing the dehydron-wrapping contributions from side chains at positions 614 and 646, the mutation destabilizes the uncomplexed S1 domain, making the dehydron G614-A647 a better promoter of the S1/S2 association. In the G614 mutant, the 614-647 BHB becomes more reliant on the contribution from P862 that occurs upon S1/S2 association (Fig. 2.16(d)) to maintain its structural integrity.

In other words, the D614G mutation promotes the S1/S2 association because: a) it destabilizes the free (uncomplexed) S1 structure through the enhanced exposure of the BHB pairing residues G614 and A647; and b) it stabilizes the S1/S2 interface as the D614G substitution decreases the intramolecular wrapping of the G614-A647 dehydron, thereby further promoting its intermolecular wrapping via the contribution from S2 residue P862 (Fig. 2.16(d)). A conservative estimate drawn from experimental data on the cost of unwrapping the BHB gives $3 \times 8\,\text{kJ/mol} = 5.73\,\text{kcal/mol}$ as the thermodynamic cost of destabilizing the S1 structure resulting from depriving the BHB 614-647 of three wrapping carbonaceous groups due to the D614G substitution. The lost wrapping contributions include one methylene group from the D $\rightarrow$ G substitution proper and two methylene groups from R646 that no longer can form the salt bridge with the glycine at position 614 (cf. Fig. 2.16(c)).

Thus, the net gain in stability (loss in free energy) for the S1/S2 complex resulting from the D614G mutation is significant and may be conservatively estimated at $\Delta\Delta G = -5.73kcal/mol$. We emphasize that the stabilization of the S1/S2 complex arises from the destabilization of the free (uncomplexed) S1 structure.

Thus, the epistructural, impact of the mutation D614G is consistent with established phenotypic differences between S^{G614} and S^{D614} in the sense that S^{G614} has a greater stability resulting from less S1 shedding and greater incorporation of the intact S protein into the pseudovirion. In this way, the epistructural analysis sheds light on the mechanistic underpinnings for the superior transmission efficiency of the G614 mutant of SARS-CoV-2.

The epistructural analysis presented rises the enticing therapeutic possibility of immunologically targeting the epitope involved in reducing S1-shedding as a means of impairing the infection efficacy of the G614 mutant SARS-CoV-2. Thus, a monoclonal antibody targeting the epitope associated with the dehydron 614-647 (Fig. 2.16(c)) could significantly promote S1 shedding and destabilize the S^{G614} phenotype to levels representing severe impairment of the viral infectivity. This therapeutic modality would not *a-priori* interfere directly with current efforts towards an immunological targeting of the RBD epitope, hence it could serve as complementary treatment.

Most current immunotherapies to mitigate the impact of COVID19 aim at impairing the cellular uptake of culprit SARS-CoV-2 mediated by human receptor ACE2. Vaccine-induced or administered antibodies focus on epitopes on the surface of the trimeric viral spike (S) protein that has proven to be significantly antigenic. These epitopes typically include RBD (receptor-biding domain), NTD (N-terminal domain), and intra or inter-subunit combinations thereof [78]. Given the epistructural analysis previously presented, we advocate a different therapeutic approach. The goal is to engineer therapeutic agents that amplify the vulnerabilities unraveled by the recent evolutionary history of the virus, more precisely by the D614G mutation in the S protein. This dominance implies a fitness advantage. Efforts to track down this advantage are underway and reveal that the G614 strain presents a more stable phenotype yielding higher transmission efficacy, as previously discussed. More specifically, the D614G substitution results in less S1 shedding following the pre-activation phase of S1/S2 junction cleavage, the latter being a necessary step in the process of membrane fusion. Our epistructural analysis of the impact of the D614G substitution is consistent with these findings. The D614G mutation destabilizes the free S protein monomers, thus stabilizing the S-protein quaternary structure (a trimer) after S1/S2 junction cleavage. More specifically, the D614G substitution creates a packing defect in S1, right at the S1/S2 association interface, by exposing the backbone to the structure-disruptive effects of hydration of the amide and carbonyl paired by the 614-647 backbone hydrogen bond (BHB). Thus, in the G614 strain, S1 becomes more reliant on its association with S2 (within the binding partner monomer) to maintain its structural integrity, especially the BHB 614-647, after S1/S2 junction cleavage. In thermodynamic (free energy) terms, the D614G mutation entails an additional stabilization of the S protein assemblage estimated at $\Delta\Delta G = -5.73\,kcal/mol$. When interpreted in terms of selective advantage, we may state that the dominant mutation D614G mitigates a structural defect in the virus. The vulnerability is given by the fragility of the S1/S2 interface in the S protein quaternary structure right at the BHB

614-647 which, in the G614 strain, is solvent-exposed in the free monomer.

This analysis prompts us design immunotherapies to amplify the vulnerability of the SARS-CoV-2 assemblage that surfaced upon examination of its recent evolutionary history. Because we aim to destabilize the S protein quaternary structure at the pre-activation juncture, we need to identify antigenic regions and epitopes in the free momomeric S subunits, rather than in the trimer assembly, as done in current therapeutic approaches. To be disruptive of the S protein quaternary structure upon antibody recognition, these epitopes should be adjacent to the evolutionarily signaled BHB D(G)614-A647, which in the G614 strain, becomes exposed to structure-disruptive hydration in the free monomeric S subunit.

We have identified B-cell epitopes to be targeted for virus destabilization using a linear epitope predictor from the public domain [79]. A practical hurdle arises as the PDB and FASTA files in PDB entry 6VXX for the SARS-CoV-2 S protein have different sequence numbering because disordered terminal residues are excluded in the structural file. Key residues D(G)614 and A647 become D(G)633 and A666 in the FASTA file for the amino acid sequence of the free monomeric S subunit inputted into the Bepipred Linear Epitope Prediction 2.0 accessible at http://tools.iedb.org/main/bcell/. With this caveat, the predicted epitopes (underlined) adjacent to BHB D(G)633-A666 (BHB-paired residues in bold) are subsumed in the minimal S-protein-derived antigen to induce S1 shedding:

$_{622}$NTSNQVAVLYQ**D**VNCTEVPVAIHADQLTPTWRVYSTGSNV
FQTR**A**GCLIGAEHVNNSYECDIPIGAGICASYQTQTNSPSGAG
SVASQ$_{709}$

The strength of the signal (residues scoring above 0.6) and the length (n > 20) of the two last epitopes 643–663, 674–709 flanking A666 attest to the reliability of the specific predictions.

These B-cell epitopes are to be targeted for destabilization of the quaternary structure of the spike protein in SARS-CoV-2, thereby overwriting the stabilizing effect of dominant D614G

(D633G) mutation. The virus-destabilizing monoclonal antibodies (mAbs) will need to be isolated from affinity selection using the free monomeric S subunit or the antigen derived thereof as bait for specific memory B-cells from COVID-19 patients.

As part of the S1/S2 association interface, the minimal antigen containing the reliably identified epitopes is not subject to immunosurveillance while the virus maintains the intact S protein quaternary structure. The antigen becomes exposed to immunosurveillance with a significant probability after the S1/S2 junction cleavage, as partial dismantling of the spike quaternary structure takes place during membrane fusion. Thus, the antigen described may be exploited to select mAbs that block the re-assemblage of the quaternary structure of the S protein. The proposed antigen with full coverage of the S1-shedding target region is also suitable for the vaccine-induced immune response geared at destabilizing the virus.

We may state that the epistructural analysis offered a concrete pathway to develop a COVID19 therapy which totally different from current efforts underway. We describe COVID19 immunotherapies geared at destabilizing the virus quaternary structure and promote S1 shedding, thus greatly reducing transmission efficacy. The approach draws from an analysis of the recent evolutionary history of SARS-CoV-2 and from an assessment of the selective advantages that result from the mutational mitigation of key structural defects. This observation inspired the proposed therapeutic modality based on the amplification of evolutionarily signaled virus vulnerabilities. Given the reliability of the predicted epitopes to tackle the "Achilles' heel of SARS-CoV-2", the proposed therapeutic intervention has a chance to be successful and it may not be far-fetched to state that, within a suitable vaccine platform, the proposed antigen may save millions of lives.

2.11 Why epistructural biology?

The last decades have witnessed the meteoric success of structural biology, and yet this success has also brought about an unrealistic picture of the protein in solution. The conventional structural-biology representation of crystallized proteins reveals a

3D structural arrangement obtained from the X-ray diffraction pattern or NMR or other spectroscopic means. Nothing in this static representation indicates how the protein relates to or interacts with its solvent environment since the solvent is simply represented as background to the structure. With more or less atomic detail, this is the picture that prevails in fundamental or applied research labs that exploit the output of structural biology. In fact, structural coordinates provide much more information than indicating the relative position of the atoms in the chain, its folding topology, or the chemical composition of specific locations on the protein surface. Firstly, the tightness of the protein hydration shell is widely modulated by structural features of the protein, so that an interfacial tension driving protein associations is established between protein solute and water solvent that is essentially determined by protein structure but not captured by the standard structural renderings. As discussed, certain structural defects in the protein structure named *dehydrons* are known to play a crucial role in promoting interfacial tension by causing water frustration at the interface, which in turn causes significant deviations from the standard dielectric picture introduced by Debye. Dehydrons widely modify the dielectric properties of the aqueous interface above and beyond the classical Debye picture, amplifying electrostatic fields in the protein. Thirdly, protein and aqueous interface are engaged in an exquisite dynamic entanglement reciprocally influencing and steering their respective motions. Finally, as explored in subsequent chapters, dehydrons functionalize interfacial water promoting a catalytic role that arises from water frustration. These interrelated aspects of the aqueous interface shaped by the protein structure pertain to *epistructural biology* and build upon information obtained from structural biology, and yet they differentiate from the latter. Thus, *the dehydron pattern of the protein enshrines the epistructural biology picture that complements the standard structural representation as it subsumes vital information on the physical and catalytic properties of the protein-water interface determined by the protein structure.* The epistructural aspects have remained vastly unexploited by drug designers and molecular engineers, with hefty consequences for the

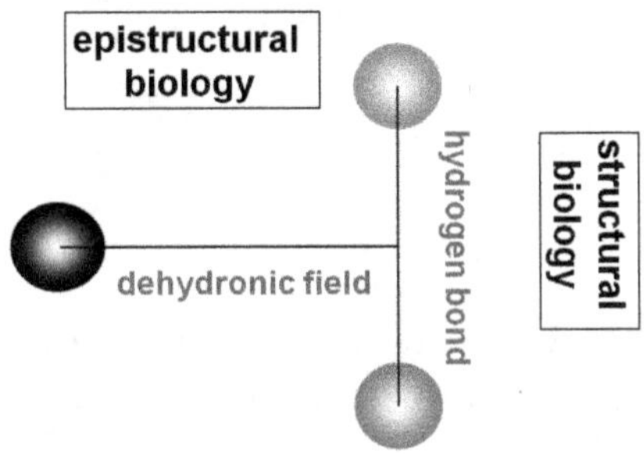

Figure 2.17. The hydrogen bond is the key feature of structural biology, while the wrapping interaction is central to epistructural biology. As shown in this chapter, the wrapping interaction is determined by the dehydronic field orthogonal to the electrostatic field that underlies the hydrogen bond.

pharmaceutical and biotechnological industries. This book is written with the intent to improve this state of affairs.

2.12 Epistructural biology versus structural biology

We may conclude by stating that the foundations of epistructural biology are to be found in the many-body nature of the hydrogen bond (Fig. 2.17). Linus Pauling raised the awareness of the relevance of the hydrogen bond as a determinant of biomolecular structure. This awareness cemented the foundations of structural biology. On the other hand, the awareness of the relevance of wrapping interactions as stabilizers of the hydrogen bond gave rise to epistructural biology. From the physicist's perspective, the electrostatic field underlying the hydrogen bond gave rise to structural biology, while the dehydronic field, orthogonal to the electrostatic field (Figs. 2.13(a), 2.17), spanned epistructural biology [80]. The hydrogen bond is a structure-defining motif, while its "stickiness" [80] places epistructural biology as a meta-discipline vis-à-vis structural biology.

At first glance, this chapter may seem disjoint from the main thrust of the book. It surely is not. It shows painstakingly that the protein epistructure is actually encoded in the structure, with a single structural feature, the dehydron, enshrining the multiscale complexity of the structure-solvent relationship. This is a crucial step in order to leverage AI, as the dehydron and its conjugate attribute, the wrapping, can be represented in tensor form, hence becoming tractable within an AI context. This is a leitmotiv of the remaining chapters.

2.13 On DeepMind's solution to the protein folding problem: Are we doing the right physics?

As discussed in Chapter 1, on November 30, 2020, DeepMind announced that their AI system AlphaFold2 had solved the "protein folding problem" [81, 82]. AlphaFold is essentially a deep learning system with a CNN trained on structural data that gets correlated in the hidden layers with inputted evolutionary information on the test amino acid sequence. The latter is obtained by alignment of the test sequence against sequences in the training set. In very much this way, AlphaFold2 is capable of predicting the 3D structure of a protein chain from its amino acid sequence.

In this chapter we have provided some of the conceptual and representational framework that will enable us to adapt an AlphaFold platform to some of the needs of the drug designer. In so doing we shall encounter a major hurdle that stems from the fact that target proteins are typically not fixed targets: they structurally adapt to the binding ligand in ways that need to be predicted. Specifically, we need to adapt AlphaFold to solve the drug-induced folding problem and even harder challenge than the protein folding problem. The goal is to steer drug design to target conformations that rely on association with the purposely designed drug to maintain their structural integrity.

The CNN of AlphaFold gets trained with PDB-reported protein structures within a multilayered architecture that generates 3D models that fit accurate predictions of distances between residue pairs. Such predictions are based on a 2D-array representation of pairwise co-evolutionary information, under the premise that two residues coevolve if and only if they are spatially related. The evolutionary information is thus subsumed in the input jointly with residue profiling including amino acid identity and secondary structure prediction. Local propagation of distance constraints from one layer to the next is achieved via progressively dilated convolutional operations (Chapter 1), where convolutional "filters" allow incorporation of features not just from neighbors of a pixel but also from further afield, incorporating surrounding context by expanding the receptive field.

The success of this AI-based inference scheme represents a towering achievement because the protein folding problem was the biggest open challenge in biology or biophysics for the last 50 years and was well on its way to be considered intractable. The big paradox is that the team that developed AlphaFold hardly had any expertise in molecular biophysics, and yet the problem they had solved is one of the paramount problems in molecular biophysics.

To solve the paradox, we emphasize that DeepMind has not tried to predict protein folding pathways that converge to the native fold as the protein chain explores conformation space in accord with physical principles. That effort would be futile. Natural proteins fold *in vivo*, not *in vitro*, and have been selected to do so, and state-of-the-art computational resources are incapable of addressing realistically the complexities of an *in vivo* environment. This situation is likely to change with the advent of AI, as illustrated in Chapter 3.

The CNN from AlphaFold is trained with sufficient structure-derived information from PDB (protein data bank) entries, and obviously, the training patterns enshrine implicitly the physics and biological complexity of the *in vivo* environment. In other words, the relevant information is incorporated in the learning phase without requiring AlphaFold developers to know about it or to introduce any *a-priori* bias. Then, through sequence alignment, the test sequence is evolutionarily related with sequences associated with structures in the training set, and the evolutionary and coevolutionary signals stemming from this alignment are inputted into the CNN in concatenation with the sequence and 1D-profile of the test protein.

The perplexing aspect of the AI method is that it is able to infer the structure without any explicit input from the physics that governed the formation of the structure. This is completely at odds with all the futile efforts reported in the literature in the past five decades. In fact, it is most likely that the feature extraction in the CNN would reveal a completely different set of physical principles tailored to the different levels of abstraction embossed in the hidden layers. The features extracted in the hidden layers probably enshrine a completely novel way of doing physics, tailored to the biology under scrutiny. In essence, AlphaFold is not in the least mindful of the way humans do physics as they address biological phenomena, much the way an extraterrestrial would deal with the problem.

Precisely these completely alien ways of solving physical problems unraveled during the feature extraction phase are likely to revolutionize physics in unfathomable ways. The dehydron and the wrapping are two relatively novel motifs coined by human intuition that may or may not emerge from feature extraction. The matter will be decided in the near future. Yet, one thing seems certain: there will be very novel unfathomable ways of doing physics that would be incommensurably more effective as AI-based approaches take the upper hand in scientific discovery.

As the AlphaFold case suggests, AI approaches will surely reveal methods and patterns that will be completely unrelated to the way we do physics today. They will literally be regarded as the working of aliens, at least for a while.

References

1. Schwede T, Peitsch M (2008) Computational structural biology. World Scientific Publishing Company, Singapore.
2. Fernández A (2016) Physics at the biomolecular interface. Springer International Publishing, Switzerland.
3. Brooks BR, Brooks III CL, Mackerell AD, Nilsson L, Petrella RJ, *et al.* (2009) CHARMM: The biomolecular simulation program. *J Comp Chem* 30:1545–1615.
4. Shaw DE, Maragakis P, Lindorff-Larsen K, Piana S, Dror RO, *et al.* (2010) Atomic-level characterization of the structural dynamics of proteins. *Science* 330:341–346.
5. Glasgow A, Glasgow J, Limonta D, Solomon P, Lui I, Zhang Y, Nix MA, Rettko NJ, Zha S, Yamin R, Kao K, Rosenberg OS, Ravetch JV, Wiita AP, Leung KK, Lim SA, Zhou XX, Hobman TC, Kortemme T, Wells JA (2020)

Engineered ACE2 receptor traps potently neutralize SARS-CoV-2. *Proc Natl Acad Sci USA* 117:28046–28055.

6. Wernet P, Nordlund D, Bergmann U, Cavalleri M, Odelius M, Ogasawara H, Näslund L, Hirsch TK, Ojamäe L, Glatzel P, Pettersson LG, Nilsson A (2004) The structure of the first coordination shell in liquid water. *Science* 304:995–999.
7. Head-Gordon T, Hura G (2002) Water structure from scattering experiments and simulations. *Chem Rev* 102:2651–2670.
8. Cheng YK, Rossky P (1998) Surface topography dependence of biomolecular hydrophobic hydration. *Nature* 392:696–699.
9. Fernández A (2013) The principle of minimal episteric distortion of the water matrix and its steering role in protein folding. *J Chem Phys* 139:085101.
10. Fernández A (2012) Epistructural tension promotes protein associations. *Phys Rev Lett* 108:188102.
11. Giovambattista N, Lopez CF, Rossky P, Debenedetti P (2008) Hydrophobicity of protein surfaces: Separating geometry from chemistry. *Proc Natl Acad Sci USA* 105:2274–2279.
12. Debye P (1929) Polar molecules. Dover Publications, New York.
13. Strekalova EG, Mazza MG, Stanley HE, Franzese G (2011) Large decrease of fluctuations for supercooled water in hydrophobic nanoconfinement. *Phys Rev Lett* 106:145701.
14. Tanizaki S, Feig F (2005) A generalized Born formalism for heterogeneous dielectric environments: Application to the implicit modeling of biological membranes. *J Chem Phys* 122:124706.
15. Stanley HE, Buldyrev SV, Kumar P, Mallamace F, Mazza MG, Stokely K, Xu L, Franzese G (2011) Water in nanoconfined and biological environments. *J Non-Cryst Solids* 357:629–640.
16. Kumar P, Han S, Stanley HE (2009) Anomalies of water and hydrogen bond dynamics in hydrophobic nanoconfinement. *J Phys Condens Matter* 21:504108.
17. Fernández Stigliano A (2013) Breakdown of the Debye polarization ansatz at protein-water interfaces. *J Chem Phys* 138:225103.
18. Fernández A (2010) Transformative concepts for drug design: Target wrapping. Springer-Verlag, Berlin.
19. Schutz CN, Warshel A (2001) What are the dielectric "constants" of proteins and how to validate electrostatic models? *Proteins-Struct Funct Gen* 44:400–408.
20. Fernández A (2014) Fast track communication: Water promotes the sealing of nanoscale packing defects in folding proteins. *J Phys Chem Condens Matter* 26:202101.
21. Wang L, Berne BJ, Friesner RA (2011) Ligand binding to protein binding pockets with wet and dry regions. *Proc Natl Acad Sci USA* 108:1326–1330.
22. Snyder PW, Mecinović J, Moustakas DT, Thomas III SW, Harder M, Mack ET, Lockett MR, Héroux A, Sherman W, Whitesides GM (2011) Mechanism

of hydrophobic effect in the biomolecular recognition of arylsulfonamides by carbonic anhydrase. *Proc Natl Acad Sci USA* 108:17889–17894.
23. Fernández Stigliano A (2015) Biomolecular interfaces: Interactions, functions and drug design. Springer-Verlag, Heidelberg.
24. Remsing RC, McKendry IG, Strongin DR, Klein ML, Zdilla MJ (2015) Frustrated solvation structures can enhance electron transfer rates. *J Phys Chem Lett* 6:4804–4808.
25. Lee M, Salsbury F, Olson MA (2004) An efficient hybrid explicit/implicit solvent method for biomolecular simulations. *J Comp Chem* 25:1967–1978.
26. Allen MP, Tildesley DJ (1989) Computer simulation of liquids. Clarendon Press, Oxford.
27. Bachmann M (2014) Thermodynamics and statistical mechanics of macromolecular systems. Cambridge University Press, Cambridge.
28. Lee MS, Olson MA (2013) Comparison of volume and surface area nonpolar solvation free energy terms for implicit solvent simulations. *J Chem Phys* 139:044119.
29. A. Fernández (2011) Nanoscale thermodynamics of biological interfacial tension. *Proc Roy Soc A* 467:559–568.
30. Clackson T, Wells JA (1995) A hot spot of binding energy in a hormone-receptor interface. *Science* 267:383–386.
31. Jaremko M, Jaremko L, Kim H, Cho M, Schwieters C, Giller K, Becker S, Zweckstetter M (2013) Cold denaturation of a protein dimer monitored at atomic resolution. *Nature Chem Biol* 9:264–270.
32. Pal SK, Peon J, Zewail AH (2002) Biological water at the protein surface: Dynamical solvation probed directly with femtosecond resolution. *Proc Natl Acad Sci USA* 99:1763–1768.
33. Li B, Liu P, Xu Z, Zhou S (2013) Ionic size effects: Generalized Boltzmann distributions, counterion stratification and modified Debye length. *Nonlinearity* 26:2899–2922.
34. Evans LC (2010) Partial differential equations. American Mathematical Society, Providence, Rhode Island.
35. Jorgensen WL, Chandrasekhar J, Madura JD, Impey RW, Klein ML (1983) Comparison of simple potential functions for simulating liquid water. *J Chem Phys* 79:926–938.
36. Sierra MB, Accordino SR, Rodriguez-Fris A, Morini MA, Appignanesi GA, Fernández Stigliano A (2013) Protein packing defects "heat up" interfacial water. *Eur Phys J E* 36:62.
37. Wang J, Wolf RM, Caldwell JW, Kollman PA, Case DA (2004) Development and testing of a general amber force field. *J Comput Chem* 25:1157–1174.
38. Darden T, York D, Pedersen LJ (1993) Particle mesh Ewald: An N· log (N) method for Ewald sums in large systems. *J Chem Phys* 98:10089–10092.
39. Ashkenazi A, Presta L, Marsters S, Camarato J, Rosenthal K, Fendly B, Capon D (1990) Mapping the CD4 binding site for human immunodeficiency virus by alanine-scanning mutagenesis. *Proc Nat Acad Sci USA* 87:7150–7154.

40. Castro MJ, Anderson S (1996) Alanine point-mutations in the reactive region of bovine pancreatic trypsin inhibitor: Effects on the kinetics and thermodynamics of binding to beta-trypsin and alpha-chymotrypsin. *Biochemistry* 35:11435–11446.
41. Kuhlmann UC, Pommer A, Moore GR, James R, Kleanthous C (2000) Specificity in protein-protein interactions: The structural basis for dual recognition in endonuclease colicin-immunity protein complexes. *J Mol Biol* 301:1163–1178.
42. Bottger V, Bottger A, Garcia-Echeverria C, Chène P, Hochkeppel HK, Sampson W, Ang K, Howard SF, Picksley SM, Lane DP (1997) Molecular characterization of the hdm2-p53 interaction. *J Mol Biol* 269:744–756.
43. Maira SM, Voliva C, Garcia-Echeverria C (2008) Class IA phosphatidylinositol 3-kinase: From their biologic implication in human cancers to drug discovery. *Expert Opin Ther Targets* 12:223–238.
44. Ihle NT, Powis G (2010) The biological effects of isoform-specific PI3-kinase inhibition. *Curr Opin Drug Discovery Devel* 13:41–49.
45. Certal V, Carry JC, Halley F, Virone-Oddos A, Thompson F, Filoche-Romme B, El-Ahmad Y, Karlsson A, Charrier V, Delorme C, Rak A, Abecassis PY, Amara C, Vincent L, Bonnevaux H, Nicolas JP, Mathieu M, Bertrand T, Marquette JP, Michot N, Benard T, Perrin MA, Lemaitre O, Guerif S, Perron S, Monget S, Gruss-Leleu F, Doerflinger G, Guizani H, Brollo M, Delbarre L, Bertin L, Richepin P, Loyau V, Garcia-Echeverria C, Lengauer C, Schio L (2014) Discovery and optimization of pyrimidone indoline amide PI3Kβ inhibitors for the treatment of Phosphatase and Tensin Homologue (PTEN)-deficient cancers. *J Med Chem* 57:903–920.
46. Anfinsen CB (1973) Principles that govern the folding of protein chains. *Science* 181:223–230.
47. Fernández A, Sosnick TR, Colubri A (2002) Dynamics of hydrogen-bond desolvation in folding proteins. *J Mol Biol* 321:659–675.
48. Chandler D (2005) Interfaces and the driving force of hydrophobic assembly. *Nature* 437:640–647.
49. Jewett A, Pande VS, Plaxco KW (2003) Cooperativity, smooth energy landscapes and the origins of topology-dependent protein folding rates. *J Mol Biol* 326:247–253.
50. Scalley-Kim M, Baker D (2004) Characterization of the folding energy landscapes of computer generated proteins suggests high folding free energy barriers and cooperativity may be consequences of natural selection. *J Mol Biol* 338:573–583.
51. Fernández A, Colubri A, Berry RS (2002) Three-body correlations in protein folding: The origin of cooperativity. *Physica A* 307:235–259.
52. Fernández A, Kostov K, Berry RS (1999) From residue matching patterns to protein folding topographies: General model and bovine pancreatic trypsin inhibitor. *Proc Natl Acad Sci USA* 96:12991–12996.
53. Fernández A, Colubri A, Berry RS (2000) Topology to geometry in protein folding: Beta-lactoglobulin. *Proc Natl Acad Sci USA* 97:14062–14066.

54. Fernández A, Kardos J, Goto J (2003) Protein folding: Could hydrophobic collapse be coupled with hydrogen-bond formation? *FEBS Letters* 536:187–192.
55. Fernández A (2001) Conformation-dependent environments in folding proteins. *J Chem Phys* 114:2489–2502.
56. Fernández A, Kardos J, Scott R, Goto Y, Berry RS (2003) Structural defects and the diagnosis of amyloidogenic propensity. *Proc Natl Acad Sci USA* 100:6446–6451.
57. Fernández A (2004) Keeping dry and crossing membranes. *Nature Biotech* 22:1081–1084.
58. Pietrosemoli N, Crespo A, Fernández A (2007) Dehydration propensity of order-disorder intermediate regions in soluble proteins. *J Proteome Res* 6:3519–3526.
59. Fernández A, Scott R (2003) Dehydron: A structure-encoded signal for protein interactions. *Biophys J* 85:1914–1928.
60. Avbelj F, Baldwin RL (2003) Role of backbone solvation and electrostatics in generating preferred peptide backbone conformations: Distributions of phi. *Proc Natl Acad Sci USA* 100:5742–5747.
61. Krantz BA, Moran LB, Kentsis A, Sosnick TR (2000) D/H amide kinetic isotope effects reveal when hydrogen bonds form during protein folding. *Nature Struct Biol* 7:62–71.
62. Fersht A (2000) Transition-state structure as a unifying basis in protein-folding mechanisms: Contact order, chain topology, stability, and the extended nucleus mechanism. *Proc Natl Acad Sci USA* 97:1525–1929.
63. Plaxco KW, Simmons KT, Baker D (1998) Contact order, transition state placement and the refolding rates of single domain proteins. *J Mol Biol* 277:985–994.
64. Fernández A, Scott LR (2003). Adherence of packing defects in soluble proteins. *Phys Rev Lett* 91:018102.
65. Fernández A, Zhang X, Chen J (2008) Folding and wrapping soluble proteins: Exploring the molecular basis of cooperativity and aggregation. *Prog Nuc Ac Res Transl Sci* 83:57–87.
66. Fernández A, Scheraga HA (2003) Insufficiently dehydrated hydrogen bonds as determinants of protein interactions. *Proc Natl Acad Sci USA* 100:113–118.
67. Fernández A, Berry RS (2003) Proteins with H-bond packing defects are highly interactive with lipid bilayers: Implications for amyloidogenesis. *Proc Natl Acad Sci USA* 100:2391–2396.
68. Deremble C, Lavery R (2005) Macromolecular Recognition. *Curr Opin Struc Biol* 15:171–175.
69. Ma B, Elkayam T, Wolfson H, Nussinov R (2003) Protein-protein interactions: Structurally conserved residues distinguish between binding sites and exposed protein surfaces. *Proc Natl Acad Sci USA* 100:5772–5777.
70. Fernández A (2003) What caliber pore is like a pipe? Nanotubes as modulators of ion gradients. *J Chem Phys* 119:5315–5319.

71. Despa F, Fernández A, Berry RS (2004) Dielectric modulation of biological water. *Phys Rev Lett* 93:228104.
72. Demetri G (2002) Efficacy and safety of imatinib mesyalte in advanced gastrointestinal stromal tumors. *N Engl J Med* 347:472–480.
73. Fernández A, Sanguino A, Peng Z, Ozturk E, Chen J, Crespo A, Wulf S, Shavrin A, Qin C, Ma J, Trent J, Lin Y, Han HD, Mangala LS, Bankson JA, Gelovani J, Samarel A, Bornmann W, Sood AK, Lopez-Berestein G (2007) An anticancer c-Kit kinase inhibitor is reengineered to make it more active and less cardiotoxic. *J Clin Invest* 117:4044–4054.
74. Korber B, Fischer WM, Gnanakaran S, Yoon H, Theiler J, *et al.* (2020) Tracking changes in SARS-CoV-2 Spike: Evidence that D614G increases infectivity of the COVID-19 virus. *Cell* 182:1–16.
75. Hu J, He CL, Gao QZ, Zhang GJ, Cao XX, *et al.* (2020) The D614G mutation of SARS-CoV-2 spike protein enhances viral infectivity and decreases neutralization sensitivity to individual convalescent sera. bioRxiv 2020.06.20.161323. DOI: https://doi.org/10.1101/2020.06.20.161323.
76. Ozono S, Zhang Y, Ode H, Seng TT, Imai K, *et al.* (2020) Naturally mutated spike proteins of SARS-CoV-2 variants show differential levels of cell entry. bioRxiv 2020.06.15.151779. DOI: 10.1101/2020.06.15.151779.
77. Zhang L, Jackson CB, Mou H, Ojha A, Rangarajan ES, Izard T, Farzan M, Choe H (2020) The D614G mutation in the SARS-CoV-2 spike protein reduces S1 shedding and increases infectivity. bioRxiv 2020.06.12.148726. DOI: https://doi.org/10.1101/2020.06.12.148726.
78. Liu L, Wang P, Nair MS, Yu J, Rapp M, *et al.* (2020) Potent neutralizing antibodies directed to multiple epitopes on SARS-CoV-2 spike. *Nature* 584:450–456.
79. Jespersen MC, Peters B, Nielsen M, Marcatili P (2017) BepiPred-2.0: Improving sequence-based B-cell epitope prediction using conformational epitopes. *Nucleic Acids Res* 45(W1):W24–W29.
80. Fernández A (2018) Stickiness of the hydrogen bond. *Ann Phys (Berlin)* 530:1800162.
81. Callaway E (2020) 'It will change everything': DeepMind's AI makes gigantic leap in solving protein structures. Nature, published online Nov. 30, 2020. doi: https://doi.org/10.1038/d41586-020-03348-4
82. Heaven WD (2020) DeepMind's protein-folding AI has solved a 50-year-old grand challenge of biology. MIT Tech Rev Nov 30, 2020 https://www.technologyreview.com/2020/11/30/1012712/deepmind-protein-folding-ai-solved-biology-science-drugs-disease/

Chapter 3

Artificial intelligence constructs *in vivo* reality to expedite protein folding

> *"Everybody takes the limits of his own vision for the limits of the world."*
>
> Arthur Schopenhauer

Natural proteins fold and have been selected to fold *in vivo*, that is in cellular environments, *not in vitro*. Likewise, therapeutic agents target dysfunctional or deregulated proteins *in vivo*, not in the test tube, where screening and affinity assays are typically performed. In regards to modeling and predictive efforts, the wanton molecular complexity of *in vivo* environments places them out of reach for investigation with molecular dynamics (MD) or other computational methods. The advent of artificial intelligence (AI) drastically changes this scenario, as shown in this chapter. Even in an *in vitro* setting, the generation of realistic protein folding pathways remains a challenge for molecular dynamics (MD) and other computational systems. This is so because for most single-domain chains, relevant timescales are inaccessible and key rare events are typically missed. Furthermore, most computational efforts have focused on *in vitro* folding, hence they are often misplaced as natural proteins have evolved to fold *in vivo*, where selective interference prevents the chain from getting kinetically trapped in misfolded states. In this chapter we empower MD by subsuming the computations within a deep learning platform that constructs an *in vivo* context shown to enhance the expediency of the folding process. To this effect, we build a convolutional neural network (CNN) trained with short MD runs that incorporate *in vivo* molecular complexity. The AI platform learns to propagate a coarse grained folding trajectory that can be decoded as an extended MD run assessing the participation of the *in vivo* context to expedite the folding process.

3.1 AI-based empowering of molecular dynamics

For decades, molecular dynamics (MD) has been adopted as a primary tool to investigate biomolecular processes *in vitro* such as protein folding [1, 2]. However, it is now recognized that such efforts may have been unrealistic and somewhat misplaced [3–6], as they may have dealt with the wrong context [6]. Proteins have evolved to fold in the cell, not *in vitro*. The fact that a few find their native structure *in vitro* is incidental, probably more the exception than the rule [6]. Through steering interference with the folding process, the *in vivo* setting prevents the protein from getting kinetically trapped in misfolded aggregation-prone states. On its own, MD is felt to be ill equipped to handle the complexities and relevant catalytic turnover timescales of an *in vivo* environment. Even in an *in vitro* context, the inadequacy of MD is usually apparent as physically relevant timescales are often inaccessible, conformation space is incompletely sampled, and rare events are typically missed [7–10].

The huge informational burden that needs to be carried over from one MD step to the next reduces the chances of MD to provide a meaningful model that can handle the complexities of *in vivo* settings. To address this problem, artificial intelligence (AI) needs to be deployed, as advocated in this work. An AI-empowered MD platform requires that we first encode the protein dynamics into a simplified representation retaining only essential topological features of the vector field that steers the MD integration process [7, 8]. First, we simplify the flow by lumping conformations within basins of attraction in potential energy and encoding the dynamics into a modulo-basin representation that averages out fast motion. Inter-basin transitions are determined by a dilated convolutional neural network (CNN) [11, 12] where the influence field on a basin transition at a residue site along the chain becomes progressively dilated in hidden network layers. Thus, the weighted influence of different contexts with different levels of locality upon each basin transition is optimized according to a loss function that contrasts network inferences against experimentally determined conformational changes. With a suitable propagation scheme obtained by training the network with big dynamic data from MD runs, this simplified AI scheme enables coverage of realistic timescales even for the *in vivo* context, while atomistic level detail is recovered through AI-empowered decoding.

To enable AI to construct an *in vivo* setting and assess its role in expediting the folding process, we incorporate the influence of specific structurally reported cellular machinery on the protein folding process. This is accomplished by training the CNN with multiple atomistic MD simulations of folding events within specific cellular molecular environments. None of the MD runs is able to cover folding timescales but together they inform the CNN on the steering influence of the *in vivo* reality.

For the sake of illustration, we adopt a training set consisting of MD runs that incorporate the influence of GroEL, a widely studied tetrameric chaperonin [3], on protein folding [4]. Inside the GroEL cavity, our atomistic MD runs showed that noncompact states with large radius of gyration (scaling with an unfolded ensemble average) interact strongly with structurally disordered residues in the GroEL C-terminus tails. These interactions disrupt the metastable states, thereby enhancing folding expediency. Thus, the influence of the *in vivo* context is incorporated through the training of the CNN in a selected environment of molecular complexity where only submicrosecond events are accessible to MD computation. The CNN generated a dynamics in which coarse grained misfolded states are levied inter-basin transitions that eventually get them dismantled, thereby preventing the protein from getting kinetically trapped. Thus, AI constructs a reality that expedites folding in a manner akin to chaperone catalysis *in vivo*.

In this way, the work describes and validates a first attempt at extending and empowering MD by exploiting the versatility of AI to absorb big data on folding events in the cell. Thus, the AI platform incorporates the feature extraction to construct an *in vivo* reality that expedites the folding process.

3.2 A CNN to empower MD computation

To reduce the informational burden in MD integration steps, we simplify the dynamics taking into account the inherent topological architecture of the MD-steering vector field. Thus we introduce an equivalence relation "$\sim$", whereby two microstates/conformations are regarded as equivalent if and only if the respective local conformations of the constitutive subunits lie in the same basins of attraction in the local potential energy surface. The "modulo basin" representation constitutes a "quotient space" made up of equivalence classes. In generic terms, if x indicates a microstate of a system of N subunits, the modulo-basin class (state) to which x belongs is denoted $\bar{x}$ and may be expressed as a Cartesian product of N basins designating the basin occupancies for the individual subunits: $\bar{x} = \prod_{n=1}^{N} b(x, n)$ where $b(x, n)$ is the basin of attraction occupied by subunit n when the system is in microstate x. Thus, for any two microstates $x, y :\ x \sim y \Leftrightarrow \bar{x} = \bar{y}$. Since the products of basins $B = \prod_{n=1}^{N} b(n)$ constitute a denumerable set, the classes/states in quotient space may be conveniently designated by encoding vectors.

Here we consider protein folding trajectories defined by the evolution of backbone torsional coordinates $\{\phi_n, \psi_n\}_{n=1,\ldots N}$. Conformation space thus becomes a 2N-dimensional torus, i. e. the product of 2N unit circles, one of each dihedral coordinate of the protein backbone [7, 8]. In this context, the modulo-basin quotient space is made up of Cartesian products of the so-called Ramachandran basins, that is, the allowed low-energy regions in the potential energy surface of each residue along the protein chain of length N (Fig. 3.1, [13, 14]). Within this mathematical construct, we may project the MD trajectory on the quotient space and then adopt deep learning to propagate the encoded "shorthand" dynamics to make computations more agile. The shorthand dynamics carry far lower information burden as conformations are lumped into classes that entail a considerable simplification of conformation space, while the transition timescale for each iteration is the minimal Ramachandran intrabasin equilibration time $\tau = 100\,\text{ps}$, considerably larger than the femtosecond integration timescales used in MD. Hence, since

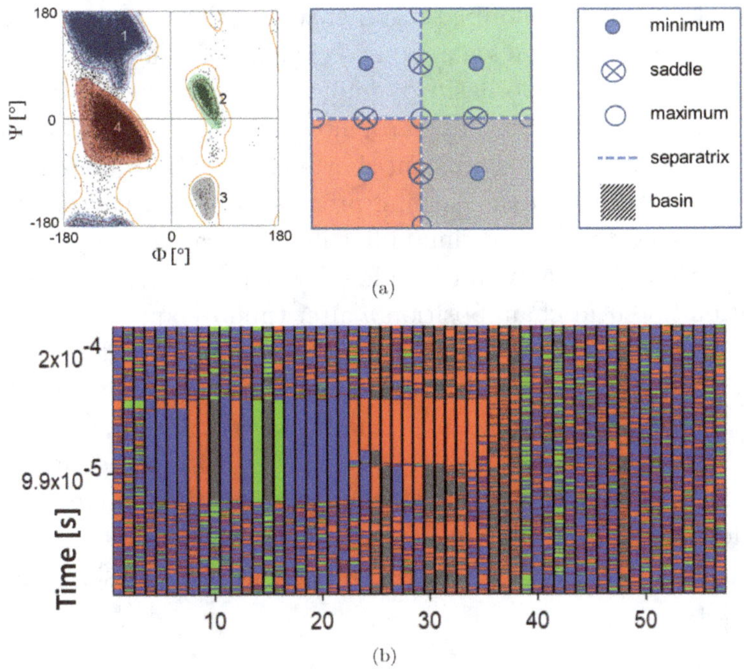

Figure 3.1. Modulo-basin simplification of the vector field integrated in MD computations generating the backbone torsional dynamics of a protein chain. **(a)** Topological representation (right panel) of the vector field steering the backbone torsional dynamics of a single residue. Opposite sides of the square are identified as per the $\pm 180°$ identification of φ, ψ dihedrals, yielding a 2-torus, or cartesian product of two circles. The four colored sectors morph topologically into the Ramachandran basins or allowed regions of potential energy (left panel). Except for glycine (G), the grey sector is energetically inaccessible to other residues due to steric clash with the side chain. Other accessibility restrictions apply to geometrically constrained proline (P) and adjacent residues. The basin topology with its distribution of critical points (minima, saddles, maxima) is compatible with the underlying 2-torus. The panel on the right describes the organization of the basins of attraction of the critical points (minima and saddles). The basins of attraction of saddles are 1-dimensional separatrices of the 2-dimensional basins of minima. **(b)** Coarse grained representation of an MD trajectory at $1\,\mu$s-resolution for the $N = 57$ chain of the B1 domain of protein G. The trajectory is subsequently extended in time using deep learning. At each time (vertical axis), the modulo-basin state of the chain is shown as a color sequence, where the basin assigned to each residue on the horizontal axis is specified following the color convention adopted in panel a. A $220\,\mu$s-folding trajectory was generated within the NPT (isothermal/isobaric, $T = 298\,$K) ensemble, selecting the timespan interval $[0, t_0 = 120\,\mu\text{s}]$ as training region and the interval $[120\,\mu\text{s}, 220\,\mu\text{s}]$ as the learning period to optimize the parametrization of the propagator Γ_τ.

intra-basin events are lumped together within the equivalence classes and the iteration timescale is five orders of magnitude longer, the propagated modulo-basin dynamics has a far better chance of capturing the infrequent or rare interbasin transitions, a highly sought after goal and a significant shortcoming in MD modeling of *in vitro* processes. The deep learning process to propagate the modulo basin dynamics, uses a maximum likelihood ansatz to train a dilated CNN so that the maximum likelihood weight, $f_\tau(n, b, b')$, for basin transition $b \to b'$ at chain position n after time τ elapsed is influenced by the amino acid identity and basin occupancy at flanking residues $(n-2, n-1, n+1, n+2)$, with an influence field progressively dilated, so that flanking positions $(n-3, n-2, n+2, n+3)$, $(n-4, n-3, n+3, n+4), \ldots, (n-8, n-7, n+7, n+8)$ with respective ranges $g = 1, 2, \ldots, 7$ also impact the transition probability. Computational cost determines that we limit the extent of dilation to maximum $g = 7$. Thus the maximum likelihood weight of the basin transition becomes:

$$f_\tau(n, b, b') = \prod_{g=1}^{7} w(n, g, A(n, g), B(n, g)) f(n, g, A(n, g), B(n, g), b, b') \tag{1}$$

Where $f(n, g, A(n, g), B(n, g), b, b')$ gives the frequency of the $b \to b'$ basin transition at position n after time τ elapsed obtained by projecting one hundred 220ns-MD runs onto a modulo-basin τ-discretized time series for chain composition $A(n, g)$ giving the amino acid identity of residues $n-g-1$, $n-g$, n, $n+g$, $n+g+1$ in the chain, and basin assignment $B(n, g)$ for residues $n-g-1$, $n-g$, n, $n+g$, $n+g+1$. The different g-influencing fields $(n-g-1, n-g, n, n+g, n+g+1)$ bearing on the basin transition at position n are weighted in accord with parameters $w(n, g, A(n, g), B(n, g))$, which are optimized vis-à-vis the loss function of the CNN.

A first stage in the training of the network yields the transition frequencies $f(n, g, A(n, g), B(n, g), b, b')$ thus following the maximum likelihood scheme. The propagation of the modulo-basin trajectory (time series) in the maximum likelihood scheme is determined by the

$b \to b'$ transition probabilities: $p_{ML}(n,b,b') = \frac{f_\tau(n,b,b')}{\sum_{b''} f_\tau(n,b,b'')}$, where b'' is any of the four basins. The destiny basin b' after a time period τ is determined by a Monte Carlo scheme taking into account the four transition probabilities at each position n along the chain.

The input in the dilated CNN is thus filtered through $7 \times 4^5 = 7168$ hidden layers in accord with range g and basin assignment $B(n,g)$ for the g-quintuples centered at each position n on the chain and influencing the basin transition at position n. The CNN input is a basin assignment for each residue along the chain, and its output is the basing assignment after time τ has elapsed. In turn, each layer contains 20^5 filters or convolution kernels in accord with amino acid identity $A(n,g)$. To convolve, a modulo-basin state for a chain of length N may be labeled with a 4N-vector $(\mathbf{b}_1|\mathbf{b}_2|\ldots|\mathbf{b}_n\ldots)$ consisting of N binary 4-tuples $\mathbf{b}_n$ $(n = 1,2,\ldots,N)$ indicating the Ramachandran basin occupancy for each residue, so the value 1 at entry m in $\mathbf{b}_n$ $(b_{nm} = 1)$ indicates that residue n occupies basin m $(m = 1,2,3,4)$ (Fig. 3.1(a)). For example, (1000|0010) indicates the coarse-grained state of a dipeptide with first residue in basin 1 and second residue in basin 3. Thus, a convolutional kernel $K(n,g,B_K(n,g))$ becomes a g-quintuple of binary 4-tuples (basin assignment $B_K(n,g)$) with range g, with the convolution operation carrying the Kronecker-delta factor $\delta_{A(n,g),A_K(n,g)}$, where $A_K(n,g)$ is the kernel amino acid assignment for positions $n-g-1$, $n-g$, n, $n+g$, $n+g+1$. Each layer $L(q,g)$ is labeled by the basin quintuple, in turn labeled by index $q = 1,\ldots,4^5 = 1024$, and range g. In each layer, the 20^5 convolution kernels are slided along the chain as stencils, and full coincidence at position n in $L(q,g)$ yields concatenation (enrichment) at position n in the (q,g)-feature map with the four attributes $f(n,g,A(n,g),B(n,g),b,b')$ for the four *a-priori* possible b' destiny basins. After processing across all 7168 hidden layers, we arrive at a full representation of the chain at layer L(1024,7), where each position n is endowed with $7 \times 4 = 28$ transition parameters $f(n,g,A(n,g),B(n,g),b,b')$, one for each influence range g and destiny basin b'. In the 7169th layer, the products $\prod_{g=1}^{7} w(n,g,A(n,g),B(n,g))f(n,g,A(n,g),B(n,g),b,b')$ are finally computed, and the four transition probabilities $p_{ML}(n,b,b')$ are obtained for each of the four *a-priori* destinies b'. Finally, in the output (7170th) layer, the destiny basin for each residue is chosen from the Monte Carlo scheme.

The optimization of the influence-defining factors $w(n, g, A(n, g), B(n, g))$ is carried out during the second training phase for the modulo-basin propagator Γ_τ defined by the Monte Carlo generator of basin transitions. To train the network in this second stage, we break up the MD trajectories spanning a time period $[0, t_f]$ into two regions, a training portion with timespan $[0, t_0]$ and an optimization portion covering the time interval $(t_0, t_f]$. With the trajectory statistics drawn for the region $[0, t_0]$ we obtain the basin-transition frequencies for triads with different stride centered at each particular residue. On the other hand, a variational optimization process during the period $(t_0, t_f]$ enables us to determine the w-parameters. Thus, the w's are obtained from a commutativity condition that reflects the compatibility of fine and coarse grained propagation of the trajectory and must be fulfilled during the period $(t_0, t_f]$. The commutativity condition is $\Gamma_\tau \circ \pi = \pi \circ M(\tau)$ as depicted by the following scheme:

$$\begin{array}{ccc} x(t) & \overset{\pi}{\rightarrow} & \overline{x(t)} \\ \downarrow M(\tau) & & \downarrow \Gamma_\tau \\ x(t+\tau) & \overset{\pi}{\rightarrow} & \overline{x(t+\tau)} \end{array}$$

Here π is the canonical projection that assigns the Ramachandran basins to each backbone torsional state of the chain and $M(\tau)$ is the molecular dynamics propagator operating on torsional states of the chain. In other words, the parametrization of the modulo-basin propagator Γ_τ is optimized to minimize the loss function $\mathcal{L}(\Gamma_\tau)$ given by

$$\mathcal{L}(\Gamma_\tau) = M^{-1} \sum_{q=1}^{M} \|\pi x(t_0 + q\tau) - [\Gamma_\tau]^q \pi x(t_0)\|^2, \tag{2}$$

where $M\tau \leq t_f - t_0 < (M+1)\tau$. We know this loss function is the correct one since $\mathcal{L}(\Gamma_\tau) = 0$ if and only if the propagator makes the diagram commutative. Once the optimal $\Gamma_\tau^* = argmin\,\mathcal{L}(\Gamma_\tau)$ has been obtained from stochastic gradient descent, the modulo-basin projected trajectory can be propagated beyond MD-accessible timescales. The set $\wp(t_0, t_f)$ of MD-generated states during the period $t_0 \leq t \leq t_f$ is sampled randomly at each iteration to compute the gradient with minibatches given by trajectory fragments spanned by randomly chosen time intervals of size $10^{-2}|t_f - t_0|$. To optimize the network connectivity that determines Γ_τ, the ADADELTA optimization protocol with learning rate 0.3 is adopted [15]. Physically meaningful timescales may be reached by computing the coarse states $\overline{x(t_f + q\tau)}$ beyond the simulation timespan t_f as $[\Gamma_\tau^*]^q\overline{x(t_f)}$.

To identify intermediate structures along an AI-generated folding pathway, the coarse-grained modulo basin trajectory needs to be decoded back to a backbone (φ, ψ)-state. This reconstruction process also requires deep learning since we need to optimize a 1-to-1 application λ: modulo-basin state $\rightarrow (\varphi, \psi) -$ state that makes the following diagram commutative in the time range $t_0 \leq t \leq t_f - \tau$:

$$\begin{array}{ccc} x(t) & \overset{\pi}{\rightarrow} & \overline{x(t)} \\ \downarrow MD & & \downarrow \Gamma_\tau^* \\ x(t+\tau) & \underset{\lambda}{\leftarrow} & \overline{x(t+\tau)} \end{array}$$

This implies that the decoder λ must be optimized to minimize the loss function:

$$\mathcal{L}(\lambda) = M^{-1}\sum_{n=1}^{M} \|x(t_0 + n\tau) - \lambda[\Gamma_\tau^*]^n \pi x(t_0)\|^2 \tag{3}$$

The choice of loss function is correct since $\mathcal{L}(\lambda) = 0$ if and only if the decoder makes the diagram commute. With the choice of decoder as $argmin\,\mathcal{L}(\lambda)$, identified with stochastic gradient descent [15], we expand the MD simulation as $\lambda[\Gamma_\tau^*]^n \pi x(t_0)$ for any $n \geq M$. In cases when in vivo reality has been incorporated, the evolution of the (φ, ψ)-state may be monitored as $\lambda\widehat{[\Gamma_\tau]}^n \pi x(t_0)$, where the *in vivo* propagator will be defined subsequently.

3.3 Injecting *in vivo* reality into the CNN to expedite protein folding

The goal is now to incorporate the role of *in vivo* settings in steering the protein chain along an expeditious folding pathway. Given computational limitations, atomistic detail on a folding trajectory in an *in vivo* context, say, in the interior of a chaperone, is hardly feasible. For example, for chaperonin GroEL, such computations are currently only accessible in hundreds-of-microseconds timescales for short substrates $N \sim 25$ with the fastest dedicated supercomputers [4]. For a typical single-domain protein ($N > 50$), such computations are not likely to yield the mechanism by which the cellular context is able to remove kinetic traps and expedite folding. To generate coarse grained *in vivo* folding trajectories, we implement a deep learning system that captures the expediency of the *in vivo* environment when trained with accessibly short (30ns) MD simulations starting at unfolded or metastable states generated *in vitro*. We need to capture the means by which the *in vivo* setting removes kinetic traps by selectively disrupting misfolded states that would be otherwise susceptible to aggregation due to high protein concentration in the cell.

Let $\widetilde{\Gamma_\tau}$ denote the modulo-basin propagator that commutes with $\widetilde{M(\tau)}$, the MD operator that steers the chain torsional dynamics in the *in vivo* setting (in our illustration, the GroEL cavity). The propagator $\widetilde{\Gamma_\tau}$ is obtained by training the CNN with many short *in vivo* runs and its domain $D(\widetilde{\Gamma_\tau})$ consists of basin assignments along the chain that undergo basin transitions (including retentions) when the chain explores conformations in the *in vivo* setting. The domain for Γ_τ^* is similarly defined *mutatis mutandis* in association with the *in vitro* setting.

To generate *in vivo* folding trajectories that span realistic timescales, a significant coverage is required of the influencing basin occupancies at positions flanking each residue along the chain placed in the *in vivo* environment. To that effect, we construct the propagator $\widehat{\Gamma_\tau}$ obtained by overwriting basin transitions yielded by Γ_τ^* in the domain $D(\Gamma_\tau^*) \cap D(\widetilde{\Gamma_\tau})$, replacing them by the transitions dictated by $\widetilde{\Gamma_\tau}$. Thus, we get $\widehat{\Gamma_\tau} = \chi_{D(\widetilde{\Gamma_\tau})}\widetilde{\Gamma_\tau} \oplus \chi_{D(\Gamma^*_\tau)\setminus[D(\Gamma^*_\tau)\cap D(\tilde{\Gamma}_\tau)]}\Gamma^*_\tau$, where χ denotes characteristic function (1 on its support, 0 elsewhere), and $D(\Gamma^*_\tau) \setminus [D(\Gamma^*_\tau) \cap D(\widetilde{\Gamma_\tau})]$ denotes the complement of $D(\Gamma^*_\tau) \cap D(\widetilde{\Gamma_\tau})$ in $D(\Gamma^*_\tau)$. Thus, the *in vivo* propagator $\widehat{\Gamma_\tau}$ commutes with $\widetilde{M(\tau)}$ in $\pi^{-1}[D(\tilde{\Gamma}_\tau)]$ and with $M(\tau)$ in $\pi^{-1}\{D(\Gamma^*_\tau) \setminus [D(\Gamma^*_\tau) \cap D(\widetilde{\Gamma_\tau})]\}$, implying that $\widetilde{\Gamma_\tau}$ overwrites Γ^*_τ in $D(\Gamma^*_\tau) \cap D(\widetilde{\Gamma_\tau})$.

3.4 Generating *in vitro* folding pathways with an MD-trained CNN

The efficacy of the dynamic DL scheme is illustrated by computing folding pathways converging to native structures. We selected an $N = 57$ chain known to fold autonomously in an *in vitro* setting: the thermophilic variant of the B1 domain of protein G from *Streptococcus* (PDB.1GB4). The thermophile was chosen over the wild type due to higher stability of the folded structure. Using the charmm package (free version of CHARMM) [2], we first generated a $220\,\mu$s-folding trajectory within the NPT (isothermal/isobaric, $T = 298\,$K) ensemble. The full MD trajectory encoded as the modulo basin version is shown in Fig. 3.1(b), with selected $t_0 = 120\,\mu s$ as training parameter and $120\,\mu s < t \leq 220\,\mu s$ as learning period to optimize the matrix propagator Γ_τ . The coarse grained trajectory is then propagated up to $t = 7500\,\mu$s (Fig. 3.2(a–c)). We note that the final state is significantly stable, prevailing since the time of its inception at $t = 3108\,\mu$s detectable on Fig. 3.2(b). Furthermore, the decoded final stable state at $t = 7500\,\mu$s (Fig. 3.3), corresponding to the eigenvector associated with eigenvalue 1 of the matrix Γ^*_τ, is topologically equivalent to the native crystallographic state (PDB.1GB4), revealing the same pattern of antiparallel and long-range parallel β-sheets with α-helix packed against the β-sheet motif. The backbone-atom RMSD is estimated at 1.91Å.

In the *in vitro* folding context, at least two metastable states can be spotted to be distinctively generated at 0.7 and 2.7 ms (Fig. 3.2), corresponding to the chain conformations displayed in Figs. 3.3(b) and 3.3(c), respectively.

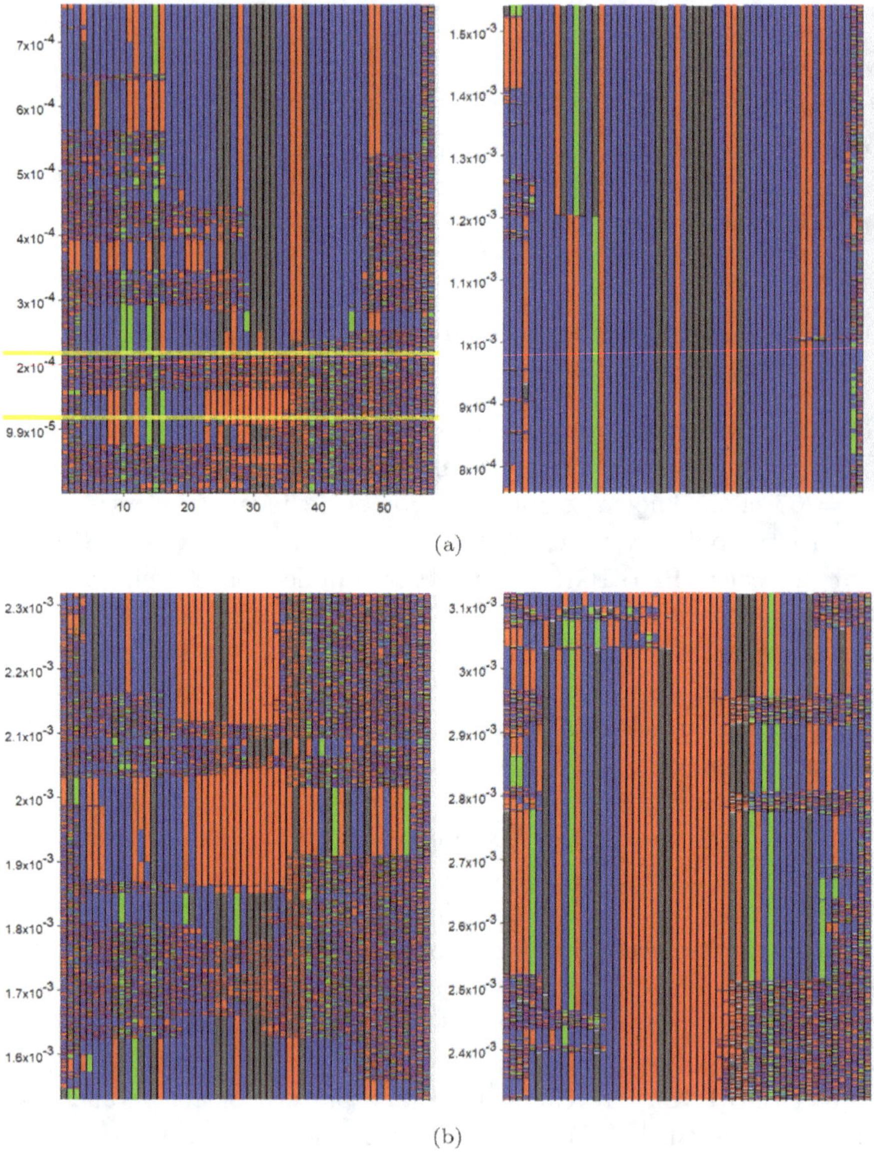

Figure 3.2. Coarse-grained propagation generated with AI of the MD trajectory shown in Fig. 3.1. **(a–c)** Key portions of the MD trajectory at 1 μs-resolution for timespan $[0, 220\,\mu\text{s}]$ and propagated to cover timespan $[0, 7500\,\mu\text{s}]$. On panel **c**, the steady state ensemble is shown for the final portion of the propagation of the trajectory (full coverage: 7500 μs). The native-like steady state begins to develop at around 3100 μs.

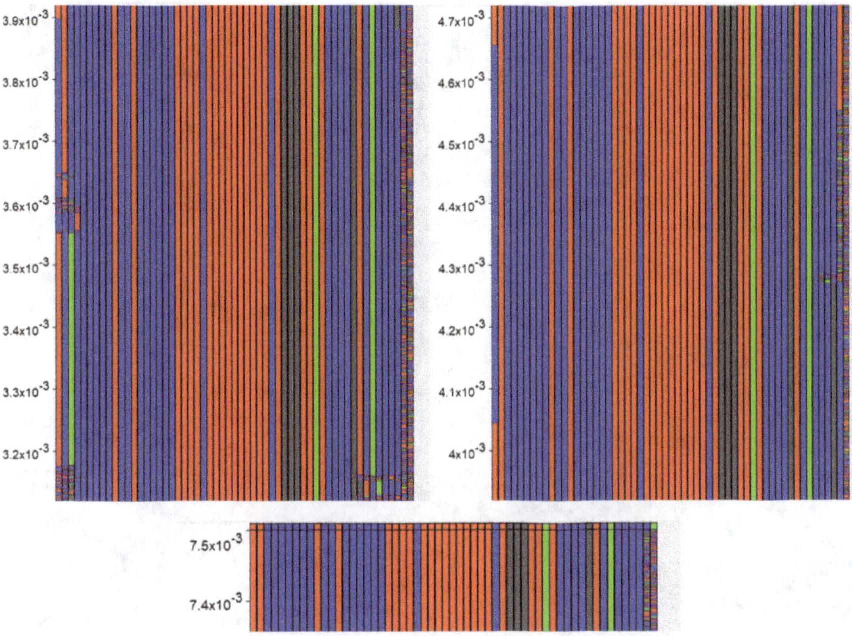

(c)

Figure 3.2. (*Continued*)

3.5 AI constructs *in vivo* reality to expedite folding pathways

To illustrate the generation of *in vivo* folding pathways, the AI platform constructed an *in vivo* reality by learning to generate the propagator $\widehat{\Gamma_\tau}$ from one hundred atomistic 30ns-MD runs of the $N = 57$ protein chain exploring conformation space within the GroEL cavity [3]. To generate atomistic level short MD-trajectories in the selected *in vivo* context, we follow standard protocol: The conformation identified with the X-ray diffraction structure of GroEL-ATP14 (PDB.1SX3) is adopted to model the GroEL cavity assumed to expedite the folding of the B1 domain of G protein. Excess Mg^{++}-complexed ATP molecules must be removed, while the 22 inherently disordered C-terminal amino acids, mainly comprised of Gly-Gly-Met repeats, are incorporated with Maestro [16]. One protein chain is

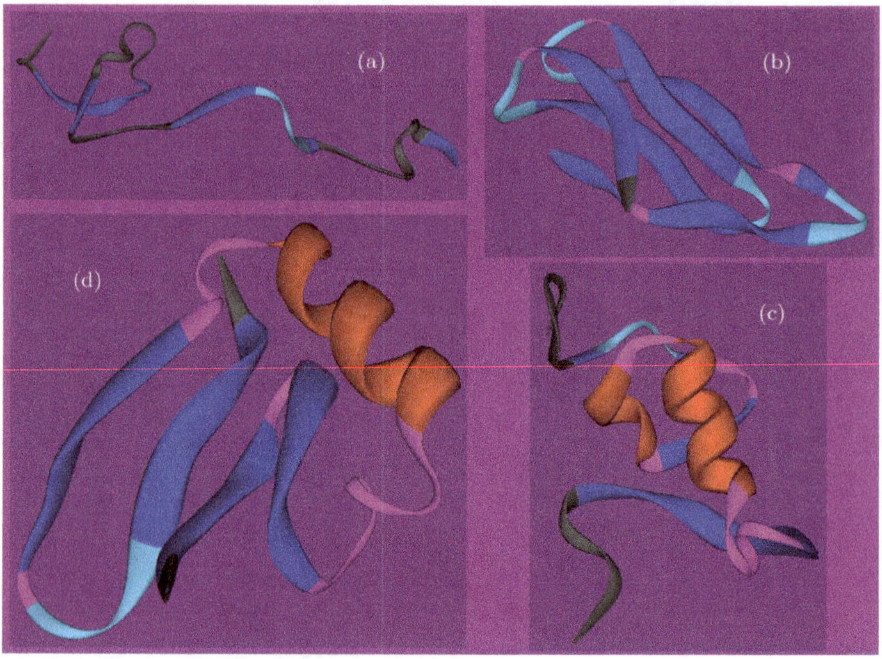

Figure 3.3. Decoded microstates in ribbon representation for the AI-enabled propagation of the MD trajectory, generated at start **(a)**, 0.7 ms (**b**), 2.7 ms (**c**), and 7.5 ms (**d**). The modulo-basin representation of the last microstate **(d)** is the eigenvector associated with eigenvalue 1 of matrix Γ_{τ}^{*} and is topologically equivalent to the native state from PDB entry 1GB4 obtained by X-ray diffraction crystallography. Conformations (b) and (c) are kinetic traps.

placed at the center of the GroEL cavity, and the system is solvated in a 200 Å × 200 Å × 200 Å water box at 120 mM KCl concentration. The final system is composed of ~1,178,000 particles. Simulations of 100ns are performed using the charmm package [2]. One hundred 100ns simulations are performed with the protein in the GroEL-ATP7 cavity. Ten runs are started in an unfolded state, ten in the protein native state (PDB.1GB4) and 90 runs are started in metastable states. The system is subject to energy minimization and equilibrated at 300 K and 1 atm with harmonic restraints on the alpha carbons. The runs are performed in the NPT ensemble with a Nosé–Hoover thermostat [17, 18] and a MTK barostat [19], with the mass of all hydrogen atoms set at 4 amu, while the time step gets fixed at 4.0 fs.

To generate *in vivo* folding trajectories, the trained CNN generates the coarse-grained propagator $\widehat{\Gamma_\tau}$ that removes kinetic traps by selectively disrupting misfolded metastable structure that would be otherwise susceptible to aggregation due to the high concentration in the cell relative to an *in vitro* environment. The CNN choreographs folding disruptions at states where $\widetilde{\Gamma_\tau}$ overwrites Γ^*_τ when the application of the latter generates metastable states characterized by the persistence of the chain in a specific basin assignment.

The CNN operationally implements the *in vivo* intervention step. Assume a substantial portion (typically 80% or more) of the basin assignment for the chain is detected to be locked at time $t_f + q_s\tau$, then the potentially disruptive propagator $\widetilde{\Gamma_\tau}$ overwrites Γ^*_τ for the step $t_f + q_s\tau \to t_f + (q_s + 1)\tau$. Thus the coarse state at $t_f + (q_s + 1)\tau$ is computed as $\widetilde{\Gamma_\tau}[\Gamma^*_\tau]^{q_s}\overline{x(t_f)}$. The disruptive propagator excludes the basin retention $b' = b$ frequency, $f_\tau(n, b, b)$, from the Monte Carlo scheme that assigns at time $t_f + (q_s + 1)\tau$ the destiny basin b' at the basin-locked chain position n. For residues that did not retained their basin assignment at time $t_f + q_s\tau$, the propagation $b \to b'$ is constructed as in Γ^*_τ We note that to generate the *in vivo* reality, full network training with 30ns atomistic MD runs and parameter optimization took approximately 18 hours on a cluster of 12 Titan RTX GPUs, while the full propagation computation required an additional 12 hours on the same resource.

The CNN-generated folding trajectory is shown in Fig. 3.4(a), while Fig. 3.4(b) shows the influence of the *in vivo* context depicted as selective interferences with basin transitions. The basin assignments implicating the *in vitro* model valid in $\mathcal{D}(\Gamma^*_\tau) \setminus [\mathcal{D}(\Gamma^*_\tau) \cap D(\widetilde{\Gamma_\tau})]$ are marked in white, those involving *in vivo* intervention in $\mathcal{D}(\widetilde{\Gamma_\tau}) \setminus [\mathcal{D}(\Gamma^*_\tau) \cap D(\widetilde{\Gamma_\tau})]$ are marked in pink, while black denotes *in vivo* overwriting of *in vitro* assignments in $\mathcal{D}(\Gamma^*_\tau) \cap D(\widetilde{\Gamma_\tau})$ and grey indicates coincidence between *in vitro* and *in vivo* assignments in $\mathcal{D}(\Gamma^*_\tau) \cap \mathcal{D}(\widetilde{\Gamma_\tau})$. The starting conformation is shown in ribbon rendering on Fig. 3.4(c). The convergence to a native fold (Fig. 3.4(d)), with RMSD = 2.1 Å relative to PDB.1GB4, occurs 750 times faster

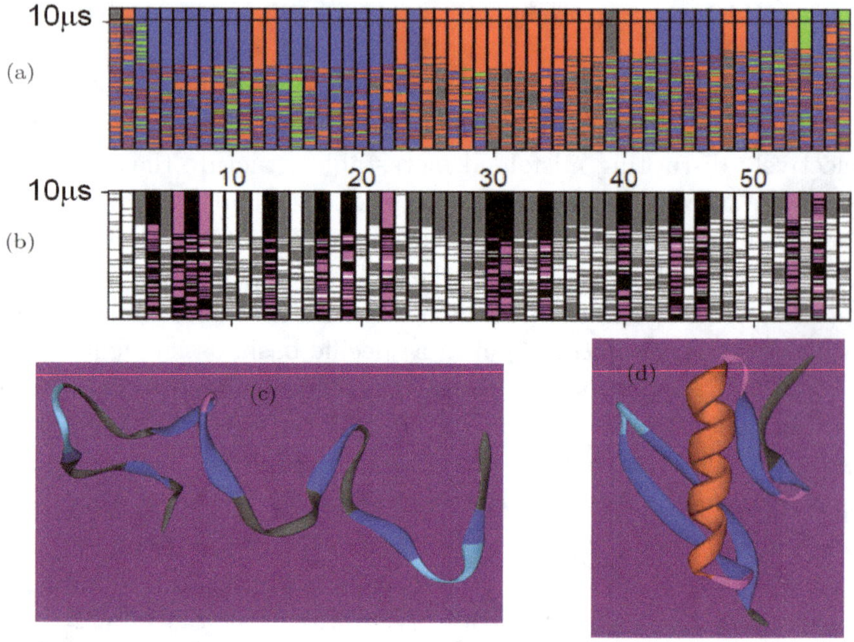

Figure 3.4. Ultra expeditious *in vivo* folding trajectory generated by AI with a CNN trained with 100 atomistic 30ns-MD runs of the chain dynamics within a GroEL environment. **(a)** Coarse grained trajectory at 0.1 μs resolution. **(b)** Influence of *in vivo* context. The basin assignments are depicted in white when implicating the *in vitro* model valid in $\mathcal{D}(\Gamma^*_\tau) \setminus [\mathcal{D}(\Gamma^*_\tau) \cap \mathcal{D}(\widetilde{\Gamma_\tau})]$, in pink when involving *in vivo* intervention in $\mathcal{D}(\widetilde{\Gamma_\tau}) \setminus [\mathcal{D}(\Gamma^*_\tau) \cap \mathcal{D}(\tilde{\Gamma}_\tau)]$, in black for *in vivo* overwriting of *in vitro* transitions in $\mathcal{D}(\Gamma^*_\tau) \cap \mathcal{D}(\tilde{\Gamma}_\tau)$ and in grey when there is coincidence between *in vitro* and *in vivo* assignments in $\mathcal{D}(\Gamma^*_\tau) \cap \mathcal{D}(\widetilde{\Gamma_\tau})$. **(c)** Initial state. **(d)** Decoded final state.

than in the *in vitro* setting (cf. Fig. 3.2), attesting to the staggering efficiency of the *in vivo* context to extricate the chain from kinetic traps.

We explored other possibilities where less *in vivo* reality is represented in the $\widehat{\Gamma_\tau}$ propagator. Strikingly, using only twenty-five 30ns-MD-runs for the chain within the GroEL cavity, a 75-factor increase in speed is achieved and no kinetic traps are apparent, as shown in Fig. 3.5, where a complete coarse-grained trajectory and the role of the *in vivo* context are displayed.

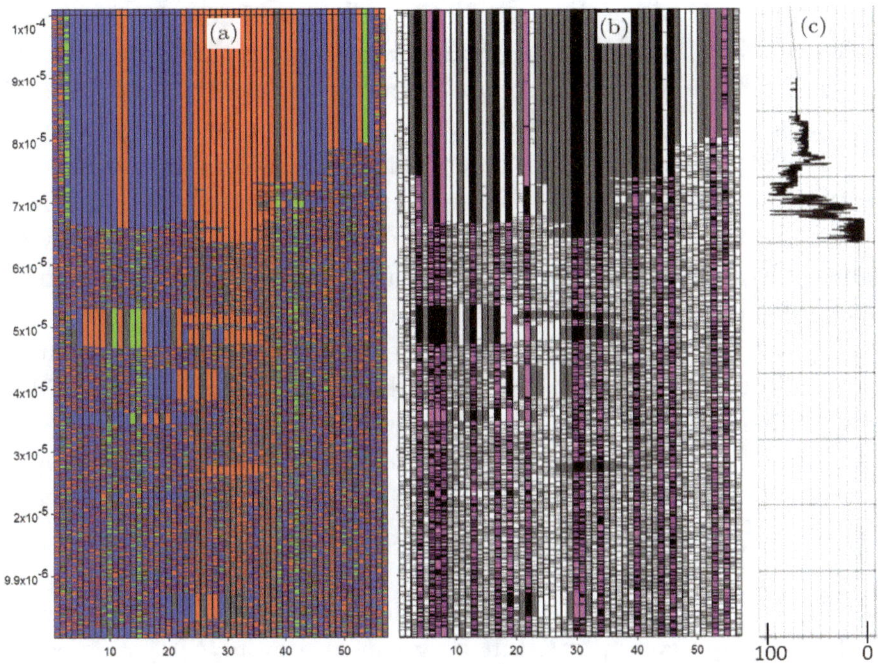

Figure 3.5. **(a)** *In vivo* folding trajectory generated by AI with a CNN trained with 25 atomistic 30ns-MD runs of the chain dynamics within a GroEL environment. **(b)** Influence of *in vivo* context on the folding process assessed by AI. Depiction of *in vivo* interventions follows the convention described in Fig. 3.4. **(c)** Number of three-body correlations corresponding to intermolecular wrapping interactions involving backbone hydrogen bonds from the protein and nonpolar groups from the flexible tails of the chaperonin.

These results invite further research to identify the minimal extent of *in vivo* intervention that would be required to ensure that folding chains are extricated from misfolded aggregation-prone states.

3.6 The nature of *in vivo* molecular cooperativity as revealed by AI

Natural proteins have been selected to fold in cellular environments, not in the test tube. Likewise, molecularly targeted therapeutic intervention to impair dysfunctional proteins is expected to be operative *in vivo*, not *in vitro*. Thus, in a general context, efforts to generate folding trajectories in an *in vitro* setting through atomistic molecular dynamics (MD) computations are probably misplaced and unrealistic. On the other hand, given the wanton complexity of the molecular settings, the generation of *in vivo* folding pathways is prohibitively expensive, prone to amplify systematic error and colossally time consuming with the computational technologies at hand. Given this dismal situation, this chapter describes a first attempt at constructing and incorporating an *in vivo* molecular reality by deploying artificial intelligence with the goal to identify the molecular underpinnings of folding expediency in a cellular environment. To this effect, we built a convolutional neural network trained with short (30 ns) MD runs to incorporate the very *in vivo* complexity that precluded MD from accessing realistic timescales and from capturing the rare events relevant to the folding process. Atomistic MD simulations are unlikely to generate realistic *in vivo* folding pathways for most single-domain proteins, even with dedicated supercomputers, but they can inform an AI system so as to enable it to incorporate the *in vivo* reality that makes folding expeditious, as shown in this chapter. Thus, the AI system learns to propagate a coarse grained folding trajectory that can be decoded as an extended MD run assessing the participation of the *in vivo* context in the folding process.

So, how exactly is the in vivo context making folding expeditious? The answer may be found in the examination of the exogenous wrapping interactions shown in Fig. 3.5. In particular, Fig. 3.5(c) shows a burst in three-body correlations corresponding to intermolecular wrapping interactions involving backbone hydrogen bonds (BHBs) from the protein and nonpolar groups from the flexible tails of the chaperonin. This burst implies extensive protection of the BHBs that eventually determine the native structure, suggesting a nucleation two-state mechanism for the expeditious folding processes that take place in vivo. *Thus, the in vivo environment intervenes cooperatively to stabilize the nucleus of the native fold.* This key intervention makes apparent the many-body nature of the folding process, as it commits the chain to fold. The native-like secondary structure in the nucleus formed at 6.85×10^{-5} s would not prevail *in vitro* without tertiary structure but is stabilized *in vivo* through cooperative interactions from within the environment.

To further explore the molecular basis of cooperativity, we need to examine the folding process from a physico-chemical perspective: With an amide and carbonyl group per residue, the backbone of the protein chain is highly polar and this molecular property imposes severe constraints on the nature of the *in vivo* intervention and on the chain composition of proteins capable of sustaining a hydrophobic collapse. Thus, the *in vivo* intervention entails the exogenous dehydration of backbone amides and carbonyls and such a process would be thermodynamically disfavored if it were not for the possibility of amides and carbonyls to engage in hydrogen bonding with each other. Hence, *not every in vivo* intervention *qualifies as being conducive to folding the protein chain: only those that ensure the formation and protection of backbone hydrogen bonds are likely to ensure an expedient folding of the chain.* On the other hand, polar-group hydration competes with intramolecular hydrogen bonds, compromising the structural integrity of proteins with a deficiently wrapped backbone, as discussed in Chapter 2. Thus, the need for formation and protection of intramolecular hydrogen bonds from water attack imposes constraints on the chain composition of an efficient folder capable of sustaining a reproducible expeditious collapse.

In accord with this picture, we may postulate that as proteins fold, the hydrogen-bond pairing of backbone amides and carbonyls is concurrent with the chaperonin wrapping burst. This fact has been rationalized taking into account that the thermodynamic cost associated with the dehydration of unpaired polar groups is relatively high, and that the wrapping hinders the backbone hydration by shielding it from water. On the other hand, the strength and stability of hydrogen bonds clearly depend on the microenvironment where they occur: The proximity of nonpolar groups to a hydrogen bond enhances the electrostatic interaction by de-screening the partial charges, and stabilizes it by hindering the hydration of the polar groups in the nonbonded state. *Thus, to guarantee the expediency of the folding process, most or at least the nucleating intramolecular backbone hydrogen bonds must be surrounded or "wrapped" by chaperonin nonpolar groups fairly thoroughly as to become significantly dehydrated during the convergence in the folding process.* On the other hand, if the intramolecular backbone hydrogen bonds fail to be properly shielded, the backbone tends to maximize its hydration level. This observation has implications at an ensemble-average level accessible to experimentalists. It may help understand the fact that single-domain proteins are likely to be two-state folders *in vivo*, with a single kinetic barrier dominating the folding process at the ensemble-average level.

The hydration propensity of amide and carbonyl and the dehydration-induced strengthening of their electrostatic association represent two conflictive tendencies, suggesting that there must be a crossover point in the dehydration propensity of a backbone hydrogen bond. If the bond is poorly wrapped by a few nonpolar groups that cluster around it, then hydration of the paired amide and carbonyl is likely to be favorable, but as the hydrogen bond becomes better wrapped, the surrounding water loses too many hydrogen bonding partnerships and thus, further removal of surrounding water is promoted. *Thus, the dehydronic field per hydrogen bond must significantly increase as hydrogen bonds get sufficiently dehydrated and this enhancement promotes further compaction of the chain and commits it fold. This switch-over behavior from backbone hydration to dehydration of backbone hydrogen bonds translated into an enhanced dehydronic field reflects the commitment to fold into a compact structure in which most backbone hydrogen bonds will be thoroughly dehydrated. This general picture is schematized in* Fig. 3.6. *The rationalization of the two-state folding kinetics of single-domain proteins in vivo is thus based on the cooperative nature of wrapping interactions with active participation of the in vivo environment.*

The crossover point in hydrogen-bond dehydration propensity may be regarded as representing a local characterization of the folding transition state if we adopt the backbone hydrogen bond dehydration as a generic folding coordinate. Once the folding process has progressed beyond the crossover point assisted by the in vivo environment (Fig. 3.5(c)), further dehydration of the backbone is

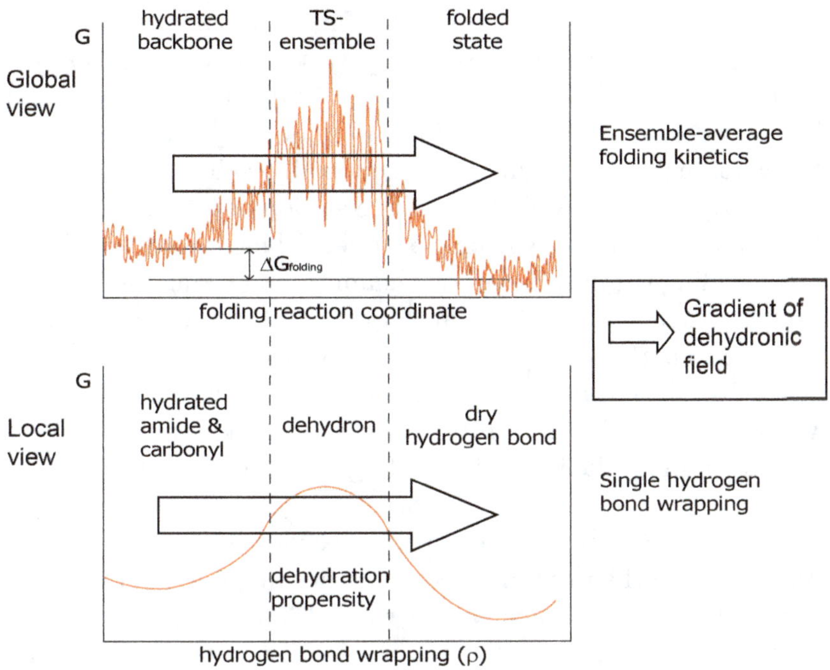

Figure 3.6. The cross-over behavior from backbone hydration to dehydration of backbone hydrogen bonds triggered by exogenous in vivo wrapping translates at the ensemble folding-kinetics level into a commitment of the chain to fold as the folding reaction progresses beyond the transition state towards hydrophobic collapse.

favored in consonance with the downhill nature of the folding process beyond the transition state. Thus, *a transition-state conformation commits the chain to fold partly because the hydrogen bonds partially wrapped by the chaperonin trigger their further desolvation, in turn promoting further chain compaction* (Fig. 3.6). This compaction is essential to augment the number of nonpolar groups within the hydrogen-bond microenvironments, thus further protecting the bonds from water attack.

3.7 Co-translational protein folding unraveled by AI

A significant portion of natural proteins initiate and advance the folding process as they are being translated in the ribosome ([20] and references therein). It is believed that about a third of the *E. coli* proteome is folded co-translationally, with comparable proportions for eukaryotes. The ribosome is a huge assemblage of protein and rRNA (ribosomal ribonucleic acid) subunits endowed with mechanical, scaffolding and enzymatic functionalities. The latter include peptidyl transferase, a tributary of translation of mRNA (messenger RNA), that performs an edit-prone sequential incorporation of amino acids extending the nascent protein chain by catalyzing the formation of peptidic linkages [20]. The translation rate for eukaryotes is about 6 amino acids per second, while for prokaryotes that number increases to about 20. Thus, it has been speculated that cotranslational folding may be a quasi-equilibrium process for those single-domain proteins that can complete their *in vitro* folding in less than $\sim$100 ms.

Most of the published results on co-translational protein folding (see for example [21]) remain mostly speculative or anecdotal. This is due mainly to the forbidding complexities in modeling the peptide exit tunnel, the nanoscale-confined water therein and the ribosomal processivity, more broadly. The tunnel is a ribosomal region, 10–20 Å wide and about 100 Å long, with rRNA lining (23S rRNA in bacteria, 28S rRNA in eukaryotes), endowed with a constriction and ending in a wide vestibule. These structural features are mainly formed by intercalating protein subunits, uL4/uL22 for the constriction, and uL23/uL24 for the vestibule, with eL39 added in eukaryotes. *Residues in the vestibule are much less conserved across orthologs than residues in other parts of the tunnel, an observation of key significance as we implement an AI system to unravel the process of co-translational folding.*

A CNN with feature extraction at the level of modulo-basin representation of the backbone torsional state of the growing chain as previously described has been implemented to capture the *in vivo* participation in the co-translational folding of human ubiquitin (UNIPROT ALIGN P0CG48), a single-domain protein with 76 amino acids. The system was trained on thousands of short (1 μs) atomistic MD runs with chains of different lengths ($4 < N \leq 76$) with the N terminus at the peptidyl transferase center and started with all residues assigned to the extended conformation basin to avoid steric hindrance. In addition, feature extraction was enhanced as the training set was enlarged to subsume compatible coarse grained structural and dynamic information from [20] and references therein. Thereafter, atomistic trajectories for the budding chains where propagated in the modulo-basin version as described in this chapter, except that chain growth at the rate of $v = 6\,\text{s}^{-1}$ was incorporated (Fig. 3.7a–c). The CNN enabled inference of the co-translational folding pathway (Fig. 3.7) with the full chain fully assembled in 355,000 steps corresponding to 12.66s $= N/v$. Each coarse step covered $35.6\,\mu$s, and a steady-state conformation at α-carbon RMSD = 1.979 Å from the native fold (PDB.1UBI) was reached in 700,000 steps or 24.976s (Fig. 3.7c).

(a)

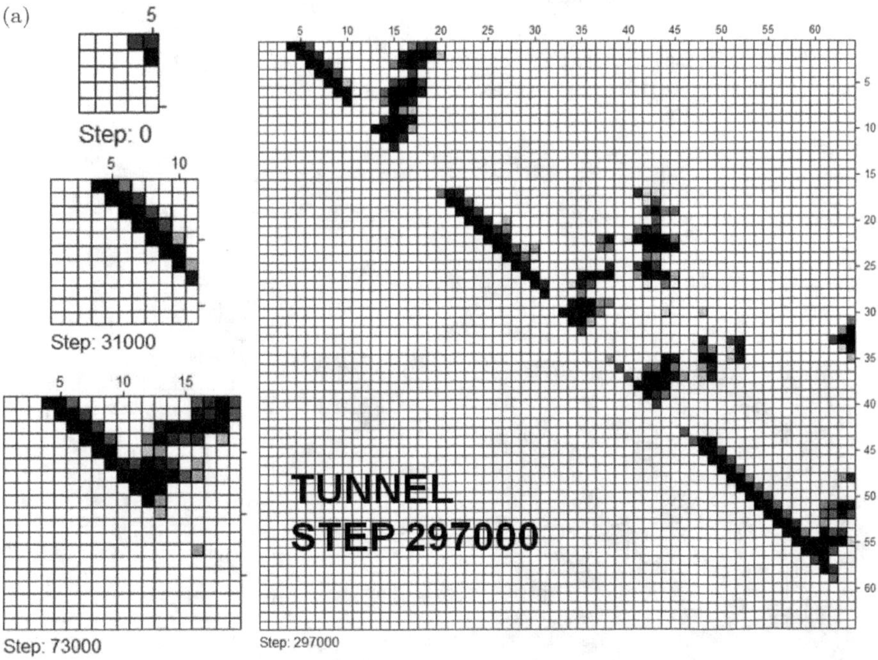

Figure 3.7. Contact matrix for the ubiquitin chain in the ribosomal peptide exit tunnel as obtained by AI-enabled propagation of a coarse grained co-translational folding pathway. Snapshots at different stages of growth and folding (**a**–**c**). A ribbon rendering of the outcome structure (**c**) is given as an aid to the eye.

(b)

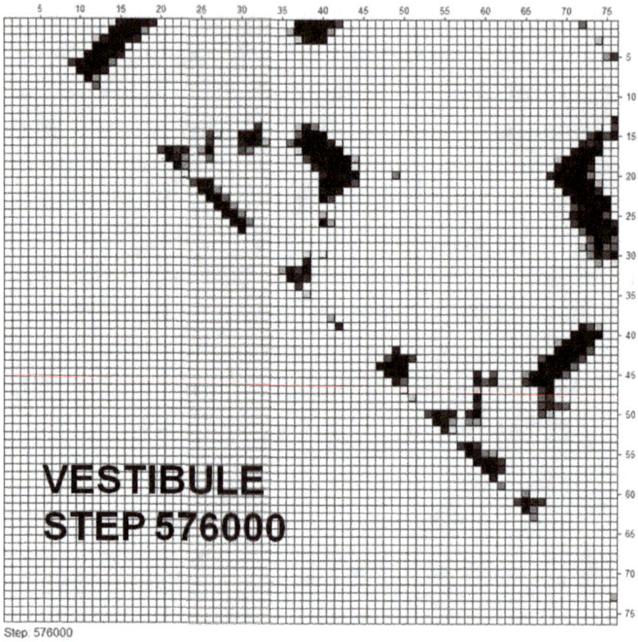

(c)

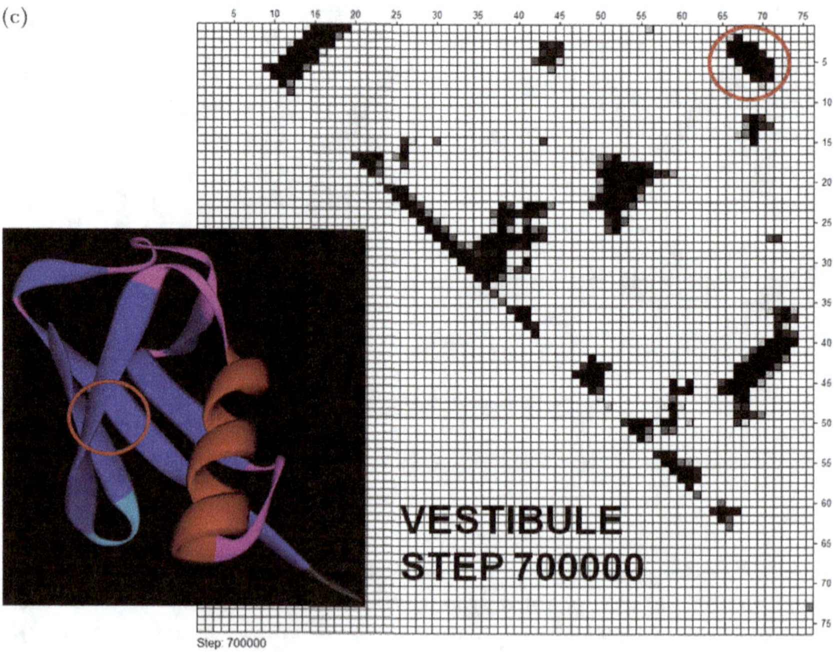

Figure 3.7. (*Continued*)

While at the tunnel, both native and nonnative secondary structure form (Fig. 3.7a,b) but no scaffolding tertiary structure forms, so the secondary structure is ephemeral even in quasi-equilibrium conditions. Essentially the tunnel prevents aggregation of misfolded structure that would otherwise take place as a result of the lack of long-range intramolecular cooperativity. The intervention of the *in vivo* context is persistent at the N-terminus for obvious reasons and, strikingly, also near the C-terminus, around residue 70 (Fig. 3.8). This implies that at the vestibule, the C-terminus, the first region to exit the tunnel, interacts very strongly, specifically and persistently with the vestibular residues and that the long-range parallel β-sheet (circle in Fig. 3.7c), which is nearly impossible to form *in vitro*, can form *in vivo* as an induced folding motif.

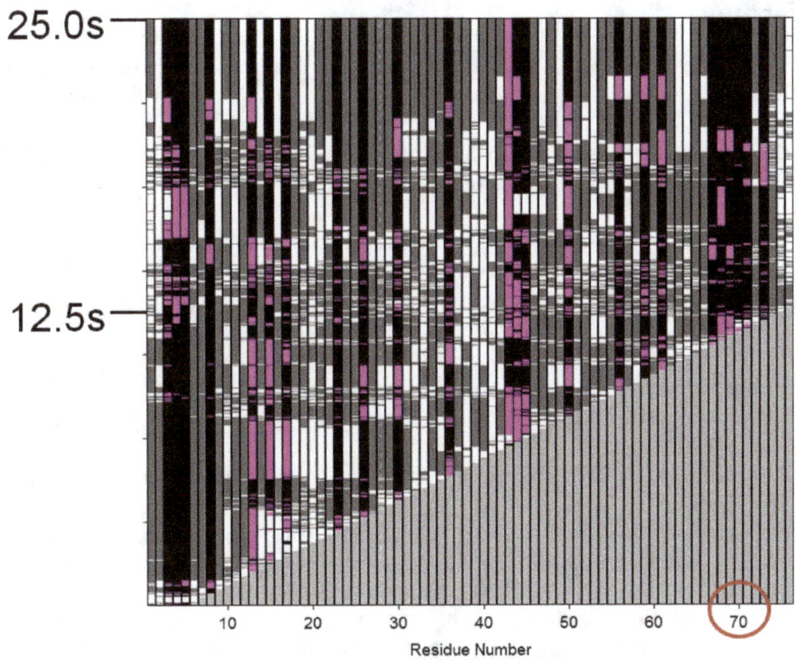

Figure 3.8. Influence of ribosomal context on the co-translational folding process assessed by AI. Depiction of *in vivo* interventions follows the convention described in Fig. 3.4.

The ribosome influences the co-translational folding process so as to turn it into an induced folding process, implicating mostly the ribosomal proteins that shape the vestibule. The *in vivo* intervention, as captured by AI, then serves two purposes: a) preclude aggregation of misfolded structure, b) cooperate to induce the long-range structural organization (i.e., the parallel β-sheet in ubiquitin). While the induced unfolding has been mentioned in previous speculations [21], none mentioned the induced folding specifically implicating the vestibular ribosomal proteins (cf. [20]).

In this way, the *in vivo* complexity that expedites co-translational protein folding can be recreated by AI in order to shed light on an otherwise intractable setting that confers long-range organization to the native structure.

References

1. Shaw DE, Maragakis P, Lindorff-Larsen K, Piana S, Dror RO, *et al.* (2010) Atomic-level characterization of the structural dynamics of proteins. *Science* 330:341–346.
2. Brooks BR, Brooks III CL, Mackerell AD, Nilsson L, Petrella RJ, *et al.* (2009) CHARMM: The biomolecular simulation program. *J Comp Chem* 30:1545–1615.
3. Clark PL, Elcock AH (2016) Molecular chaperones: Providing a safe place to weather a midlife protein-folding crisis. *Nature Struct Molec Biol* 23:621–3.
4. Piana S, Shaw DE (2018) Atomic-level description of protein folding inside the GroEL cavity. *J Phys Chem B* 122:11440–11449.
5. Thommen M, Holtkamp W, Rodnina MV (2017) Co-translational protein folding: Progress and methods. *Curr Opin Struct Biol* 42:83–89.
6. Sorokina I, Mushegian A (2018) Modeling protein folding in vivo. *Biology Direct* 13:13.
7. Fernández A (1999) Folding a protein by discretizing its backbone torsional dynamics. *Phys Rev E* 59:5928–5934.
8. Fernández A, Colubri A, Berry RS (2000) Topology to geometry in protein folding: Beta-lactoglobulin. *Proc Natl Acad Sci USA* 97:14062–14066.
9. Singhal N, Pande VS (2005) Error analysis and efficient sampling in Markovian state models for molecular dynamics. *J Chem Phys* 123:204909.
10. Zimmerman MI, Bowman GR (2015) Fast conformational searches by balancing exploration/exploitation trade-offs. *J Chem Theory Comput* 11:5747–5757.
11. Schmidhuber (2015) Deep learning in neural networks: An overview. *Neural Netw* 61:85–117.

12. Fernández A (2020) Artificial intelligence teaches drugs to target proteins by tackling the induced folding problem. *Mol Pharm (ACS)* 17:2761–2767.
13. Fernández A (2016) Physics at the biomolecular interface. Springer International Publishing, Switzerland.
14. Fernández A, Shen M, Colubri A, Sosnick TR, Berry RS, Freed KF (2003) Large-scale context in protein folding: Villin headpiece. *Biochemistry* 42: 664–671.
15. Zeiler MD (2012) ADADELTA, an adaptive learning rate method. arXiv:1212.5701 https://arxiv.org/abs/1212.5701.
16. Lippert RA, Predescu C, Ierardi DJ, Mackenzie KM, Eastwood MP *et al.* (2013) Accurate and efficient integration for molecular dynamics simulations at constant temperature and pressure. *J Chem Phys* 139:164106.
17. Nosé S (1984) A unified formulation of the constant temperature molecular-dynamics methods. *J Chem Phys* 81:511–519.
18. Hoover WG (1985) Canonical dynamics: Equilibrium phase-space distributions. *Phys Rev A* 31:1695–1697.
19. Martyna GJ, Tobias DJ, Klein ML (1994) Constant pressure molecular dynamics algorithms. *J Chem Phys* 101:4177–4189.
20. Liutkute M, Samatova E, Rodnina MV (2020) Cotranslational folding of proteins on the ribosome. *Biomolecules* 10:97.
21. O'Brien EP, Christodoulou J, Vendruscolo M, Dobson CM (2011) New scenarios of protein folding can occur on the ribosome. *J Am Chem Soc* 133:513–526.

Chapter 4

Epistructural meta-analysis of functional genomics repositories: Towards an AI platform to infer amyloidogenic propensity

The PDB (protein data bank) constitutes an information repository on proteins with reported structure. This chapter offers a meta-analysis of the PDB where structures are examined vis-à-vis the aqueous surrounding solvent. We address the issue of enriching the field of structural bioinformatics by incorporating information on protein-water interfaces subsumed in reported protein structures. That is, we apply the methods of epistructural biology and machine learning to carry out a meta-reading of the PDB that will ultimately become helpful for drug design pursuits. As shown in Chapter 2, protein epistructure is encoded in protein structure and this chapter decodes this information.

Soluble proteins maintain their structural integrity by shielding their backbone hydrogen bonds from competing hydration of the paired backbone amides and carbonyls. Thus, a *dehydron* constitutes a structural defect, since it promotes structure-disruptive hydration. In this chapter we describe the functional properties of dehydron-rich proteins with high dehydron density. We show that dehydron clusters represent structural singularities belonging to an order-disorder twilight zone that generates a sharp local quenching of the dielectric permittivity of the surrounding medium. The functional roles of such singularities are assessed. Special emphasis is placed on the molecular etiology of aberrant amyloidogenic aggregation arising in dehydron-rich soluble proteins with large deviations from the empirical laws that govern the molecular architecture of stable soluble proteins. The order-disorder twilight arising from high dehydron concentration at the protein surface is shown to be a marker for dysfunctional misfolding. We also show how to predict such regions solely from sequence information using a machine learning approach. Finally, equipped with the conceptual and representational arsenal described, the chapter concludes by delineating an AI platform to infer amyloidogenic propensity at a genome-wide level.

4.1 Dehydron clusters and disordered proteins

As noted in the preceding chapters, the structural integrity of a soluble protein is contingent on its capacity to exclude water from its amide-carbonyl hydrogen bonds [1,2]. Thus, under-wrapped intramolecular hydrogen bonds or dehydrons, constitute structural singularities representing packing defects that have been extensively characterized as implicated in protein associations and macromolecular recognition [2–13]. The strength and stability of dehydrons may be modulated by an external agent. More precisely, intramolecular hydrogen bonds which are not "wrapped" by a sufficient number of nonpolar groups may become stabilized and strengthened by the attachment of a ligand or binding partner that further contributes to their dehydration.

In this chapter we construct a meta-reading of the PDB based on epistructural biology. The analysis is enabled by the fact that the epistructure is encoded by the structure. In particular, we identify functional indicators of PDB-reported soluble proteins with clusters of dehydrons. Such regions, rich in structural vulnerabilities, may be characterized as belonging to a "twilight zone" between order and native disorder [4]. This characterization is already suggested by a strong correlation between wrapping of intramolecular hydrogen bonds (ρ) and propensity for structural disorder (f_d), as shown in Fig. 4.1. The correlation reveals that the inability to exclude water intramolecularly from pre-formed hydrogen bonds is causative of the loss of structural integrity.

The disorder propensity may be accurately quantified by a sequence-based score generated by the program PONDR-VLXT

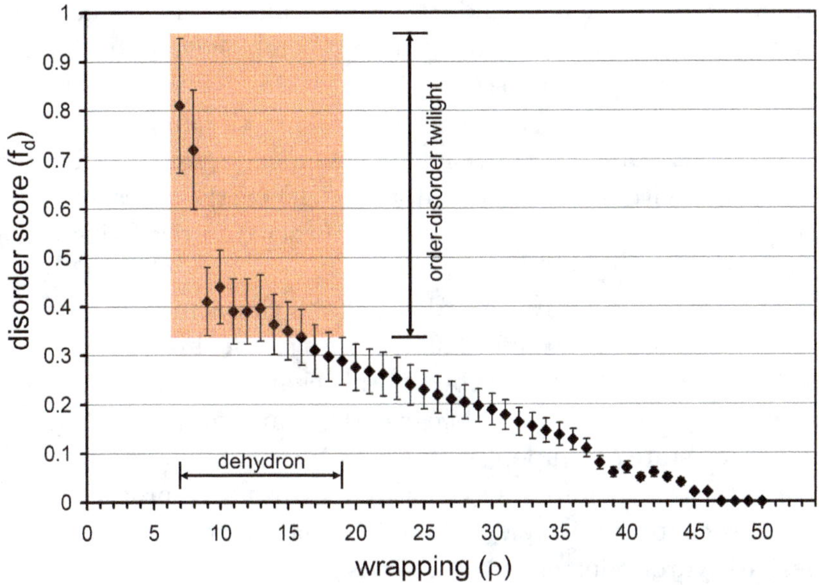

Figure 4.1. Correlation between the disorder score of a residue and the extent of wrapping (ρ) of the backbone hydrogen bond engaging that particular residue (if any). The disorder score on each individual residue was obtained for 2,806 nonredundant nonhomologous PDB domains. Residues have been independently grouped in 45 bins of 400 residues each, according to the extent of wrapping ($7 \leq \rho \leq 52$). The average score has been determined for each bin (square), and the error bars represent the dispersion of disorder scores within each bin. The strong correlation between the disorder score and the extent of wrapping and the dispersions obtained imply that dehydrons can be safely inferred in regions where the disorder score is $f_d > 0.35$. The red rectangle represents the region of order-disorder twilight where the existence of dehydrons may be inferred from disorder score with absolute certainty. No hydrogen bond in monomeric domains reported in PDB was found to possess less than 7 wrappers, implying a threshold for structural sustainability in soluble proteins. Reprinted from [19], copyright 2007 with permission from the American Chemical Society.

[14–16], a predictor of native disorder that takes into account residue attributes such as hydrophilicity, aromaticity, and their distribution within the window interrogated. The disorder score ($0 \leq f_d \leq 1$) is assigned to each residue within a sliding window, representing the predicted propensity of the residue to be in a disordered region ($f_d = 1$, certainty of disorder; $f_d = 0$, certainty of order). Only 6% of 1,100 nonhomologous PDB proteins gave false positive predictions of disorder in sequence windows of 40 amino acids. The strong correlation (over 2,806 nonredundant nonhomologous PDB domains, Fig. 4.1) between disorder score of a residue and extent of wrapping of the hydrogen bond engaging the residue (if any) implies that clusters of dehydrons correspond to extended regions of structural vulnerability within a structured domain. Hence, the characterization of dehydron clusters as belonging to an order-disorder twilight zone appears to be warranted.

Both order and native disorder are well characterized structural attributes of protein chains [16]. However, the highly vulnerable regions in a soluble fold described in this chapter belong to the novel category of "tamed disorder" because they can acquire and maintain a structured state only upon association. Neither order nor disorder is an adequate category to describe such dehydron-rich protein regions.

In this chapter we explore the functional role of regions with the largest dehydron clusters. A cluster is defined as the maximal set of dehydrons with intersecting desolvation domains or overlapping microenvironments. These regions actually belong to an order-disorder twilight and are shown to be strong dielectric modulators, i.e. quenchers of the local dielectric permittivity, thus providing a local enhancement of Coulomb fields nearby. This property arises since clusters of packing defects promote local dehydration of the protein interface promoted by a significant reduction in hydrogen-bonding partnerships of solvating water molecules.

These discrete effects relating to local water structuring around packing defects cannot be captured properly by existing continuous models of the interfacial electrostatics [17]. This is mainly because such models are based on mean-force potential approximations to solvent interactions, where solvent degrees of freedom are averaged out, and this is clearly an inappropriate *ansatz* to deal with cavities of the size of solvent molecules themselves, as shown in chapter 2.

4.2 Interfacial dielectrics and structural defects

The dehydrons in a soluble protein ($\rho \leq 19$, for desolvation radius 6 Å) are partially exposed to solvent. As previously shown, these bonds promote the removal of hydrating molecules to enhance the underlying polar-pair electrostatics. Furthermore, the resulting bond stabilization overcomes the amount of work needed to remove solvating water molecules [3,5]. To describe this dehydration propensity, we first compute the extent of constraint of interfacial water molecules. This parameter is identified with the thermal average of g, denoting the average number of hydrogen-bond partnerships involving water molecules within the desolvation domain of each residue along the chain ($0 \leq g \leq 4$, Fig. 4.2). As an illustration we focus on the DNA-binding domain of antitumor gene p53 [18]. This domain was selected because it contains three of the largest dehydron clusters to be found in the PDB (Fig. 4.3). The functional significance of these clusters relates to their interplay with the electrostatics of DNA recognition by this transcription factor [19].

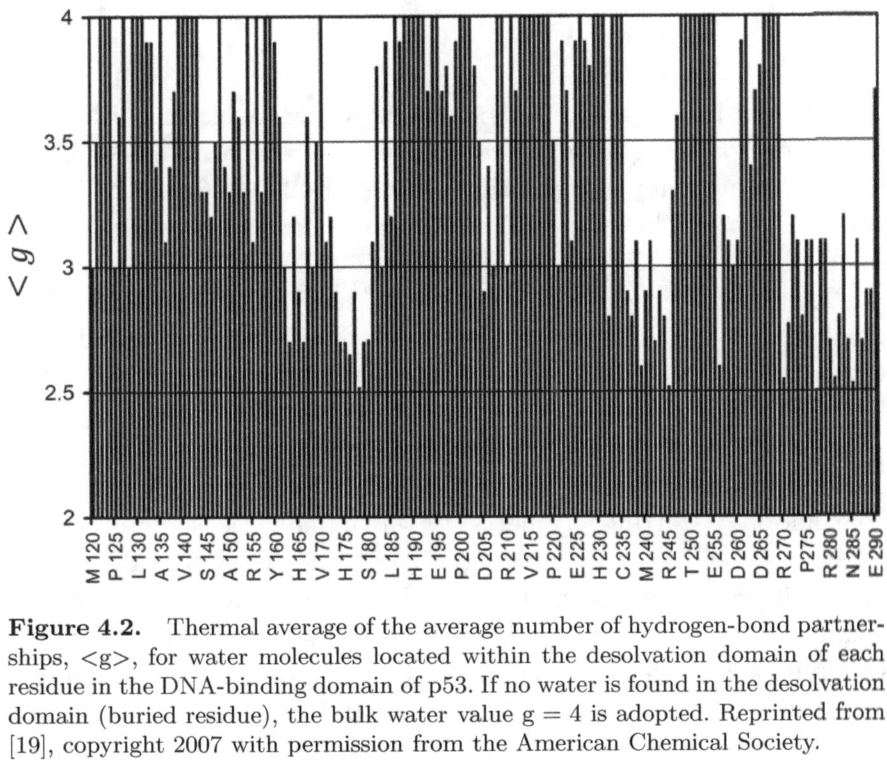

Figure 4.2. Thermal average of the average number of hydrogen-bond partnerships, <g>, for water molecules located within the desolvation domain of each residue in the DNA-binding domain of p53. If no water is found in the desolvation domain (buried residue), the bulk water value $g = 4$ is adopted. Reprinted from [19], copyright 2007 with permission from the American Chemical Society.

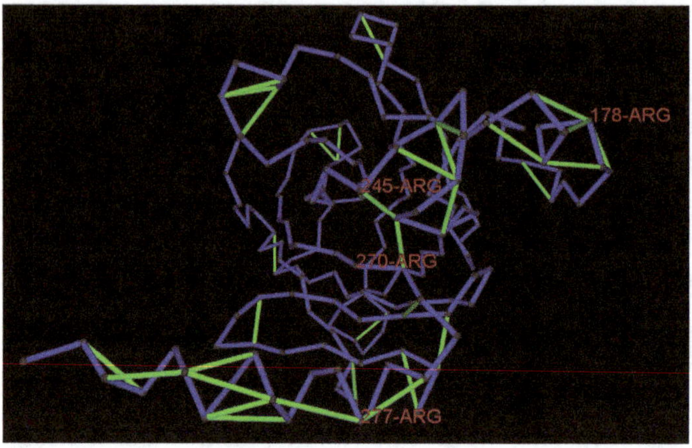

Figure 4.3. Dehydrons for p53 DNA-binding domain. The backbone is indicated by blue virtual bonds joining α-carbons and dehydrons are shown as green segments joining the α-carbons of residues paired by backbone hydrogen bonds. Reprinted from [19], copyright 2007 with permission from the American Chemical Society.

Fig. 4.2 shows the thermal average, $<g>$, of the average number of hydrogen-bond partnerships involving water molecules within the desolvation domain for each residue. Three dehydration hot spots are apparent, comprising residues 171–181, 236–246 and 270–289, respectively. The location of these hot spots corresponds to the three major dehydron clusters shown in Fig. 4.3.

The thermal average, $<g>$, of the number of hydrogen-bond partnerships involving water molecules hydrating the p53 DNA-binding domain was obtained from classical trajectories generated by 5 ns molecular dynamics (MD) simulations (see chapter 2). The g-values were determined for each water molecule within a 6 Å-radius spherical domain centered at the α-carbon of the residues. The adopted starting geometry is the monomeric structure from PDB entry 2GEQ. The starting conformation was embedded in a pre-equilibrated cell of explicitly represented water molecules and counterions [19]. The entire system was initially equilibrated for 5 ns. Computations were performed by integration of Newton's equations of motion with time step 2fs [20] in the NPT ensemble with box size $8 \times 8 \times 8\,\text{nm}^3$ and periodic boundary conditions (Chapter 2).

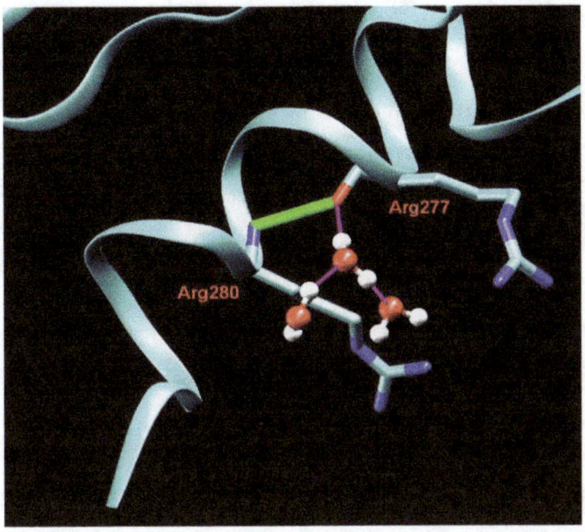

Figure 4.4. Selected snapshot (after 1 ns of MD) of a solvating water molecule and its hydrogen bond partnerships (purple bonds) within the desolvation domain of Arg277 in the DNA-binding domain of tumor antigen p53 (ribbon representation, fragment). The backbone amide-carbonyl dehydron Arg277–Arg280 is shown in green. Reprinted from [19], copyright 2007 with permission from the American Chemical Society.

This computation was repeated to include representatives of the three major fold topologies: all-β (SH3 domain, N = 55, 2 dehydrons, PDB.1SRL), all-α (λ-repressor, N = 86, 26 dehydrons, PDB.1LMB) and α/β (ubiquitin, N = 76, 16 dehydrons, PDB.1UBI). Consistency with the p53 calculation was obtained, as dehydrons proved to become the dehydration hot spots on the protein interface [19].

The confinement of solvating water determined by a packing defect is illustrated in Fig. 4.4. The figure displays a snapshot of a water molecule within the desolvation domain of Arg277, a residue paired by a dehydron to Arg280. This water molecule has 3 hydrogen-bond partners, two with vicinal water and one with the Arg277 backbone carbonyl. A 3.6 Å-threshold is adopted for hydrogen bond distance between the heavy atoms. The snapshot was extracted after 1ns of MD simulations equilibrating the protein chain with surrounding water. Due to the incomplete wrapping of dehydron (Arg277, Arg280) in the p53 domain, the closest water molecule is found at a distance 2.8 Å between carbonyl and water oxygen atoms.

While electrostatically engaged with the Arg277 backbone carbonyl, this water molecule is deprived of one hydrogen bond partnership when compared with bulk water (Fig. 4.3, 4.4).

In order to determine a generic relation between ρ and g, three additional single-domain folds representative of protein topologies were also analyzed: SH3-domain; ubiquitin, and λ-repressor, as indicated above.

The correlation between wrapping and dehydration propensity (Fig. 4.5) has the following characteristics: a) dehydrons ($\rho \leq 19$) generate g-values in the range $2 \leq g \leq 3.6$; b) the upper wrapping bound, $\rho = 28$ corresponds to bulk-like water ($g = 4$) in the desolvation domain; and c) all solvating water is excluded from the desolvation domain for $\rho > 28$.

Using the analytical methods described in chapter 2, we may derive the Debye dielectric permittivity as a function of g (or the frustration). Fig. 4.6 displays the rigorously derived g-dependence of the dielectric permittivity $\varepsilon^{||}$. The dielectric quenching is extreme upon moderately small losses in hydrogen-bond partnerships. Thus,

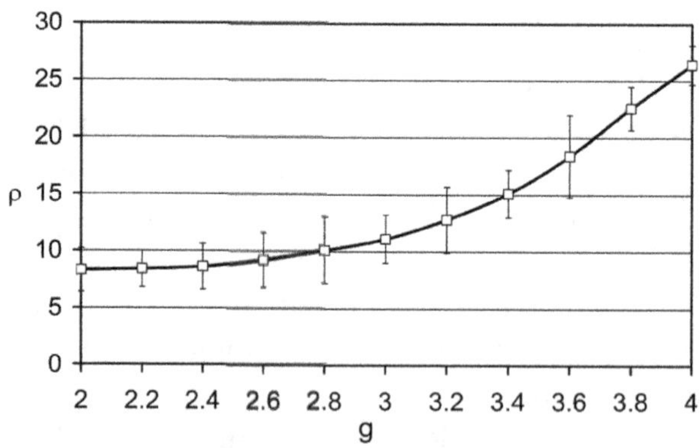

Figure 4.5. Correlation between hydrogen-bond wrapping ρ and wetting parameter g. Each residue is assigned a ρ-value averaged over all backbone hydrogen bonds in which it is engaged. The data was extracted from the wetting computation on the p53 DNA-binding domain and three additional folds: the SH3 domain (N = 55, 2 dehydrons, PDB.1SRL); ubiquitin (N = 76, 16 dehydrons, PDB.1UBI), and λ-repressor (N = 86, 26 dehydrons, PDB.1LMB). Reprinted from [19], copyright 2007 with permission from the American Chemical Society.

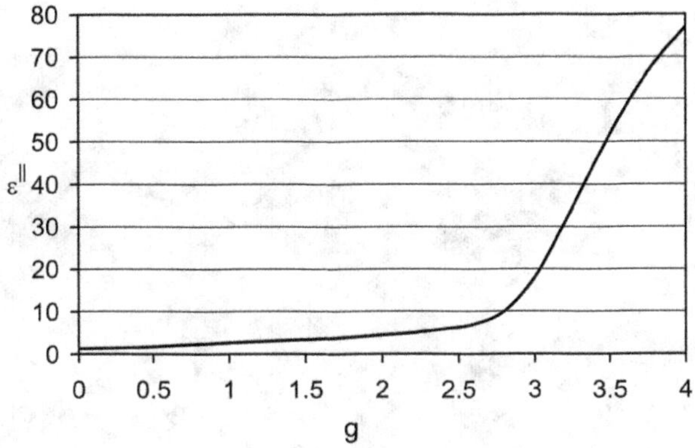

Figure 4.6. Dependence of the Debye dielectric permittivity on the parameter g.

the most dramatic decrease is marked by a drop in $\varepsilon^{||}$-values from 50 to 7 as g is reduced from 3.5 to 2.5.

Taken together, Figs. 4.5, 4.6 lead us to the conclusion that *clusters of packing defects act as dramatic enhancers of the electric fields generated at the protein interface.* The typical loss in hydrogen bonding partnerships associated with dehydron solvation puts g in the range: $2 \leq g \leq 3.5$. This range contains the region of most dramatic dielectric quenching (Fig. 4.6), decreasing the Debye component of the permittivity by an order of magnitude with respect to bulk water. In turn, this effect translates in an order of magnitude increase for electrostatic interactions, hence rationalizing the functional role of dehydron-rich regions.

4.3 Dielectric modulation by dehydrons in the p53 DNA-binding domain

The functional significance of the three dielectric modulators in the DNA-binding domain of p53 can now be understood by examining its dimeric state and its role as transcription factor. Thus, a major cluster involving the 5 dehydrons (173, 176), (174, 178), (175, 178), (176, 179) and (178, 180) is found at the dimer interface (Fig. 4.3, 4.7). This cluster fosters dimerization in accord with the dehydration

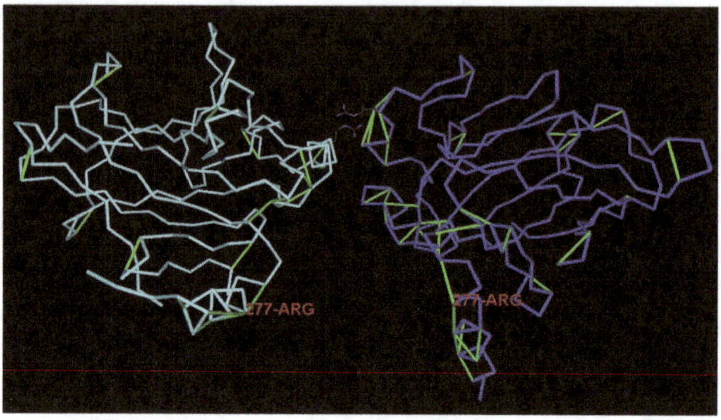

Figure 4.7. Backbone/dehydron representation of the dimmer interface for the DNA-binding domain of p53 (PDB.2GEQ). The side chains of the Arg178 of each monomer involved in a resonance pair are shown. Reprinted from [19], copyright 2007 with permission from the American Chemical Society.

propensity of dehydrons and their role as promoters of protein associations [2,5,10–13]. The dimerization involves a resonant pairing of the Arg178 from each monomer (Fig. 4.7) likely, to promote supramolecular charge delocalization with distal charge separation at all times. Significantly, <g> reaches a minimum precisely at Arg178 (Fig. 4.2), in accordance with the low dehydration penalty for the guanidinium ion[21] and with the fact that the Arg-Arg resonant association requires guanidinium dehydration (cf. Fig. 4.7).

Besides Arg 178, there are three additional minima in <g>, corresponding to residues Arg245, Arg270 and Arg277 (Fig. 4.2). The latter three arginines play a pivotal role in DNA recognition [18], as discussed below. Residue Arg245 is engaged in the dielectric quenching region 236–246 and is part of the dehydron cluster involving pairs (236, 239), (237, 245), (237, 271), (239, 242), (239, 244), (240, 242) (Fig. 4.3). Residues 270 and 277 lie within the dielectric quenching region 270–289 and are part of the dehydron cluster involving pairs (237, 271), (274, 277), (277, 281), (280, 284), (281, 285), (282, 285), (285, 288) (Figs. 4.3, 4.8). The latter cluster is one of the largest to be found in a PDB-reported soluble protein.

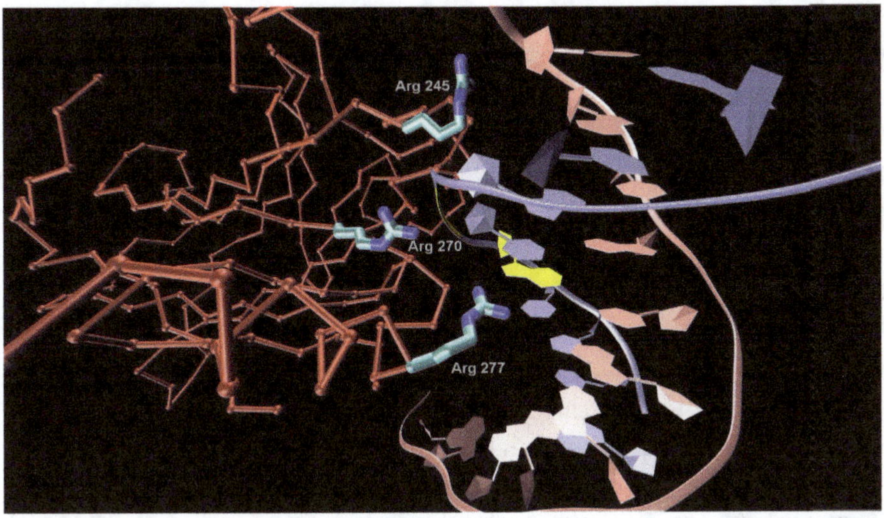

Figure 4.8. Protein-DNA complex of the DNA-binding domain of p53 (PDB.2GEQ). Side chains of the key residues directly implicated in DNA recognition, Arg245, Arg270 and Arg277 are shown. The pyridine base recognized by Arg277 is shown in yellow, while the individual DNA strands are shown in lilac and light magenta. Reprinted from [19], copyright 2007 with permission from the American Chemical Society.

Direct examination of the protein-DNA complex (PDB.2GEQ), reveals that the three residues directly implicated in DNA recognition are precisely Arg245, Arg270 and Arg277 (Fig. 4.8). Residue Arg277 acts as intra-base intercalator, while the other two interact with the negatively charged backbone phosphates (Fig. 4.8). The electrostatics of protein-DNA recognition is not merely the result of matching charges along the geometrically compatible interfaces, otherwise ion pairs would prevail in water. Rather, electrostatic recognition of the DNA polyelectrolyte requires a device to promote dehydration at the protein-nucleic acid interface. The large dehydron clusters surrounding the three arginines directly implicated in the protein-DNA association (Fig. 4.3, 4.8) provide such an expedient, as they quench the local dielectric (Fig. 4.2), thus enhancing the electrostatic recognition. Thus, the fact that the three arginines involved in DNA recognition are also dehydration hot spots satisfies a functional imperative for the transcription factor.

4.4 Machine learning methods to obtain epistructural information in the absence of structure: The Twilighter

When a protein has no reported structure, a dehydron prediction from protein sequence is required. This imperative becomes particularly pressing for drug designers that often face the problem of a lack of structural information on the target protein. As noted in section 4.1, dehydron-rich regions entail a significant exposure of the protein backbone that translates into a significant propensity for native structural disorder. Thus, sequence-based predictors of disorder can provide the signal for identifying dehydrons in the missing structure. The publicly available Predictor for Native Disorder PONDR® is a tool of choice to infer dehydrons from protein sequence. At the time when this book is being composed, PONDR may be freely accessed at the URL: http://pondr.com.

PONDR provides a coarse resolution, generating a smeared-out plot resulting from prediction of disorder propensity on a sliding sequence window. We need to deconvolute the smeared-out signal to obtain individual amino-acid values of disorder propensity, as described below. When using PONDR, one can only report averaged trends over sequence windows, not individual disorder propensities. This is so because the dehydron prediction with PONDR is only a statistical inference over a sliding window. The broad disorder regions ($f > 0.5$) without disorder certainty usually have a fine-grained saw-like structure embedded in them with many order-disorder twilight zones rich in dehydrons. This fine structure is usually missed in a PONDR reading because the latter provides a coarse-grained picture which is adequate to predict large disorder regions (PONDR's intent) but not adequate for obtaining detailed dehydron prediction at the residue-level resolution that is necessary for the drug designer. In PONDR's broad signals we are looking at the envelope of a saw-like structure, and in the reported envelope we are missing the dehydron-rich twilight regions.

A protocol of how to resolve PONDR signals to the level of fine graining needed to infer specific dehydrons is provided subsequently. The raw data uses PONDR to infer dehydrons but uses also structural information (templates in a training set for supervised learning) to get the level of resolution needed to generate dehydron predictions. In other words, the output from a structure-based dehydron calculator (Appendix 1) is needed to infer dehydrons from PONDR. The dehydron calculator enables one to construct a training set that is used to "learn to infer dehydrons" from PONDR plots through learned resolution enhancement (LRE). Once a smeared-out (window-averaged) PONDR signal is obtained, the signal has to be resolved at the amino acid level in order to identify the twilight regions rich in dehydrons. This process of LRE is implemented by developing a computational resource, hereby named *Twilighter*, based on supervised learning technology trained with [sequence/PONDR-score/(# of dehydrons)] windows extracted from the PDB and from the PONDR plots generated for PDB-reported proteins. Once trained, the Twilighter maps the number of dehydrons onto a sequence/PONDR-score compound window. A goal is to generate the wrapping parameter ν = D/H (D = number of dehydrons, H = number of backbone hydrogen bonds) subsumed in the smeared-out PONDR plot.

Since dehydrons are local features and disorder predictions cannot be resolved to the level of locality required to infer the presence of individual dehydrons, a scale or resolution problem arises when PONDR is used for dehydron inference. The twilight regions corresponding to dehydrons are often smeared out as the window is slid along the sequence, and often the dehydron microstructure embedded in the PONDR signal is lost due to poor resolution.

This problem is akin to probing reaction kinetics at different temperatures and finding different orders for the chemical reaction depending on the temperature. Fine-grained features of the potential energy surface that are smeared out at high temperature become important when thermal fluctuations scale down, dramatically altering the observable kinetics of the reaction.

In our particular context of interest, a helical structure with "frayed ends", rich in dehydrons (cf. helix 25–35 in ubiquitin, Fig. 2.2(b,c)), will be typically "read" by PONDR as a broad disorder signal with no certainty of disorder, unless the length of the helical region is incommensurately larger than the length of PONDR sliding window. The resolution problem is solved exploiting unsupervised learning technology to interpret and de-convolute the broad signals generated by PONDR. Here we describe the supervised learning algorithm that we have aptly named Twilighter that de-convolutes PONDR-signals to identify dehydrons by learned resolution enhancement (LRE) [4].

Twilighter is easily implemented and adopts as training set the direct dehydron identification obtained using Dehydron Calculator (Appendix 1) for a large proportion (typically 66%) of the proteins reported in the PDB combined with the PONDR plot output on the protein sequences for the same PDB-entries. Each PONDR signal is discretized as a 9-tuple of disorder propensities corresponding to a typical PONDR-sliding window and the training data is represented by combining the outputs of PONDR and Dehydron Calculator into an 19-tuple: 9 entries for amino acid sequence window, 9 entries for PONDR scores, and 1 entry for number of dehydrons obtained from Dehydron Calculator. In this way, the learning machine is trained to interpret each PONDR signal from a PDB reported protein as containing a well determined number of dehydrons that would not be identifiable from direct reading of the PONDR plot. This training is then used to make sequence-based dehydron inferences based on 9-tuples of PONDR scores for 9-amino acid sequence windows.

The testing set for this machine is the rest (approx. 33%) of PDB-reported proteins, where we can directly contrast a PONDR-based learned dehydron prediction assigning # dehydrons to each 18-tuple (window sequence identity + the 9 respective PONDR scores) with the actual identification of dehydrons obtained using Dehydron Calculator.

A training set amounting to roughly 66% of PDB (40,719 entries) gives a prediction accuracy of 93%, with most outliers being small floppy peptides ($N < 35$) with structure determined from NMR.

This tool is needed to extract wrapping information from sequence-based disorder prediction, since the latter is an attribute averaged over a sliding sequence window, while dehydrons pair two specific residues, thus requiring fine resolution at the single amino acid level. Thus, a learned resolution enhancer (LRE) was required to translate PONDR signals into dehydron patterns. A feedforward neural network resource can be built trained with the wrapping and PONDR-based disorder scores from PDB-represented proteins in order to infer wrapping patterns of foldable proteins with unknown or unreported structure.

The network may be trained with information on proteins with PDB representation. The training data is represented as a vector $(\mathbf{s},\mathbf{w},\mathrm{F}) = (\mathbf{X},\mathrm{F})$, where $\mathbf{s}$ is the protein sequence window of length $\mathrm{N} = 9$, $\mathbf{w}$ is the 9-vector of "raw" PONDR scores in the window, $\mathbf{X} = (\mathbf{s},\mathbf{w})$, and F is the number of residues within the window that are paired by dehydrons. The F-values for proteins in PDB (training set) are computed using Dehydron Calculator (Appendix 1).

The inference is then defined by input $\mathbf{X}$ and output $\mathrm{F} = \mathrm{F}(\mathbf{X})$ for a protein with unknown structure, for which $\mathbf{X}$ is determined using PONDR. Thus, learned resolution enhancement (LRE) is simply an *in silico* lens used to get information from a smeared signal. The exact work flow of the LRE is described in Figure 4.9.

The LRE uses the standard learning strategy. The idea is to generate the function $\mathrm{F}(\mathbf{X})$ = (# residues paired by dehydrons) from a data representation $\mathbf{X} = (\mathbf{s}, \mathbf{w})$. For simplicity, we discretized the single amino acid score f in three ranges: low (1/3) $0 < \mathrm{f} < 0.35$; medium (2/3): $0.35 < \mathrm{f} < 0.8$ ("dehydron range") and high (1): $\mathrm{f} > 0.8$.

We defined the training set H as the set of $\mathbf{X}$-vectors obtained from PDB-reported proteins and their PONDR scores. We define the standard metric d in sequence space and the standard metric d in the space of ternary w-vectors. We of course know the $\mathrm{F}(\mathbf{Y})$ values for all $\mathbf{Y}$s in H, because we can compute them directly from structure using the Dehydron Calculator.

For crude inferences, given an $\mathbf{X}$ not belonging to H, we infer the value $\mathrm{F}(\mathbf{X})$ by defining the set $H(\mathbf{X})$ as the set of vectors in the training set H that are "closest" to $\mathbf{X}$. The set $H(\mathbf{X})$ is constructed using the BLAST tool (available at the US National Library of Medicine site http://blast.ncbi.nlm.nih.gov/Blast.cgi).

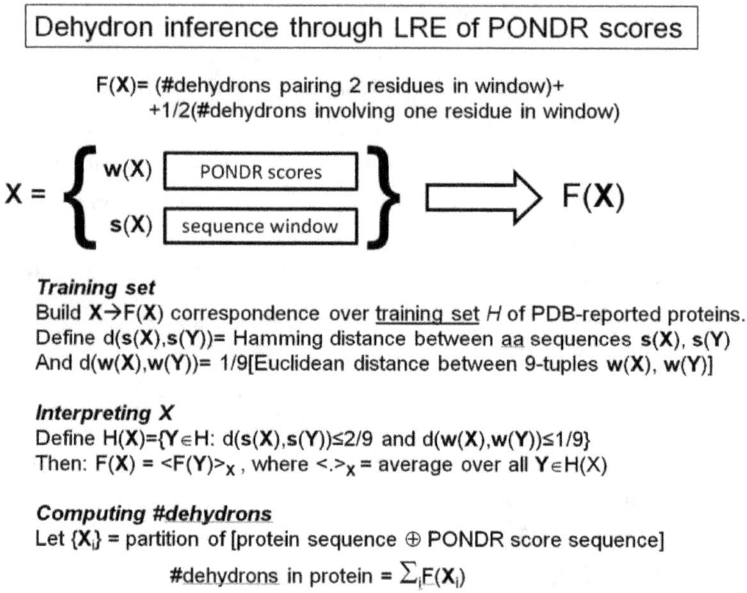

Figure 4.9. Work flow of the learned resolution enhancement (LRE) machine "Twilighter" used in [4] to infer dehydrons from sequence-based predictions of disorder propensity.

Then, we estimate $\mathrm{F}(\mathbf{X})$ as the [integral part] of the average of $\mathrm{F}(\mathbf{Y})$ over all $\mathbf{Y}$'s in $H(\mathbf{X})$.

To get the exact result $\mathrm{F}(\mathbf{X})$, we exploit a basic property of the network: For any two vectors $(\mathbf{X}_1,\mathrm{F}_1)$ and $(\mathbf{X}_2,\mathrm{F}_2)$ in the training set, F satisfies the strong "continuity" relation:

$$\mathrm{F}_1 - \mathrm{F}_2 = \mathrm{q}[\mathrm{d_w}(\mathbf{s}_1, \mathbf{s}_2) + (3/2)\mathrm{d_{PONDR}}(\mathbf{w}_1, \mathbf{w}_2)], \tag{1}$$

where $\mathrm{d_w}$ is the wrapping quasi-distance between the two sequence windows, defined as the difference in the number of carbonaceous side-chain nonpolar groups; $\mathrm{d_{PONDR}}$ is the compound difference in the PONDR scores (residue-by residue) in the window, and $\mathrm{q} = 0.16$ is a constant. The value $\mathrm{q} = 0.16$ (approx.$1/(4+2)$) is obtained by noting that $\underline{1}$ new dehydron is created when the number of wrappers in the window decreases by $\underline{4}$ and $\underline{2}$ residues qualitatively raise their discretized PONDR score $(1/3 \to 1)$ as defined above. Thus, $\mathrm{F}(\mathbf{X})$

is "continuous" in the sense that $\mathrm{F}(\mathbf{X}_2) - \mathrm{F}(\mathbf{X}_1) = \mathrm{q}\Delta(\mathbf{X}_2, \mathbf{X}_1)$, where

$$\Delta(\mathbf{X}_2, \mathbf{X}_1) = [\mathrm{d_w}(\mathbf{s}_1, \mathbf{s}_2) + (3/2)\mathrm{d_{PONDR}}(\mathbf{w}_1, \mathbf{w}_2)] \tag{2}$$

Then the rigorous way to infer the # dehydrons in a window takes advantage of the "continuity" relation for the neural network output F. Thus, for $\mathbf{X}$ not in H we get:

$$\mathrm{F}(\mathbf{X}) = \mathrm{F}(\mathbf{X}^*) + \mathrm{q}\Delta(\mathbf{X}, \mathbf{X}^*), \tag{3}$$

where $\mathbf{X}^*$ belongs to H (hence $\mathrm{F}(\mathbf{X}^*)$ can be computed with certainty using Dehydron Calculator) and is obtained by blasting $\mathbf{X}$ in H ($\mathbf{X}^*$ realizes the minimum distance between $\mathbf{X}$ and H).

To summarize, dehydron predictions can be adequately generated from sequence-based disorder propensity inference using supervised learning technology trained with PDB-reported structures, their structure-based dehydron pattern and their PONDR plots. The computational toolbox presented in this section is extremely useful for the design of drugs targeting proteins with unreported or unknown structure and to build pharmacoinformatics platforms, as shown in the subsequent chapters.

4.5 Epistructural biology defines the molecular architecture of soluble proteins

This section introduces a basic design principle that can be rationalized through an analogy. Just like defiance of gravity in building engineering requires buttressing to preserve the integrity of the building, protein design allowing for backbone hydration (the force counteracting structural cohesion) requires disulfide bridges to maintain the structural integrity of the protein. In this regard, this section unravels two constants that define a fundamental architectural constraint in soluble proteins: after suitable normalization, a single disulfide bond stabilizes *five* structural deficiencies, and every soluble protein has a *20%*-baseline level of structural deficiency. These constants define a design principle.

The baseline structural deficiency Y = 20 represents the maximum of a tight distribution (standard deviation $\sigma = 2.25$) of Y-values for the structural deficiency of soluble proteins with no disulfide bridges. This baseline Y-value implies that soluble proteins are not perfectly packed and maintain at least 20% of unburied backbone hydrogen bonds. Since such structural deficiencies locally promote backbone hydration, they belong to an intermediate region between order and disorder and hence represent markers of structural flexibility. Thus, because of its universality, the Y = 20 constant may be interpreted as the baseline flexibility needed for protein function.

In this section, dehydrons are characterized purely as structural deficiencies (Chapter 2). These deficiencies are of a special kind: they indicate loci for backbone hydration and hence, destabilize the native structure. On the other hand, disulfide bonds preformed in the denatured state reduce the structure-destabilizing conformational entropy cost associated with the folding process, hence stabilizing the native structure. Thus, it should be generally expected that the two major and opposite contributors to native-structure destabilization would be correlated, as revealed by the balance equation described in this section.

This relation is hence likely to assist the molecular engineering of soluble proteins. Furthermore, since disulfide bridges can be formed or dismantled in accord with redox environmental conditions, the relation presented is likely to enable the type of design fine tuning that may be required for an environmental modulation of the protein function.

As the dehydron/disulfide organizational principle is established and shown to hold for soluble proteins, we cannot fail to notice that it also introduces a new set of problems stemming from a basic question: *what is in physical terms the fate of a soluble protein whose structure significantly violates the architectural constraints defined by the balance equation?* This issue will be explored in the next section.

Wrapping defects in soluble proteins represent local weaknesses of the native structures and have received little attention, especially by the drug design community. The protein structure may be inherently weak at sites where hydration of the backbone is locally hampered by formation of an intramolecular hydrogen bond which in turn is not stabilized through complete burial within a hydrophobic environment. This section explores the architectural implications stemming from the existence of these vulnerabilities. Thus, the unburied backbone hydrogen bonds or *dehydrons*, are shown to be compensated by disulfide bridges that are needed to maintain the structural integrity in extracellular environments. Examination of all reported soluble structures reveals that the number of disulfide bonds correlates tightly with the number of dehydrons in a 1:5 ratio. The results have implications for biomolecular design as they introduce universal constraints in the architecture of water-soluble proteins.

Backbone hydration, prevalent in the unfolded state of a polypeptide chain, is often hindered in a soluble folded state as backbone amides and carbonyls are paired through hydrogen bonds [22, 23]. Yet, the thermodynamic cost of dehydration is not always compensated, especially if the backbone hydrogen bond is not completely sequestered from solvent. In soluble proteins, such bonds may be readily identified from the structural coordinates by determining the number of nonpolar groups within the bond microenvironment [2, 6, 19]. These unburied backbone hydrogen bonds constitute structural deficiencies and represent markers for protein associations [2]. In turn, these associations are required to maintain the structural integrity of the protein through intermolecular protection of the preformed hydrogen bonds.

A thorough examination of the PDB singles out toxin peptides with picomolar affinity for the Kv1.3 potassium channel [24], such as HsTX1 (PDB.1QUZ), as having the highest extent of structural deficiency. The unburied hydrogen bonds in such proteins can make up to 100% of the backbone hydrogen bonds. This observation immediately suggests a reason for the extremely high target affinity of neurotoxins: we expect a huge *dehydronic field* for such biomolecules.

A separate analysis reveals that such proteins contain an inordinately large number of disulfide bonds, with an average of 11 when normalized to 100 amino acids. These observations prompt us to investigate the relation between structural deficiency and disulfide bonds in search for a balance equation that reflects a statistical correlation between structural strengths and vulnerabilities of soluble proteins and polypeptides. The balance equation unraveled in this chapter is likely to impact the design of soluble proteins and enable a better control of their functional modulation in relation to environmental redox conditions.

A comprehensive wrapping analysis of the PDB yields the structural deficiencies of an exhaustive nonredundant set of 2,989 monomeric uncomplexed soluble proteins or peptides with disulfide links and 8,975 proteins without disulfide links [25]. These data is compiled as illustrated in Table 4.1 for some selected PDB entries. Peptide chains were excluded from the analysis if their structural integrity required prosthetic groups or cation coordination. In order to compare protein or peptide chains of different lengths, two normalized parameters were used to characterize a protein structure: Y = number of structural deficiencies per 100 backbone hydrogen bonds, and X = number of disulfide bonds per 100 amino acids. Proteins were binned according to their X-value in integer groups with $\mathrm{n} = 0, 1, \ldots, 18$, where proteins with no disulfide bonds ($X = 0$) belong to group $\mathrm{n} = 0$ and proteins with X in the range $\mathrm{n} < X \leq \mathrm{n} + 1$ belonged to group $\mathrm{n} + 1$. The mean Y-value and standard deviation were computed for each n-group and the results are shown in Fig. 4.10(a). A tight $X - Y$ linear correlation ($\mathrm{R}^2 = 0.96$) results and is further corroborated by the raw X-Y-trendline generated by linear regression on all (X, Y) data points (Fig. 4.10(b)). Taken together, the results from Fig. 4.10 unambiguously reveal a simple balance relation $Y = 5X + 20$. *This statistical relation introduces a 1:5 ratio to buttress vulnerable proteins and allows for a 20%-baseline in structural deficiency.*

To illustrate the role of this relation in defining protein structure we focus on specific examples of proteins with widely diverse levels of structural deficiency. Figs. 4.11(a,b) shows the structural deficiencies of the alpha-amylase inhibitor HOE-467A (PDB.1HOE; length N = 74; 2 disulfide bonds). This protein contains 23 fully buried backbone hydrogen bonds (5 are double bonds, with each paired residue contributing both proton donor and acceptor, and 13 are single bonds) and 11 structural deficiencies (2 double bonds, 7 single

Table 4.1. Structural parameters for few selected monomeric uncomplexed soluble proteins with disulfide bridges lacking prosthetic groups and scaffolding cation coordination.

PDB entry	Disulfide bonds	Chain length	Structural deficiencies	Backbone HBs	X	Y	Non alpha/ Beta residues (%)
2PNE	2	81	37	37	2.47	100.00	100.00
1M4F	4	25	8	8	16.00	100.00	68.00
1EZG	8	81	33	48	9.87	68.75	77.78
1HOE	2	74	11	34	2.70	32.35	54.05
2Z9T	1	100	10	40	1.00	25.00	50.00
135L	4	129	35	109	3.10	32.11	63.57
153L	2	185	38	185	1.08	20.54	48.65
154L	2	185	39	194	1.08	20.10	48.65
172L	1	164	47	188	0.61	25.00	30.49
1A2J	1	189	57	196	0.53	29.08	39.15
1A39	9	402	69	250	2.24	27.60	59.70
1A3P	2	45	9	18	4.44	50.00	82.22
1A43	1	87	22	67	1.15	32.84	49.43
1A67	2	108	20	62	1.85	32.26	48.15
1A7M	3	180	37	155	1.67	23.87	41.67
1AC5	3	483	91	370	0.62	24.59	51.76
1ACJ	3	537	77	404	0.56	19.06	50.09
1ACW	3	29	18	18	10.34	100.00	41.38
1ACX	2	108	20	44	1.85	45.45	56.48
1ADX	3	40	5	7	7.50	71.43	100.00
1ADZ	3	71	11	35	4.23	31.43	76.06
1AE5	4	225	33	123	1.78	26.83	62.22
1AEC	3	218	33	155	1.38	21.29	55.96
1AFH	4	93	39	74	4.30	52.70	46.24
1AG2	1	103	15	80	0.97	18.75	43.69
1AGG	4	48	11	14	8.33	78.57	87.50
1AGI	3	125	18	82	2.40	21.95	48.80
1AGY	2	200	43	158	1.00	27.22	51.50
1AH1	2	129	15	51	1.55	29.41	60.47
1AHK	3	129	13	43	2.33	30.23	80.62
1AHL	3	49	6	14	6.12	42.86	87.76
3DHM	1	100	10	50	1.00	20.00	52.00
3DIH	7	122	35	97	5.74	36.08	52.46
3EGP	1	108	8	37	0.93	21.62	58.33
3EHS	3	476	93	359	0.63	25.91	40.34
3EMY	1	329	44	198	0.30	22.22	49.85

(*Continued*)

Table 4.1. (*Continued*)

PDB entry	Disulfide bonds	Chain length	Structural deficiencies	Backbone HBs	X	Y	Non alpha/ Beta residues (%)
3ENG	7	213	34	119	3.29	28.57	66.67
3EO5	1	171	47	125	0.58	37.60	48.54
3EOW	2	221	21	75	0.90	28.00	70.14
3ETP	2	187	22	89	1.07	24.72	51.87
3EXD	4	129	35	113	3.10	30.97	63.57
3EZM	2	101	31	57	1.98	54.39	42.57
3GF1	3	70	25	53	4.29	47.17	77.14
3LYM	4	129	36	109	3.10	33.03	63.57
3LZ2	4	129	32	91	3.10	35.16	64.34
3MAN	1	302	58	252	0.33	23.02	50.99
3PTE	1	349	70	297	0.29	23.57	50.43
3RAT	4	124	28	81	3.23	34.57	49.19
3RSD	4	124	25	78	3.23	32.05	49.19
3SEB	1	238	27	153	0.42	17.65	50.00
3SSI	2	113	26	69	1.77	37.68	59.29
3TGF	3	50	13	34	6.00	38.24	68.00
3TGL	3	269	42	221	1.12	19.00	49.81
4AIT	2	74	13	35	2.70	37.14	54.05
4APE	1	330	49	195	0.30	25.13	47.88
4CMS	3	323	53	203	0.93	26.11	42.72
4ENG	7	210	34	119	3.33	28.57	67.14
4RAT	4	124	29	82	3.23	35.37	49.19
4TGL	3	269	36	204	1.12	17.65	50.19
4TSV	1	150	15	70	0.67	21.43	50.67
5LYT	4	129	32	102	3.10	31.37	62.79
5LYZ	4	129	29	90	3.10	32.22	64.34
5PEP	3	326	51	200	0.92	25.50	46.01
5RAT	4	124	28	79	3.23	35.44	49.19
5RNT	2	104	21	62	1.92	33.87	64.42
6HIR	3	65	10	13	4.62	76.92	90.77
6LYT	4	129	32	103	3.10	31.07	62.79
6LYZ	4	129	27	95	3.10	28.42	62.79
7LYZ	4	129	24	88	3.10	27.27	62.79
7RAT	4	124	28	81	3.23	34.57	49.19
8PTI	3	58	10	29	5.17	34.48	65.52
8RAT	4	124	25	76	3.23	32.89	49.19
9RAT	4	124	28	76	3.23	36.84	49.19

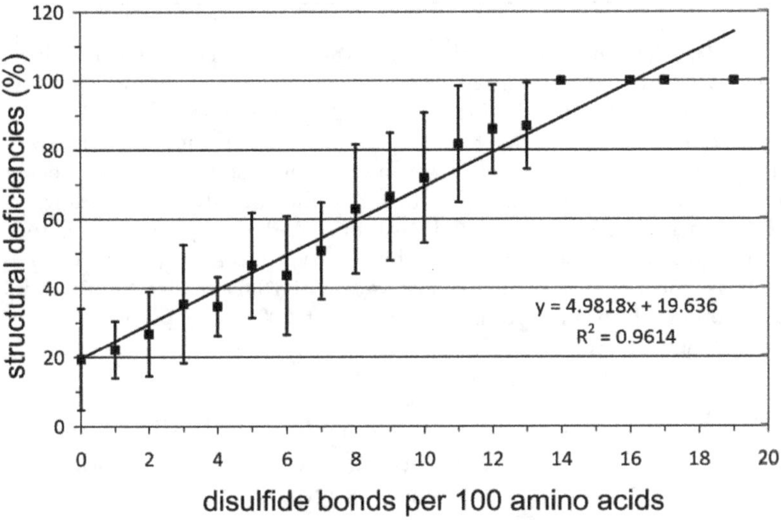

(a)

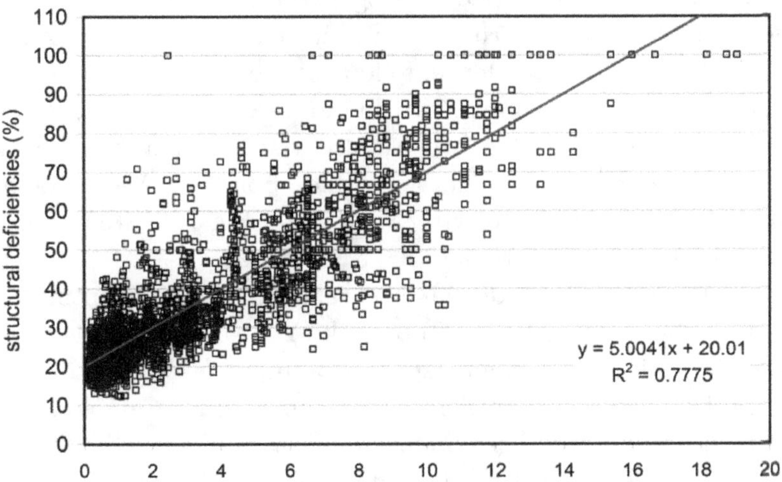

(b)

Figure 4.10. (*Continued*)

Figure 4.10. (*Continued*) Number of structural deficiencies (unburied backbone hydrogen bonds) normalized to 100 backbone hydrogen bonds (Y) plotted against number of disulfide bonds normalized to 100 amino acids (X) for PDB-reported soluble proteins. **(a)** Mean Y-value (square) and standard deviation (error bar) for proteins grouped according to their number of disulfide bonds. Proteins were binned according to their X-value in integer groups with $n = 0, 1, \ldots, 18$, where proteins with no disulfide bonds ($X = 0$) belong to group $\mathrm{n} = 0$ and proteins with $\mathrm{n} < X \leq \mathrm{n}+1$ belong to group n+1. **(b)** All (X, Y)-data points from the nonredundant exhaustive set of PDB-entries for uncomplexed soluble proteins. Reprinted from [25], copyright 2009 with permission from the American Chemical Society.

bonds). Hence, its parameters are $Y = 11 \times 100/(11 + 23) = 32.35$; $X = 2 \times 100/74 = 2.70$. Applying the balance relation, we get the estimate $Y = 5 \times 2.7 + 20 = 33.5$, differing in less than 1% from the real Y-value. Beta2-microglobulin (PDB.2Z9T, N = 100, $X = 1$), has 30 fully buried hydrogen bonds (9 double bonds, 12 single bonds), and 10 structural deficiencies (1 double bond), as shown in Figs. 4.11(c,d). Hence, following the balance equation, Y is estimated at $5 \times 1 + 20 = 25$, which agrees exactly with the actual value $Y = 10 \times 100/(10 + 30)$. Finally, the antimicrobial hormone hepcidin (PDB.1M4F, N = 25, 4 disulfide bonds or $X = 16.00$) has a fully defective structure with $Y = 100$ (Figs. 4.11(e,f)), fitting exactly the balance equation $100 = 5 \times 16 + 20$.

The dehydron/disulfide balance relation clearly identifies proteins with excess ($\mathrm{Y} > 5\mathrm{X} + 20$) or lack ($\mathrm{Y} < 5\mathrm{X} + 20$) of structural deficiencies, with the former likely to be more favorably denatured than the latter under equivalent redox and denaturation conditions. To test this prediction, thermodynamic data on thermal denaturation (Table 4.2) was obtained for an exhaustive set of proteins for which structural information was also available [25]. Thus, the thermal denaturation free energy change, $\Delta\mathrm{G}$, under reducing conditions and comparable temperatures [25, 26] was obtained for monomeric uncomplexed PDB-reported proteins with disulfide bonds and lacking prosthetic groups or ion coordination. A significant anticorrelation was found ($\mathrm{R}^2 = 0.72$, Fig. 4.12) between the deviation from the balance equation, measured as $\mathrm{Y} - (5\mathrm{X} + 20)$, and the thermal

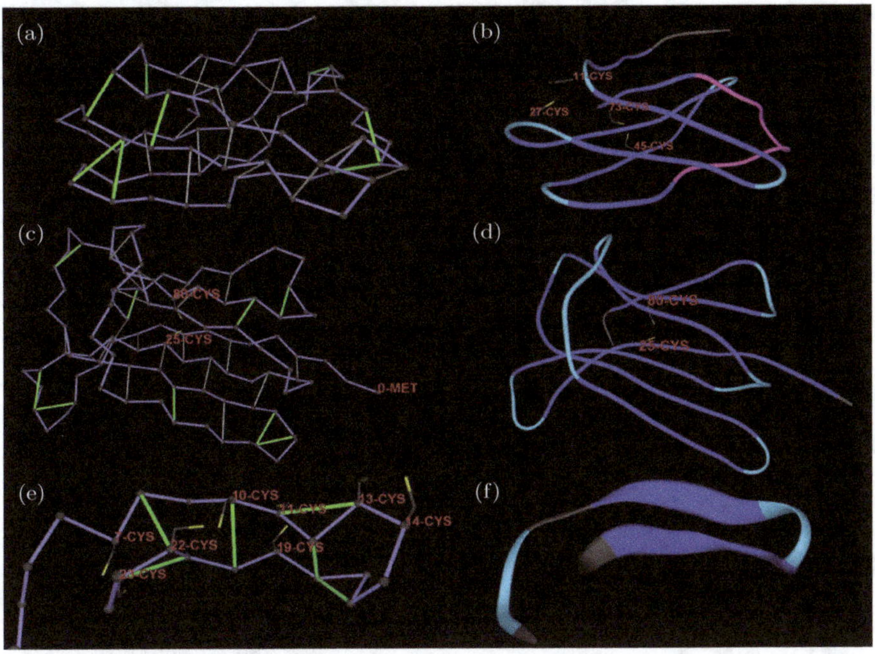

Figure 4.11. Structural deficiencies in soluble proteins. The protein backbone is shown as virtual bonds (blue) joining consecutive α-carbons in the peptide chain. Light-grey segments joining α-carbons represent completely buried backbone hydrogen bonds, and green segments represent structural deficiencies (unburied backbone hydrogen bonds). A tube/ribbon representation is added for visual aid. Cysteines involved in disulfide bonds are identified by side-chain display. Structural deficiencies (**a, c, e**) and tube/ribbon representation (**b, d, f**) respectively of alpha-amylase inhibitor HOE-467A (PDB.1HOE) (**a, b**), beta-2 microglobulin (PDB.2Z9T) (**c, d**) and antimicrobial hormone hepcidin (PDB.1M4F) (**e, f**). Reprinted from [25], copyright 2009 with permission from the American Chemical Society.

denaturation free energy (ΔG). This tight anticorrelation provides a thermodynamic validation of the balance equation.

The 5:1 rule may be justified on thermodynamic grounds. Thus, Doig and Williams [27] addressed the inconsistencies in Flory's treatment of the entropic contribution to protein denaturation, calculating $\Delta\Delta$G for denaturation for a cross-linked protein versus its non-cross-linked counterpart. At physiological temperature 300 K, they estimated $\Delta\Delta G \approx 4.4\,\text{kcal/mol}$. This value is essentially

Table 4.2. *Thermodynamic and structural parameters of soluble proteins.* Thermal denaturation free energy change, ΔG, under reducing conditions and comparable temperatures for an exhaustive set of monomeric uncomplexed proteins with disulfide bonds and without prosthetic groups or ion coordination [25]. Deviations from the balance relation are measured by Y − (5X + 20), and shown to anticorrelate tightly ($R^2 = 0.72$) with the denaturation free energies.

PDB entry	Y−(5X + 20)	ΔG (kcal/ mol)	T (C)	pH	Reference
1BSQ	−9.83	11.10	40.00	7.00	INT J BIOL MACROMOL 38, 9–17 (2006)
1RTB	−5.00	10.10	25.00	8.40	BIOPHYS CHEM 127, 51–63 (2007)
4LYZ	−3.30	9.02	26.85	7.00	BIOPOLYMERS 85, 264–273 (2007)
1CX1	−3.26	5.38	24.85	7.09	BIOCHEMISTRY 37, 3529–3537 (1998)
1QG5	1.13	8.80	40.00	7.00	INT J BIOL MACROMOL 38, 9–17 (2006)
2AIT	2.39	6.70	25.00	5.00	J MOL BIOL 223, 769–779 (1992)
3SSI	8.82	4.07	20.00	7.00	J MOL BIOL 249, 625–635 (1995)
1HIC	25.58	5.02	25.00	7.00	EUR J BIOCHEM 202, 67–73 (1991)
1PMC	38.33	1.10	20.00	3.00	NAT STRUCT BIOL 3, 45–53 (1996)

independent of protein length and loop size and best represents the insensitivity of experimental values to loop size-dependent configurational entropies [28].

This 4.4 kcal/mol constant agrees reasonably well with the free energy contribution associated with the native-state destabilization brought about by five structural deficiencies. If we take into account that −0.93 kcal/mol is the free energy change associated with complete dehydration of an unburied backbone hydrogen bond [3, 6], we may estimate the net destabilization effect promoted by 5 structural deficiencies at $0.93\,\text{kcal/mol} \times 5 = 4.65\,\text{kcal/mol}$. This value is in close proximity to the Doig-Williams constant. The thermodynamic

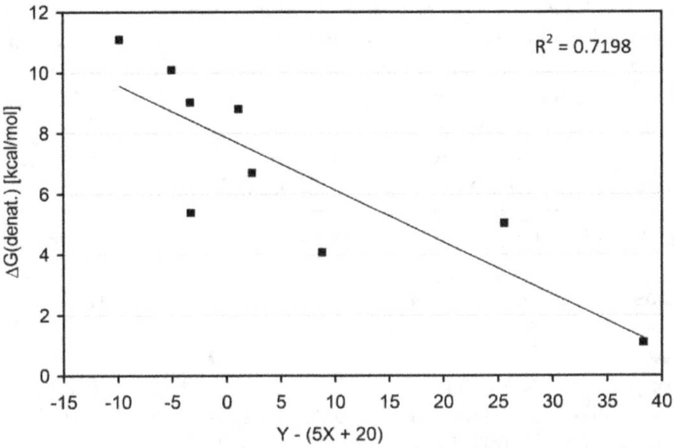

Figure 4.12. Anticorrelation between denaturation free energy (ΔG) and excess structural defects with respect to the balance relation, measured by Y − (5X + 20). The exhaustive set of monomeric uncomplexed proteins with disulfide links and the respective denaturation conditions are given in Table 4.2. The coefficient $R^2 = 0.72$ for the linear fit was obtained by linear regression. Reprinted from [25], copyright 2009 with permission from the American Chemical Society.

agreement supports the 5:1 golden ratio for protein buttressing arising from structural analysis.

Since the evolutionary axis is germane to any biological analysis, the following question naturally arises: Is the architectural constraint defined by the dehydron/disulfide balance equation respected by evolution? Bioinformatics evidence on orthologous proteins (homologs across species) supports the tenet of evolutionary conservation. Thus, we may compare the structural deficiency and normalized number of disulfide bonds across 1105 homolog pairs that differ in at least one disulfide bond (one homolog may have no disulfide bond). The changes in X and Y (ΔX, ΔY) were obtained for homolog pairs identified by their respective PDB accessions and the deviation from ideality was measured as $\Gamma = \Delta Y - 5\Delta X$. For all homolog pairs we obtained $\Gamma/Y < 11\%$, with Y associated with either homolog. Table 4.3 illustrates the tightest evolutionary conservation of the architectural constraint across homolog pairs with nontrivial buttressing differences.

Table 4.3. Evolutionary conservation of the balance relation Y = 5X + 20. (*) SCOP: structural classification of proteins (Murzin AG, Brenner SE, Hubbard T, Chothia C (1995) SCOP: a structural classification of proteins database for the investigation of sequences and structures. *J Mol Biol* 247:536–540).

SCOP family*	Sequence identity	ΔY−5ΔX	ΔX	ΔY	Homolog 1	Homolog 2
Fibronectin type II module	63.125	−0.1	0.21	0.95	1QO6	1E8B
beta-glycanases	40	−0.1	0.31	1.45	1FH8	1I1X
beta-glycanases	42.13836478	−0.1	0.31	1.45	1E0V	1B30
C-type lysozyme	57.69230769	−0.09	0.79	3.86	1KXY	1LHM
C-type lysozyme	58.46153846	−0.09	0.79	3.86	1JIS	1LHM
Ribonuclease A-like	30.23255814	−0.09	0.79	3.86	1RUV	1B1E
Ribonuclease A-like	31.00775194	−0.09	0.79	3.86	1RUV	1H52
Acetylcholinesterase-like	30.82437276	−0.07	0.18	0.83	2CKM	1K4Y
C-type lysozyme	67.69230769	−0.07	0.79	3.88	1LMP	2BQM
C-type lysozyme	56.92307692	−0.07	0.79	3.88	1LSM	2BQK
Eukaryotic proteases	31.47410359	−0.07	0.29	1.38	1EX3	1DST
Snake venom toxins	32.89473684	−0.07	0.4	1.93	1TXA	1ERA
Pepsin-like	40	−0.06	0.31	1.49	1PSN	1FQ6
Ribonuclease A-like	31.74603175	−0.06	0.73	3.59	1RTB	1K5B
C-type lysozyme	59.23076923	−0.05	0.79	3.9	1IR7	1HNL
C-type lysozyme	59.23076923	−0.05	0.79	3.9	1XEK	1HNL
C-type lysozyme	59.23076923	−0.05	0.79	3.9	1UIH	1HNL
Ribonuclease A-like	31.00775194	−0.05	0.79	3.9	4RAT	1K5A
C-type lysozyme	58.46153846	−0.05	0.79	3.9	2HS7	2BQK
Plant proteinase inhibitors	47.74774775	−0.04	0.34	1.66	1TIH	1FYB
Papain-like	70.21943574	−0.03	0.84	4.17	1ITO	2PBH
beta-glycanases	36.36363636	−0.03	0.31	1.52	2XYL	1B3X
C-type lysozyme	84.72222222	−0.03	1.02	5.07	3LZ2	1LSG
Ribonuclease A-like	31.00775194	−0.03	0.79	3.92	1RHB	1K5A

4.6 Epistructural etiology of protein misfolding and aberrant aggregation

In the previous section we investigated the architectural constraints imposed by the extent of under-wrapping of a soluble protein. In view of the characterization of proteins with large dehydron clusters given in the previous section, time is ripe to pose the question: *What is physically the fate of a soluble protein with a large dehydron cluster and with* $Y \gg 5X + 20$, *that is, with poor disulfide-bridge buttressing relative to the high level of structural deficiency?* The answer obviously depends on the extent to which the protein is capable of recruiting binding partners to maintain its structural integrity. As noted in section 4.5, the worse wrapped proteins are potassium channel neurotoxins but their buttressing is actually adequate for an extracellular protein with such a level of structural deficiency.

On the other hand, the cellular form of the human prion (PDB.1QM0) is very poorly buttressed for its extensive underwrapping, belongs to the reducing cytosolic space, contains spots of large dehydron density and makes no obligatory complex. We know that prions misfold and aggregate aberrantly into highly organized amyloidogenic fibrils. Is this then a generic behavior of proteins sharing the same molecular attributes? This question prompts us to investigate the amyloid phase more closely.

There is significant evidence supporting the view that amyloidogenic aggregation is a generic phase of peptide chains [29–31]. The term generic phase refers to a three dimensional organization dominated by main-chain interactions which is essentially insensitive to the information encoded in the primary sequence. Such intermolecular associations appear to be dominated by a basic structural motif: the cross-β structure [32], an intermolecular sheet-pleated pattern ubiquitous in fibrillogenic aggregation. This assertion remains conjectural, as no crystal of the fiber for natural prions has been obtained. By contrast, the folded state of the peptide chain is relatively well understood: natural soluble proteins tend to adopt single-molecule conformations of marginal stability.

While the folding process and its final stable outcome are crucially dependent on the amino-acid composition of the chain, the amyloid state appears to be fairly insensitive to this information: At first sight, amyloidogenic aggregation does not seem to require an "aggregation code", as some recent claims would have it [29–31]. But further analysis reveals that it must place severe constraints on the primary sequence, as some proteins tend to be prone to aggregate under physiological conditions [8], while others require extreme conditions to do so or simply do not aggregate reproducibly [29, 33]. In addition, negative-design features of the folded state purposely encoded in the protein primary sequence may avert aggregation [34]. *Thus, it is not entirely correct to characterize the aberrant aggregation as a "polymer physics phase", shared by polypeptides with arbitrary, suboptimal or random sequence, in contrast with the folded state, determined unambiguously by the primary sequence.*

Proteins are subject to selection pressure and adapt to become good folders, i. e., expeditious structure seekers with a reproducible and stable soluble structure. This optimization is needed to prevent the functionally competent fold from reverting to a primeval amyloid phase. On the other hand, certain sequences are better optimized to escape aggregation than others even under conditions known to sustain the native fold [8].

While amyloidogenic aggregation has been shown to be always plausible provided sufficiently stringent denaturation conditions are applied [29–33], a marked amyloidogenic propensity has been detected on a number of proteins even under physiological or near-physiological conditions, particularly if the monomeric folding domain is deprived of its natural interacting partners [8]. *Such findings imply that not all soluble structures have been optimized to the same degree in order to avert aggregation, and that the more reliant the structure is on binding partnerships or complexations, the more vulnerable it becomes in regards to reverting to the primeval phase.* Thus, an over-expression of a folding domain with high complexation requirements *in vivo*, or the modification of its binding partners as a result of genetic accident, or any factor that distorts its natural interactive context is likely to bolster a transition to an amyloidogenic state.

These observations lead us to the following question: *What type of deficiency in the native fold constitutes a signal for aberrant aggregation?* A recent assessment of the *wrapping* of soluble structure might prove critical to address this problem. For highly underwrapped proteins (~50% dehydrons or more), densities higher than

4 dehydrons per 1000 Å^2 on the protein surface become inducers of protein aggregation [8].

Thus, the condition of "keeping the structure dry in water" becomes a requirement to preserve the structural integrity of soluble proteins and imposes a severe building constraint (and thereby an evolutionary pressure) on such proteins. It is expected that the optimization of the structures resulting from this type of evolutionary constraint would be uneven over a range of soluble proteins, resulting in marked differences in aggregation propensity.

This wrapping analysis clarifies the physical picture put forth by Dobson [29–31], in which amyloidogenic propensity depends crucially on the fact that main-chain interactions become dominant in detriment of the amino-acid sequence that encodes the folded state. Precisely, main-chain interactions may dominate as the main chain of the folded state is not properly protected from water attack.

It is instructive to compare this statement with the local analysis of Avbelj and Baldwin [35] in the sense that backbone solvation is a determinant of β-sheet propensity. Thus, an over-exposed backbone hydrogen bond in the native fold is an indicator of a failure in folding cooperativity, as it reveals an inability to remove water from an interactive polar pair by means of a many-body correlation, and at the same time, it is a signal enabling the diagnosis of amyloidogenic propensity. Thus, the wrapping concept enables us to discern why some soluble proteins may have been better optimized to avoid amyloidogenic aggregation than others.

Direct inspection of the pattern of desolvation of the main chain clearly reveals that the cellular fold of the human prion [19, 36] is too vulnerable to water attack and at the same time too sticky to avert aggregation. Clearly, its sequence has not been optimized to "keep the backbone hydrogen bonds dry" in the folded state. In fact, *their extent of exposure of backbone hydrogen bonds is the highest among soluble proteins in the entire PDB*, with the sole exception of some toxins whose stable fold is held together by a profusion of disulfide bridges. This discussion leads us to identify proteins with amyloidogenic propensity as significant outliers in

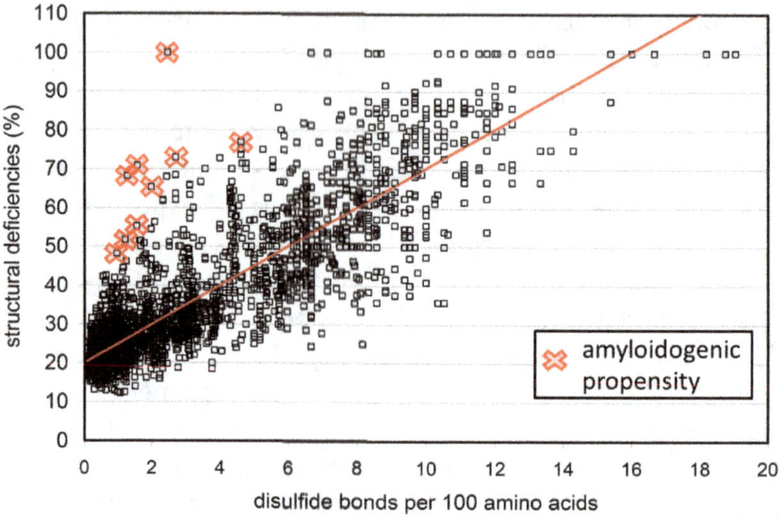

Figure 4.13. Distribution of proteins with known or established amyloidogenic propensity in the X-Y plane (Y = ordinates = %dehydrons, X = abscissas = number of disulfide bridges every 100 amino acids) with datapoints lineraly fitted to the architectural golden rule Y = 5X + 20.

flagrant violation of the X-Y architectural golden rule, as described in Fig. 4.13.

It is suggestive that an inability to protect the main chain is precisely the type of deficiency that best correlates with a propensity to reverse to a primeval aggregation phase determined by main-chain interactions. The actual mechanism by which such defects induce or nucleate the transition is still opaque, although the inherent adhesiveness of packing defects obviously plays a role.

An atomic-detail structure of a fibrillogenic aggregate, with its β-sheets parallel to the main axis and the strands perpendicular to it, was reported and revealed a tight packing of β-sheets [37]. The cross-β spine of the fibrillogenic peptide GNNQQNY reveals a double parallel β-sheet with tight packing of side chains leading to the full dehydration of intra-sheet backbone-backbone and side-chain-side-chain hydrogen bonds. However, *there is not a single pair-wise interaction between the β-sheets, no hydrogen bond and no hydrophobic interaction*. Instead, a direct examination of the crystal

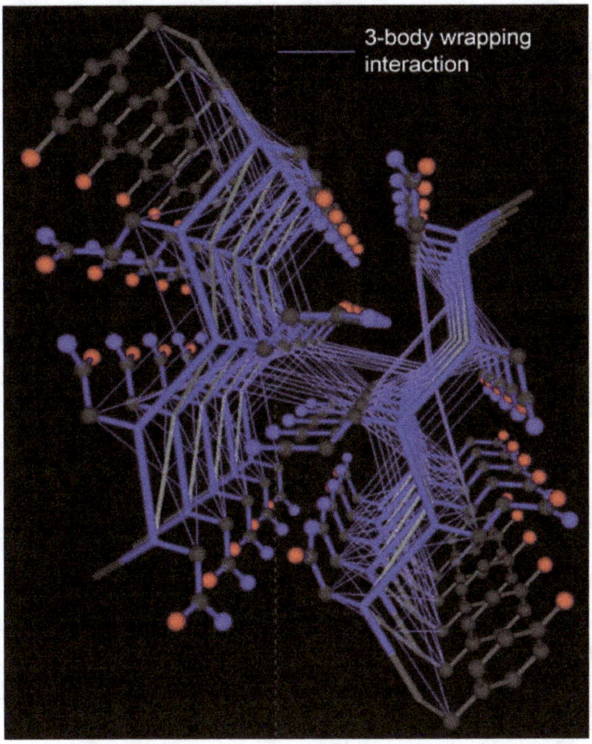

Figure 4.14. Pattern of inter-sheet wrapping of backbone–backbone hydrogen bonds in the fibrillogenic state of peptide GNNQQNY. The strand backbone is represented as virtual bonds (blue) joining α-carbons, and backbone hydrogen bonds are displayed as light grey lines joining the α-carbons of the paired residues. A thin blue line from the β-carbon of a residue to the barycenter of a hydrogen bond indicates wrapping of the bond by the residue: at least one non-polar group from the residue is contained in the desolvation sphere of the bond.

structure reveals that the association is driven by the dehydration propensity of pre-formed intra-sheet dehydrons, as depicted in Fig. 4.14.

This discussion naturally leads us to some evolutionary considerations. A paradigmatic discovery in biology revealed that folds are conserved across species to perform specific functions. However, the wrapping of such folds is clearly not conserved [4]. This fact suggests how complex physiologies may be achieved without dramatically expanding genome size, a standing problem in biology. Considerable network complexity may be achieved by actually fostering a higher level of complexation or binding partnership, as promoted by a more precarious wrapping of the isolated protein domains. According to our previous analysis, such complex design also entails an inherent danger: the reversal of highly under-wrapped folding domains to an amyloidogenic phase even under physiological conditions. Amyloidosis is thus likely to be a consequence of high complexity in proteomic connectivity, as dictated by the structural fragility of highly interactive proteins (cf. Fig. 4.13).

4.7 AI platform for genome-wide prediction of amyloidogenic propensity

When predicting amyloidogenic propensity, the researcher is faced with a big conundrum. This may appear surprising at first glance since dehydron patterns may be derived from protein structure (Chapter 2) and the protein folding problem has been solved, as announced by DeepMind, a Google company: https://deepmind.com/blog/article/alphafold-a-solution-to-a-50-year-old-grand-challenge-in-biology.

The solution to the protein folding problem would imply in principle that the dehydron pattern be directly obtained from structural coordinates, whether experimentally determined or predicted by AlphaFold2 (the latest DeepMind predictor) following the simple arithmetic described in Chapter 2. Then, the inference of amyloidogenic propensity would simply require the additional computation of the extent of deviation from the architectural constraints described in this chapter, another straightforward calculation relating number of dehydrons and number of intramolecular disulfide linkages. However, most aggregation-prone proteins are unable to sustain a stable fold under the conditions where current folding predictions are made. They are so underwrapped that their structure, if any, can only be induced in a structural adaptation upon binding to a partner or under aggregation conditions at high protein concentration. This implies that amyloidogenic propensity, although a structure-derivative attribute, cannot be inferred using

AI in the same way that AI is used to infer protein structure from sequence.

The forays into the subject described in this chapter shed light on the matter. The key is that the representation of the data must include as input a prediction of disorder propensity, an attribute that is absent from the representational scheme subsumed in the TensorFlow of the AI systems AlphaFold and AlphaFold2. Furthermore, the underlying CNN must be trained with a relational dataset where dehydrons are determined from structures in the training set but also related to disorder propensity computations on the sequences associated with the structures in the training set. In essence, AlphaFold2 and other structure predictors cannot handle the conflictive signals that are naturally incorporated in the Twilighter, as those signals clash with the existence of the very object they try to predict.

For these reasons, the prediction of amyloidogenic propensity becomes unyielding to current efforts to predict protein structure: the structure predictors must input a signal for the *absence* of structure. The AI platform for predicting amyloidogenic propensity is subsumed in the architectures described in Chapters 11 and 12, which reconcile the incorporation of a signal for missing structure with the extraction of the dehydron as structure-derivative feature. Thus, the platform in Chapter 12 is ideally suited to compute the susceptibility to induced folding, that is, to infer dehydrons that only occur when the chain adapts to binding partners. In the case of amyloids, or other aggregation prone proteins, the folding of the chain is induced by binding to a copy of itself.

Reconciling the conflicting signals for presence and absence of structure and the incorporation of the twilight region in the training data is thus the hallmark of the next generation of AI platforms, as described in detail in Chapters 11, 12.

References

1. Fernández A, Sosnick TR, Colubri A (2002) Dynamics of hydrogen-bond desolvation in folding proteins. *J Mol Biol* 321:659–675.

2. Fernández A, Scheraga HA (2003) Insufficiently dehydrated hydrogen bonds as determinants of protein interactions. *Proc Natl Acad Sci USA* 100:113–118.
3. Fernández A, Scott LR (2003) Adherence of packing defects in soluble proteins. *Phys Rev Lett* 91:018102.
4. Fernández A, Lynch M (2011) Nonadaptive origins of interactome complexity. *Nature* 474:502–505.
5. Fernández A, Scott RL (2003) Dehydron: A structurally encoded signal for protein interaction. *Biophys J* 85:1914–1928.
6. Fernández A (2004) Keeping dry and crossing membranes. *Nature Biotech* 22:1081–1084.
7. Fernández A, Scott RL, Berry RS (2006) Packing defects as selectivity switches for drug-based protein inhibitors. *Proc Natl Acad Sci USA* 103:323–328.
8. Fernández A, Kardos J, Scott R, Goto Y, Berry RS (2003) Structural defects and the diagnosis of amyloidogenic propensity. *Proc Natl Acad Sci USA* 100:6446–6451.
9. Fernández A, Berry RS (2003) Proteins with hydrogen-bond packing defects are highly interactive with lipid bilayers: Implications for amyloidogenesis. *Proc Natl Acad Sci USA* 100:2391–2396.
10. Deremble C, Lavery R (2005) Macromolecular recognition. *Curr Opin Struc Biol* 15:171–175.
11. Ma B, Elkayam T, Wolfson H, Nussinov R (2003) Protein-protein interactions: Structurally conserved residues distinguish between binding sites and exposed protein surfaces. *Proc Natl Acad Sci USA* 100:5772–5777.
12. Ma B, Pan Y, Gunasekaran K, Venkataraghavan RB, Levine AJ, Nussinov R (2005) Comparison of the protein-protein interfaces in the p53-DNA crystal structures: Towards elucidation of the biological interface. *Proc Natl Acad Sci USA* 102:3988–3993.
13. Rajamani D, Thiel S, Vajda S, Camacho CJ (2004) Anchor residues in protein-protein interactions. *Proc Natl Acad Sci USA* 101:11287–11292.
14. Dunker AK, Cortese MS, Romero P, Iakoucheva LM, Uversky VN (2005) Flexible nets: The roles of intrinsic disorder in protein interaction networks. *FEBS J* 272:5129–5148.
15. Iakoucheva LM, Dunker AK (2003) Order, disorder, and flexibility: prediction from protein sequence. *Structure (London)* 11:1316–1317.
16. Dunker AK, Obradovic Z (2001) The protein trinity-linking function and disorder. *Nature Biotech* 19:805–806.
17. Wade RC, Gabdoulline RR, Lüdemann SK, Lounnas V (1998). Electrostatic steering and ionic tethering in enzyme-ligand binding: Insights from simulations. *Proc Natl Acad Sci USA* 95:5942–5949.
18. Ho WC, Fitzgerald MX, Marmorstein R (2006) Structure of the p53 core domain dimer bound to DNA. *J Biol Chem* 281:20494–20502.
19. Pietrosemoli N, Crespo A, Fernández A (2007) Dehydration propensity of order-disorder intermediate regions in soluble proteins. *J Prot Res* 6:3519–3526.

20. Lindahl E, Hess B, Van der Spoel D: GROMACS 3.0: A package for molecular simulations and trajectory analysis. *J. Mol. Modeling 2001* 7:302–317.
21. Mason PE, Neilson GW, Dempsey CE, Barnes AC, Cruickshank, JM (2003) The hydration structure of guanidinium and thiocyanate ions: Implications for protein stability in aqueous solution. *Proc Natl Acad Sci USA* 100:4557–4561.
22. Baldwin RL (2003) In search of the energetic role of peptide hydrogen bonds. *J Biol Chem* 278:17581–17588.
23. Powers ET, Deechongkit S, Kelly JW (2006) Backbone-backbone H-bonds make context-dependent contributions to protein folding kinetics and thermodynamics: Lessons from amide-to-ester mutations. In: Peptide solvation and H-bonds, Baldwin RL and Baker D, eds, *Adv Prot Chem* 72:40–79.
24. MacKinnon R, Reinhart PH, White MN (1988) Charybdotoxin block of Shaker K^+ channels suggests that different types of K^+ channels share common features. *Neuron* 1:997–1001.
25. Fernández A, Berry RS (2009) Golden rule for buttressing vulnerable soluble proteins. *J Proteome Res* 9:2643–2648.
26. Kumar MD (2006) ProTherm and ProNIT: Thermodynamic databases for proteins and protein-nucleic acid interactions. *Nuc Ac Res* 34:D204–D206.
27. Doig AJ, Williams DH (1991) Is the hydrophobic effect stabilizing or destabilizing in proteins: The contribution of disulfide bonds to protein stability. *J Mol Biol* 217:389–398.
28. Betz SF (1993) Disulfide bonds and the stability of globular proteins. *Protein Science* 2:1551–1558.
29. Dobson CM (1999) Protein misfolding, evolution and disease. *Trends Biochem Sci* 24:329–332.
30. Dobson CM (2001) The structural basis of protein folding and its links with human disease. *Philos Trans R Soc Lond Ser B* 356:133–145.
31. Fändrich M, Dobson CM (2002) The behavior of polyamino acids reveals an inverse side chain effect in amyloid structure formation. *EMBO J* 21:5682–5690.
32. Sunde M, Blake CCF (1998) From the globular to the fibrous state: Protein structure and structural conversion in amyloid formation. *Q Rev Biophys* 31:1–39.
33. Dobson CM (2002) Protein misfolding diseases: Getting out of shape. *Nature* 418:729–730.
34. Richardson JS, Richardson DC (2002) Natural β-sheet proteins use negative design to avoid edge-to-edge aggregation. *Proc Natl Acad Sci USA* 99:2754–2759.
35. Avbelj F, Baldwin RL (2003) Role of backbone solvation and electrostatics in generating preferred peptide backbone conformations: Distributions of phi. *Proc Natl Acad Sci USA* 100:5742–5747.
36. Prusiner SB (1998) Prions. *Proc Natl Acad Sci USA* 95:13363–13383.
37. Nelson R, Sawaya M, Balbirnie M, *et al.* (2005) Structure of the cross-beta spine of amyloid-like fibrils. *Nature* 435:773–778.

Chapter 5

Molecular evolution from the perspective of epistructural biology

The protein-water interface constitutes a unique marker for molecular evolution. This fact endows epistructural biology with a vantage point to explore the evolutionary axis, which is essential to understand and manipulate biological phenomena. A key result emerging from such forays is that dehydron patterns are not conserved across homologous proteins. Drug designers can take advantage of this fact to create specific targeted agents. As described previously, dehydrons may be targeted by wrapping ligands that serve as leads to therapeutic drugs. Thus, the evolutionary insights obtained from epistructural analysis have implications for the drug designer. Homologous proteins typically share the same fold and this structural similarity introduces problems for molecular targeted therapy since it leads to undesirable cross reactivities with hazardous off-target effects. As shown in this chapter, while the topology of a protein fold is conserved across homologs, the wrapping patterns are substantially different, enabling the wrapping drug to funnel its impact on clinically relevant targets. The evolutionary root of the differences in dehydron pattern across homologs is established across species and within the human species. Wrapping variations across homologs can be exploited to considerable advantage as we aim at engineering target-specific and species-specific therapeutic agents and build meaningful animal models for disease. In delineating the evolutionary forces that promote epistructural differences across orthologs, we discovered that random genetic drift plays an operational role in promoting dehydron enrichment. This structural degradation enhances the propensity for protein interactivity and becomes more pronounced in species with low population, where mildly deleterious mutations resulting from random drift have a higher probability of getting fixed in the population. The fitness consequences of this evolutionary strategy are assessed for humans, and reveal their high exposure to fitness catastrophes.

5.1 The evolution of epistructure investigated with AI

No biological object can be fully understood or manipulated without incorporating the evolutionary axis. This book is about designing protein-ligand interfaces for therapeutic purpose and hence cannot escape that dictum. Accordingly, this chapter addresses the question: how do protein interfaces evolve? Since ligands displace water as they bind proteins, the question must be complemented with a tributary question: how do protein-water interfaces evolve?

As we address these questions, we become acquainted with the conceptual richness of epistructural biology. This is so because the dehydron, the key defining feature of epistructure, is a marker for evolution as well as a targetable feature. That the deydron is drug-targetable is a property we are already acquainted with since reading Chapter 2. However, the role of the dehydron as evolutionary marker still needs to be ascertained, and that is precisely the purview of this chapter. And why should that property of dehydrons matter to the drug designer? Because, as markers for evolution, dehydron patterns cannot be fully conserved across human proteins of common ancestry (paralogs). Indeed they are not, as shown in this chapter, and hence dehydrons may be regarded as filters for drug specificity. This is an observation with far reaching, almost unfathomable, consequences for the pharmaceutical industry and a recurrent theme in the rest of the book.

Investigating the evolution of dehydron patterns may seem a straightforward matter. Since proteins with common ancestry share a common fold, or are structurally similar, the alignment of their structures should be feasible and so should be the alignment of dehydrons within the structures. Dehydrons may be represented in

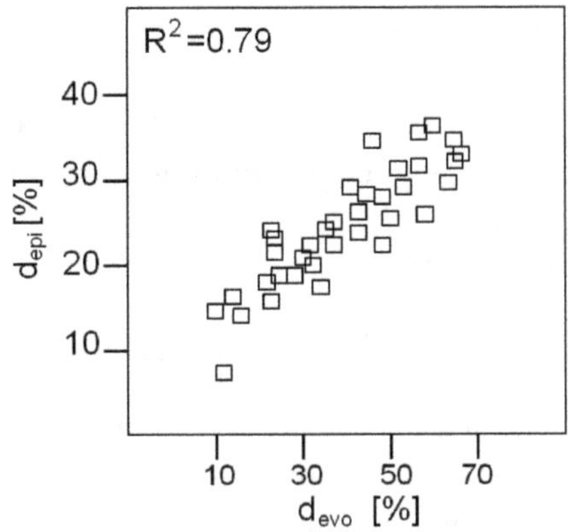

Figure 5.1. Epistructural versus evolutionary distance for the 36 pairs of kinase paralogs in the SRC family.

matrix form, with binary ij-entry $= 1$ if residues i and j are paired by a dehydron, and $= 0$ otherwise. This matrix representation of the dehydron patterns in paralogs naturally enables us to define an epistructural distance, $\mathrm{d_{epi}}$, as simply the eucidean distance between the two binary 2D-arrays. Then, $\mathrm{d_{epi}}$ may be contrasted against the well defined $\mathrm{d_{evo}}$, the standard evolutionary distance defined as percentage of sequence identity.

Indeed both distances are correlated, as suggested by Fig. 5.1, where the two distances for the 36 pairs from the nine paralogous kinases in the SRC family (SRC, LCK, YES, FYN, FGR, HCK, FRK, LYN, BLK) are plotted against each other. This sort of analysis including all family members often encounters a major hurdle: protein structures are very much underreported relative to protein sequences. In other words, we have many more protein sequences than structures. As shown in Chapter 11, the advent of AI changes dramatically this state of affairs. That is so because AI enables us to infer the dehydron matrix even in the absence of protein structure, in so far as the structure-based training of the CNN may be cast in terms compatible with TensorFlow (Chapter 1), that is, in tensor-based representation.

Since dehydrons are also functional markers, as demonstrated in Chapter 6, we may conclude that dehydrons must be vehicles for functional innovation as needed to segregate proteins following a gene duplication event in order to avoid dosage imbalance. This analysis is pursued in this chapter, and again, AI is likely to play a significant role in extending this analysis to sequence databases, as shown in Chapter 11.

5.2 Molecular evolution for the drug designer

From a structural biology perspective, one of the most striking observations regarding protein evolution is the uncanny similarity of the 3D structure of proteins with a common ancestry (Fig. 5.2). This similarity across homologous proteins is often quantified by a RMSD < 1.5 Å for the aligned backbone atoms and holds even at low levels of sequence identity ($\sim$25%), that are nevertheless sufficient to establish protein homology.

From the perspective of a drug designer, this structural similarity across homologs of the protein target is in principle troublesome. Major goals in drug design are related or entangled with this evolutionary aspect. They are: a) the control of drug specificity; b) the engineering of species-selective therapeutic impact in the treatment of infectious diseases; and c) the building of insightful animal models to properly assess drug efficacy. In all three contexts, the existence of homologs of the protein target within the species (paralogs) or across species (orthologs) can introduce undesired cross reactivities due to their high level of structural similarity with the target. These cross reactivities, in turn, can result in adverse and even health-threatening side effects or can render inconsequential or irrelevant the animal models for a particular disease or malignancy.

The fold may be highly conserved across homologs, but as shown in this chapter, the wrapping or dehydron pattern is not conserved, and neither is the regulation of the expression pattern across homologs. As described below, we should distinguish orthologs from paralogs when assessing the evolutionary origins of these dissimilarities. Thus, in the case of orthologs, the variations arise mostly from differences in the level of efficiency of natural selection across different species. On the other hand, in paralogs the dissimilarity is

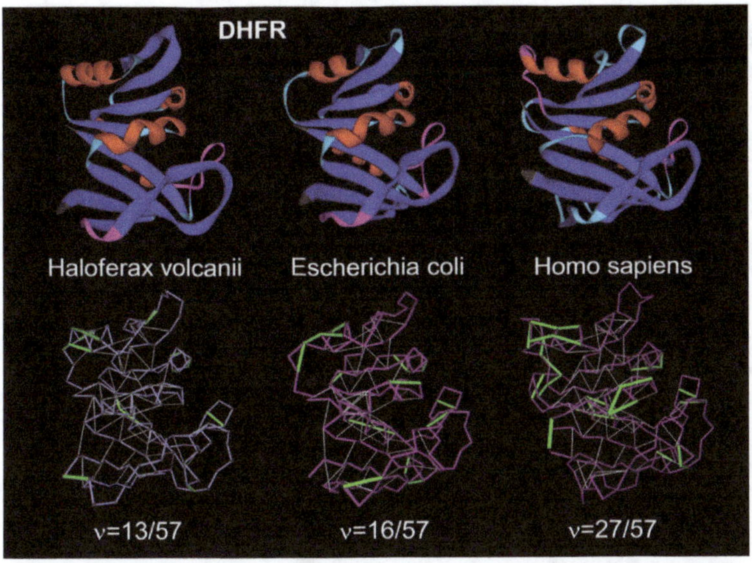

(a)

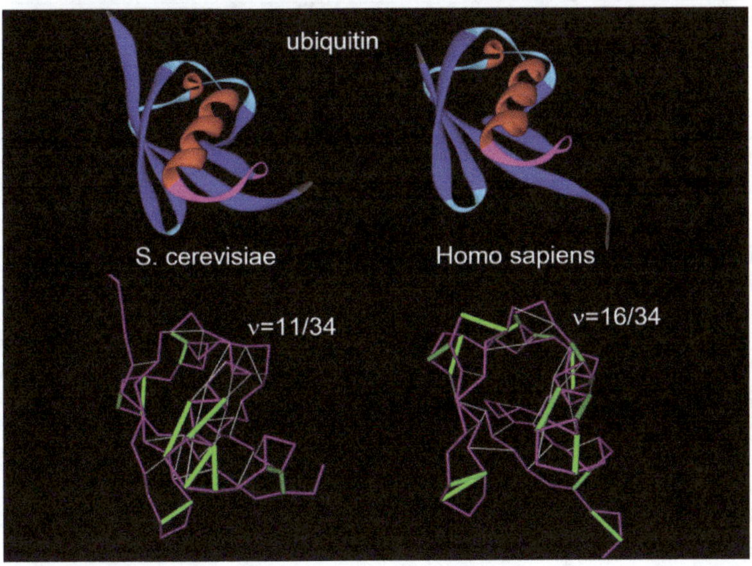

(b)

Figure 5.2. (*Continued*)

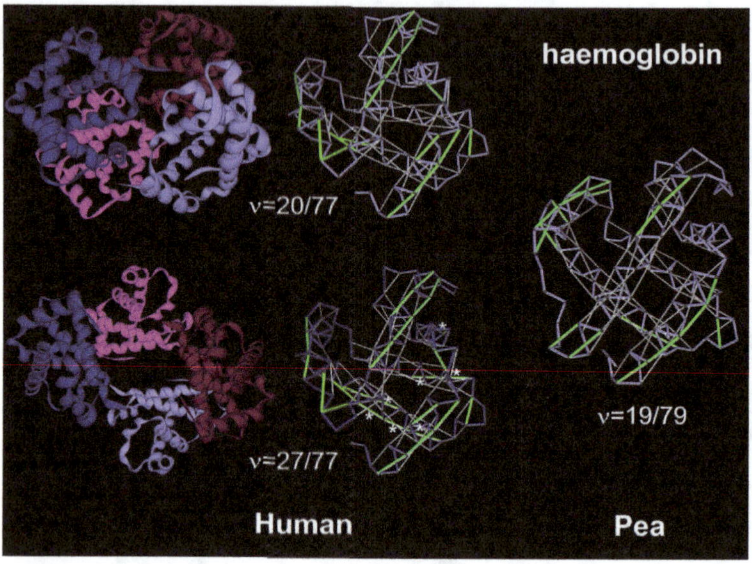

(c)

Figure 5.2. (*Continued*) **(a)** Under-wrapping of three orthologous versions of dehydrofolate reductase (DHFR) from three kingdoms of life archea, bacteria and eukarya, represented by species *Haloferax volcanii*, *Escherichia coli* and *Homo sapiens*, respectively. **(b)** Wrapping patterns of ubiquitin from *Saccharomyces cerevisiae (yeast)* and *Homo sapiens*. **(c)** Wrapping patterns of haemoglbin in human and of its ortholog leghaemoglobin in pea (*Pisum sativum*). In human, the monomer within the tetramer (upper left panels) contains less dehydrons that the monomer in isolation (lower left panels) due to intermolecular wrapping. As the monomer is taken in isolation, seven additional dehydrons (marked by asterisks) occur. These dehydrons promote the quaternary structure and become well wrapped hydrogen bonds in the homomeric complex. By contrast the pea leghaemoglobin ortholog is better wrapped and lacks the dehydrons that would trigger oligomerization and promote allostery.

rooted in the imperative to curb dosage imabalances that would arise if two copies of the same gene would be retained undifferentiated. As shown in the subsequent chapters, these subtle variations of proteins that essentially share the same 3D-fold have paramount consequences to engineer drugs that can fulfill the three goals described above.

The picture that emerges from this chapter is essentially that wrapping constitutes a biological dimension utilized by evolution to promote complexity and at the same time, that wrapping differences within a fold offer escape routes to the fitness consequences introduced by paralog retention. Both evolutionary aspects will be leveraged in subsequent chapters, especially in Chapter 7 as we herald the new generation of wrapping-based drugs.

As we explored the evolutionary forces that sculpt differences in the dehydron patterns across orthologous proteins, we came to realize that random genetic drift is the main factor causing dehydron enrichment in species with low population. Because dehydrons are markers for protein association (Chapter 2), this type of structural degradation promotes higher protein interactivity which becomes more pronounced in species with low population, such as humans. This is because dehydron-generating mildly deleterious mutations resulting from random genetic drift have a higher probability of getting fixed in the relatively low population of the human species. As shown in this chapter, the fitness consequences of nature's "evolutionary gambit" reveal the high exposure of the human species to fitness catastrophes resulting from aberrant protein aggregation.

5.3 Epistructural analysis of orthologous proteins reveals nonadaptive traits

Since proteins with common ancestry tend to share the same fold or at least the same structure topology [1, 2], we may state that essentially the same molecular machinery is operative in organisms that diverged from each other billions of years ago. For example, the metabolic enzymatic function "dehydrofolate reductase" (DHFR) is exerted by a molecular machinery that has hardly changed in structure as we compare species in different kingdoms of life, like *archea* (i.e. *Haloferax volcanii*), bacteria (i.e. *Escherichia coli*) and higher eukaryotes (i.e. *Homo sapiens*). When closely examined, the wrapping of the DHFR has gotten worse (richer in dehydrons) in species with small population size, that is, those where natural selection became less efficient [3] (Fig. 5.2(a)). This trend is apparent even when examining highly conserved protein domains, such as ubiquitin: *There is a progressive enrichment in dehydrons as the species population decreases* (Fig. 5.2(b)).

For operational reasons, the under-wrapping or packing deficiency of a protein may be defined as ν = % dehydrons in the set of backbone hydrogen bonds. As we focus on any functionally competent fold, the anectdotal examples we harvested suggest a clear trend: ν(archea) $<$ ν(bacteria) $<$ ν(unicellular eukaryotes) $< \cdots <$ ν(higher eukaryotes). This trend probably follows from the fact that mildly deleterious mutations have a better chance to prevail and get fixed in species with smaller populations [3]. In this regard, the reader should note that most mutations are detrimental and hardly ever beneficial. Thus it is more likely that a mutation will loose up the fold (create a dehydron), rather than tighten it. These mildly detrimental mutations that prevail manage to degrade the wrapping of the protein, enriching its dehydron content, thereby making the protein more reliant on binding partnerships to maintain its structural integrity [1,2]. *Thus, as protein interactivity, regulation and allostery increases with decreasing species population, one may say that complexity is in this sense promoted by nonadaptive forces.*

An illustration of the probable nonadaptive origin of allostery is furnished by the wrapping of haemoglobin across orthologs in species with vastly different population size. Thus, this protein becomes richer in dehydrons and more prone to oligomerization in species with smaller population, with the majority of the new dehydrons located at the interface that promotes the quaternary structure of the homomer (Fig. 5.2(c)).

5.4 Natural selection of epistructural interfaces

Dosage imbalances occur when protein concentration levels at specific locations in tissues or metabolic/developmental phases do not fit the stoichiometry of the complexes in which the proteins are involved [4–6]. The complexes may be transient, adventitious or obligatory with regards to maintaining the structural integrity of the protein [7] and hence the effects of the imbalances may vary widely. Therefore, dosage sensitivity, that is, the impact of dosage imbalances on fitness, must be influenced not only by whether the protein is part of a complex but also by the extent of reliance of the protein on its binding partners to maintain structural integrity and functional competence.

While overexpression, gene duplication, misfolding and self-aggregation may all cause dosage imbalance, the structural or molecular properties determining the magnitude of the resulting effects remain largely unknown. For example, as we focus on gene duplication, we notice that paralog proteins, identical when they initially diverge, are subject to higher or lower selection pressure depending on their dosage sensitivity [5].

Cross examination of genetic and structural information revealed that the under-wrapping or packing deficiency of a protein, ν, is a molecular quantifier of dosage sensitivity [5] precisely because it constitutes a measure of the reliance of the protein on binding partnerships to maintain the integrity of the native fold. As expected, a deficiently packed protein is more likely to be engaged in an obligatory complex [7] and its concentration imbalances relative to the complex stoichiometry are more likely to impact fitness than those of a well packed protein.

In unicellular organisms, the packing quality (100-ν) of soluble gene products correlates with the number of paralogs or family size [5]. That is, the better the packing quality, the less likely that gene duplication would introduce a fitness disadvantage, hence the higher the chance that the duplicate gene would be retained. However, this correlation becomes less significant in higher eukaryotes, as shown in Fig. 5.3. Thus, paralog survival is dependent on the packing quality of protein structure with $P < 10^{-16}$ in *Escherichia coli* and $P < 6.7 \times 10^{-3}$ in human [5]. This contrast between simple and complex organisms is hard to interpret due to wide differences at the proteome level. However, alternative measures point to a similar trend. For example, the average difference in packing deficiency between singletons and duplicate genes is 18% in *E. coli*, 6% in worm (*Caenorhabditis elegans*), and ~2% in human (*Homo sapiens*).

In human, this insensitivity to dosage imbalance may be attributed in part to selection inefficiency arising from smaller population size [3], implying that the selection pressure exerted on

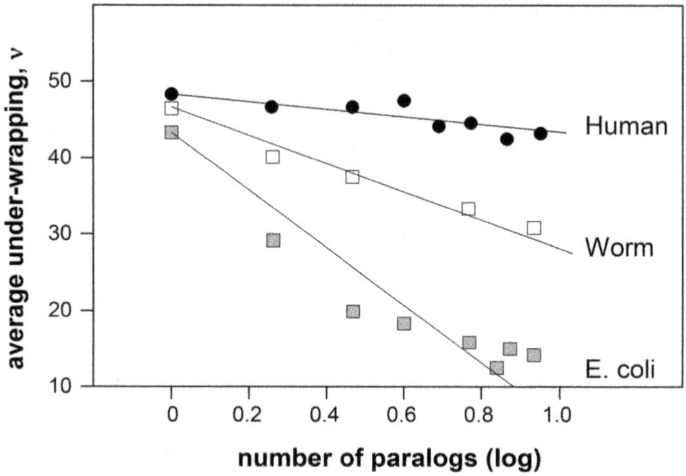

Figure 5.3. Negative correlation between protein under-wrapping, ν, and gene duplicability or family size represented by the number of paralogs in the gene family. Structural and genetic information was obtained for different species and ν-values were averaged over all families with a fixed number of paralogs, as described in ref. [5].

paralogs of deficiently packed proteins has simply not become operative. Alternatively, the higher complexity of expression regulation in higher eukaryotes may introduce a tolerance to dosage imbalance not found in unicellular organisms. This chapter explores this latter possibility, focusing on evolution-related dosage imbalances and the mechanisms that humans possess to cope with the troubling aspects of selection inefficiency.

5.5 Epistructural analysis reveals inefficient selection in humans

If selection is indeed inefficient in humans and this inefficiency enabled duplicate genes to stay around awaiting further specialization, significant dosage imbalances must have occurred during human evolution. How did we cope with such imbalances, which are likely to be significant when the gene products are very under-wrapped? The key to this problem lies in the ability of humans to regulate the expression of both gene copies dissimilarly through a plausible process that involves random deleterious mutations.

To address this problem, we first assess the selection pressure on gene duplicates exerted as paralogs are co-expressed at the mRNA (messenger RNA) level and hence are likely to compete for their interactive partners. Then we relate packing deficiency (ν) with differences in post-transcriptional regulation patterns within families. Thus, we investigate how differences in miRNA-target patterns [8], telling apart paralogs through different patterns of translational repression, impinge on the selection pressure on duplicate genes by mitigating dosage imbalances. In human these patterns are significantly dissimilar across paralogs of poorly packed proteins while nearly coincident across paralogs of well packed proteins [17], thus underscoring a means to buffer dosage imbalance effects arising from gene duplication.

This miRNA-based capacitance is not expected to be nearly as significant in species with larger effective population size due to the higher efficiency of evolutionary forces in such organisms when compared with human [3]. Thus, the selection pressure affecting the retention of gene duplicates is likely to be more efficient in these organisms promoting adaptation through functional innovation or purifying selection.

The next two sections are devoted to provide further evidence in support of the claim that protein wrapping quality is a determinant of dosage sensitivity while upholding the view that resilience to dosage imbalance is achieved in human by diversifying miRNA-regulatory patterns across paralogs.

5.5.1 *Evolutionary strategies to segregate paralog proteins*

As indicated in Chapter 2, soluble proteins may further protect their backbone hydrogen bonds and improve packing quality through binding partnerships by increasing the number of nonpolar groups in their hydrogen-bond microenvironments [7, 9]. Hence, the extent of intermolecular protection determines whether the complex is obligatory, ephemeral or adventitious, and thus packing quality may be recognized as an important factor in determining dosage sensitivity [5].

Gene duplication introduces dosage imbalance and the resulting selection pressure on paralogs [6, 10, 11] appears to depend on the packing deficiency of the parental gene [5]. This trend is clear in *E. coli* and *S. cerevisiae*, but not so apparent in higher eukaryotes. This observation suggests that expression dissimilarities at the mRNA level and at post-transcriptional levels may be exploited to separate paralogs and avoid competition for the binding partners of the parental gene. Thus, to study human capacitance to dosage imbalance arising from gene duplication, we examined families with paralog coexpression at the mRNA level [12] and assessed post-transcriptional microRNA (miRNA) regulation patterns in relation to the packing quality of the proteins in the family.

To assess the role of miRNA regulation in the human capacitance to dosage imbalance, we selected human genes from an exhaustive set of 583 non-singleton families for which genetic [13], evolutionary [14], structural [5], expression [12] and post-transcriptional [15,16] data is available for at least two paralogs (Table 5.1). We obtained human gene information from the Ensembl Genome Database (NCBI36). Using the Ensembl gene family annotation [13], 22,357 human genes were grouped into 12,394 families [17]. Gene expression data were obtained from Novartis Gene Expression Atlas [12] in the form of expression levels across a panel of 73 normal human tissues. We then mapped the putative miRNA-target patterns for each classified gene. Putative conserved target sites in the 3'UTR (untranslated region) of each gene for 156 conserved microRNA families were identified using TargetScanS (version 5.1). Thus, to determine co-expression and co-regulation patterns across paralogs, each gene i is represented by two vectors:

a) A normalized mRNA-expression vector $\Phi_i/||\Phi_i||$, where the vector Φ_i has 73 entries indicating mRNA expression levels in 73 normal tissues and $||\Phi_i||$ is the norm of the vector.
b) A normalized miRNA vector $\Psi_i/||\Psi_i||$ of 156 entries representing the pattern of miRNA-related repression efficacy on gene i, with

Table 5.1. PDB representation of selected human gene families of different sizes. Human gene information is from Ensembl Genome Database (NCBI36).

Ensembl ID	Family size	Swiss prot ID	Gene name	PDB ID
>ENSF00000000393	7	Q05066	SRY	1HRY_A
>ENSF00000000393	7	P48431	SOX2	1O4X_B
>ENSF00000000784	4	P08048	ZFY	1KLR_A
>ENSF00000002256	4	Q8IUE1	TGIF2LX	2DMN_A
>ENSF00000000640	6	Q9HC56	PCDH9	2EE0_A
>ENSF00000000504	6	P38919	EIF4A3	2HXY_A
>ENSF00000000661	16	Q01105	SET	2E50_A
>ENSF00000001155	23	Q15414	RBMY1B	2FY1_A
>ENSF00000001155	23	Q14011	CIRBP	1X5S_A
>ENSF00000000702	5	P17612	PRKACA	2GU8_A
>ENSF00000000530	19	P13501	CCL5	1B3A_A
>ENSF00000000530	19	O00175	CCL24	1EIG_A
>ENSF00000001027	4	Q92565	RAPGEF5	1WGY_A
>ENSF00000000301	14	Q05923	DUSP2	1M3G_A
>ENSF00000000301	14	Q16690	DUSP5	2G6Z_A
>ENSF00000001036	2	O00763	ACACB	2DN8_A
>ENSF00000002731	2	P61923	COPZ1	2HF6_A
>ENSF00000000164	18	Q9Y3D6	CLDN15	1NZN_A
>ENSF00000000212	11	Q9UHX3	EMR2	2BO2_A
>ENSF00000002211	2	Q8WUA7	TBC1D22A	2QFZ_A
>ENSF00000002844	2	Q8IWR0	ZC3H7A	2D9M_A
>ENSF00000001386	3	Q9UQB8	BAIAP2	1WDZ_A
>ENSF00000001211	4	P01100	FOS	1A02_F
>ENSF00000000285	19	Q8NHL6	LILRB1	1G0X_A
>ENSF00000001565	4	P50616	TOB1	2D5R_B
>ENSF00000002661	2	Q6XZF7	DNMBP	1UG1_A
>ENSF00000000647	6	P55201	BRPF1	2D9E_A
>ENSF00000001800	2	O96006	DHRSX	2CT5_A
>ENSF00000000849	6	Q9H8S9	MOBK1B	1PI1_A
>ENSF00000000030	2	P03999	OPN1SW	1KPN_A
>ENSF00000000192	21	P15157	TPSB2	1LTO_A
>ENSF00000000192	21	P20231	TPSAB1	1A0L_A
>ENSF00000000254	9	Q14832	GRM3	1S8M_A
>ENSF00000000521	7	Q05586	GRIN1	2NR1_A
>ENSF00000000521	7	Q13224	GRIN2B	1S11_A
>ENSF00000001623	2	P30291	WEE1	1X8B_A
>ENSF00000000001	458	Q8WTR7	ZNF473	2EMB_A

(*Continued*)

Table 5.1. (*Continued*)

Ensembl ID	Family size	Swiss prot ID	Gene name	PDB ID
>ENSF00000000001	458	Q96SE7	ZNF347	2EMA_A
>ENSF00000000001	458	Q8NHY6	ZFP28	2EM2_A
>ENSF00000000001	458	Q9H4T2	ZSCAN16	2COT_A
>ENSF00000000822	3	Q86UL8	MAGI2	1UEP_A
>ENSF00000001433	3	Q9H2H8	PPIL3	1XYH_A
>ENSF00000000610	5	P84022	SMAD3	1MHD_A
>ENSF00000000610	5	Q15797	SMAD1	1KHU_A
>ENSF00000000153	12	Q96JP2	MYO15B	2DLP_A

$||\Psi_i||$ = vector norm. This representation is in accord with the identified target sites for the 156 conserved miRNA families (broadly conserved, intermediately conserved and mammalian specific) in 17,444 human genes [8, 15]. The n-th entry in Ψ_i is $\Psi_i(\mathrm{n}) = 1 - 2^{\mathrm{s(i,n)}}$, where $\mathrm{s(i,n)} \leq 0$ is the context score of conserved miRNA-binding site n in the 3'UTR of gene i [18]. Thus, $\Psi_i(\mathrm{n}) = 1$ indicates full repressive efficacy of the nth miRNA conserved site on gene i ($\mathrm{s(i,n)} = -\infty$), while $\Psi_i(\mathrm{n}) = 0$ (or $\mathrm{s(i,n)} = 0$) indicates absolute lack of repressive regulatory power. The context score is known to correlate tightly with the post-transcriptional downregulation efficacy, $2^{\mathrm{s(i,n)}}$, of the predicted binding site for the nth miRNA family within the 3'UTR of gene i [18]. Thus, $2^{\mathrm{s(i,n)}} \approx \mathrm{g(i)/g(i,n)}$, where g(i) is the translation level for gene i and $\mathrm{g(i,n)}$ is the i-translation level with knockout of the nth miRNA family. If the n-site in not predicted in the 3'UTR of gene i, $\mathrm{g(i)} = \mathrm{g(i,n)}$ and therefore $\mathrm{s(i,n)} = 0$.

Only paralogs that are significantly co-expressed are likely to produce dosage imbalances if the genes have not diverged significantly. Thus, similarities between mRNA expression profiles of two genes i, j will be assessed by the Pearson correlation coefficient $\eta(i, j)$ of their expression vectors Φ_i and Φ_j. In general, for two expression vectors $\boldsymbol{X}$ and $\boldsymbol{Y}$, the Pearson coefficient is given by

$$\eta(\boldsymbol{X},\boldsymbol{Y}) = \frac{<(X - <X>)(Y - <Y>)>}{\sqrt{<X^2> - <X>^2}\sqrt{<Y^2> - <Y>^2}}, \tag{1}$$

where X, Y are generic coordinates in the vectors $\boldsymbol{X}$ and $\boldsymbol{Y}$ respectively, and $<\,>$ indicates mean over cell types.

For paralogs with significant coexpression, a tolerance to dosage imbalance may still arise through differences in translational repression patterns. Thus, orthogonal miRNA-repression patterns for paralogs with high dosage sensitivity may introduce an escape route to the selection pressure introduced by the dosage imbalance. To test this hypothesis, we introduce the extent of miRNA-target coincidence $\tau(i,j)$, defined as the scalar (dot) product of the two miRNA-target vectors: $\tau(i,j) = \Psi_\mathrm{i}/||\Psi_\mathrm{i}||.\Psi_\mathrm{j}/||\Psi_\mathrm{j}||$.

To determine the dosage sensitivity we calculated the packing deficiency of each gene-encoded protein based on its PDB coordinates, if available. Otherwise, packing deficiency was determined based on homology-threaded structure coordinates adopting as templates PDB-reported paralogs [19]. The input for the computation consists of the set of constraints applied to the spatial structure of the amino acid sequence to be modelled and the output is the 3D structure that best satisfies these constraints.

The resulting homology model was validated by comparing its inferred dehydron pattern with the dehydron pattern predicted from a sequence-based computation of disorder score, as described in the previous chapter [17]. The inability of an isolated protein fold to protect specific intramolecular hydrogen bonds from water attack may lead to a structure-competing backbone hydration with concurrent local or global dismantling of the structure. This view of under-wrapping implies a strong correlation between the degree of solvent exposure of intramolecular hydrogen bonds and the local propensity for structural disorder. Hence, the latter parameter was used to validate the former.

5.5.2 *Dehydron enrichment increases interfacial tension enhancing dosage imbalance*

To assess the selection pressure imposed by dosage imbalance we first consider an exhaustive set of 457 non-singleton human gene families with paralog co-expression at the mRNA level: $<\eta>>0$, $<>=$ family average. This condition is essential since paralogs expressed in different cell types cannot introduce dosage imbalance, regardless of their extent of identity. The families with paralog co-expression are selected to discern the factors that buffer dosage imbalance caused by gene duplication. Thus, the selection pressure may be assessed at the post-transcriptional level in terms of dissimilarities in miRNA-targeting patterns across paralogs.

The families with significant mRNA co-expression were deemed likely to generate dosage imbalance. To assess how these imbalances impinge on the degree of divergence in post-transcriptional repression patterns across paralogs, we must compare families with similar divergence time of gene duplicates. This is so since significant regulatory dissimilarities across paralogs may simply result from long divergence times. Thus, we adopt K_s, the synonymous nucleotide divergence [14], as a proxy for divergence time [20] and bin human families with $<\eta> > 0$ according to their respective maximum K_s over paralog pairs. Each class contains families whose duplicate divergence is located in time vis-a-vis particular speciation events. Thus, we construct four classes of human families with significantly coexpressed paralogs [17]: class I: $K_s > 2.98$ (378 families); class II: $2.98 > K_s > 1.48$ (68 families); class III: $1.48 > K_s > 1.11$ (6 families) and class IV: $K_s < 1.11$ (5 families), in accord with the K_s values between human and orangutan (*Pongo pygmaeus*) ($K_s = 2.98$), human and gorilla (*Gorilla gorilla*) ($K_s = 1.48$) and human and chimpanzee (*Pan troglodytes*) ($K_s = 1.11$) [21]. All K_s values are given as percentages and the data for each orthology class is compiled in Table 5.2.

The conservation-based reliability of miRNA site prediction [8] is the highest in class I and decreases with lower divergence times for duplicate genes. This is so since the condition: K_s (duplicate genes) >

Table 5.2. Dataset of evolutionary, expression, miRNA-based regulation and structural information on human families binned in different K_s-classes.

Ensembl ID	Size	max. K_s	Expression correlation	miRNA-target coincidence	Packing deficiency
Class I. Representative families from 378 with $K_s > 2.98$					
>ENSF00000000529	7	4.7368	0.092	0	58.611
>ENSF00000000100	20	4.3361	0.105	0	57.905
>ENSF00000000139	4	3.5898	0.009	0	57.905
>ENSF00000001722	3	4.5429	0.112	0	57.235
>ENSF00000001167	4	4.257	0.031	0.100156612	49.166
>ENSF00000000095	26	4.8626	0.091	0.100505579	41.711
>ENSF00000001308	3	4.5669	0.137	0.100723554	53.574
>ENSF00000000711	4	4.0037	0.058	0.100919215	43.801
>ENSF00000000137	10	5.618	0.054	0.146230992	40.942
>ENSF00000000284	10	4.2759	0.099	0.146538636	41.175
>ENSF00000001426	4	3.7137	0.026	0.183940909	31.682
>ENSF00000000564	5	4.4951	0.052	0.184436777	38.162
>ENSF00000002030	3	4.5383	0.032	0.203391736	44.664
>ENSF00000001001	2	3.1208	0.201	0.204847727	41.439
>ENSF00000001947	3	4.5458	0.355	0.206692562	44.336
>ENSF00000000469	6	4.2126	0.369	0.207894326	47.726
>ENSF00000001542	3	4.9462	0.088	0.20806405	33.63
>ENSF00000001394	3	4.4438	0.185	0.215967149	40.265
>ENSF00000000676	4	5.1652	0.052	0.220155165	32.679
>ENSF00000000750	4	4.555	0.032	0.249786777	31.144
>ENSF00000000662	6	4.1415	0.148	0.252284504	33.377
>ENSF00000000678	3	4.398	0.077	0.259919421	29.562
>ENSF00000001387	4	4.6489	0.132	0.265183678	33.705
>ENSF00000001289	2	3.2296	0.234	0.289453099	37.129
>ENSF00000002412	2	3.5859	0.504	0.291411364	34.575
>ENSF00000000546	7	4.4044	0.314	0.29621157	37.76
>ENSF00000001974	3	5.605	0.116	0.301903926	31.719
>ENSF00000001090	4	3.8111	0.092	0.30237686	38.952
>ENSF00000002334	3	4.0352	0.117	0.305980165	26.024
>ENSF00000001936	2	5.4117	0.076	0.309117355	26.752
>ENSF00000000747	3	4.4318	0.239	0.326588636	39.481
>ENSF00000001530	3	4.1787	0.1	0.326981198	36.141
>ENSF00000001820	2	3.007	0.048	0.337169628	34.925
>ENSF00000001225	3	4.5539	0.042	0.436954752	35.533
>ENSF00000004001	2	3.5857	0.042	0.467541529	21.877
>ENSF00000001160	3	3.8174	0.393	0.746814463	19.7721

(*Continued*)

Table 5.2. (*Continued*)

Ensembl ID	Size	max. K_s	Expression correlation	miRNA-target coincidence	Packing deficiency
Class II. The 68 human families with $2.98 > K_s > 1.48$					
>ENSF00000001825	2	2.9144	0.041	0	58.601
>ENSF00000001266	2	2.6079	0.155	0	57.999
>ENSF00000000708	2	1.7241	0.157	0	58.999
>ENSF00000003280	2	2.9426	0.201	0	57.981
>ENSF00000001173	3	2.6772	0.23	0	56.613
>ENSF00000001409	3	2.0711	0.473	0	56.132
>ENSF00000004229	2	2.0857	0.062	0	55.729
>ENSF00000000656	5	2.736	0.471	0	55.62
>ENSF00000001587	2	2.6153	0.452	0	55.192
>ENSF00000000881	2	2.4164	0.12	0	54.574
>ENSF00000000675	5	2.4562	0.009	0	54.434
>ENSF00000001679	2	2.3438	0.48	0	54.33
>ENSF00000001375	4	2.2318	0.217	0	54.074
>ENSF00000001081	2	2.864	0.392	0	54.036
>ENSF00000000178	7	1.9737	0.146	0	53.456
>ENSF00000000572	2	2.1986	0.045	0	53.121
>ENSF00000003334	2	1.7844	0.035	0	52.671
>ENSF00000002313	2	1.8049	0.018	0	52.216
>ENSF00000000436	5	2.8531	0.29	0	51.945
>ENSF00000000074	21	2.7213	0.061	0	51.689
>ENSF00000003192	3	2.3561	0.4	0	51.646
>ENSF00000001401	3	2.8501	0.041	0	51.446
>ENSF00000000271	16	2.2647	0.292	0	51.438
>ENSF00000001153	4	2.6993	0.155	0	51.215
>ENSF00000001694	3	2.0918	0.258	0	51.198
>ENSF00000003861	2	1.6126	0.243	0	50.846
>ENSF00000001802	2	1.6984	0.537	0	50.768
>ENSF00000000847	4	2.8478	0.376	0	50.687
>ENSF00000001880	2	1.9662	0.219	0	50.687
>ENSF00000003481	2	1.8106	0.446	0	50.687
>ENSF00000003653	2	2.2285	0.183	0	50.332
>ENSF00000001645	3	2.2403	0.206	0	50.135
>ENSF00000000637	8	1.9319	0.041	0	50.062
>ENSF00000002038	2	1.8469	0.109	0	52.797
>ENSF00000002767	2	2.2562	0.07	0	52.795
>ENSF00000001162	5	2.0596	0.097	0	53.704
>ENSF00000001747	2	1.7805	0.019	0	52.532
>ENSF00000000570	6	2.1163	0.013	0	52.377

Table 5.2. *(Continued)*

Ensembl ID	Size	max. K_s	Expression correlation	miRNA-target coincidence	Packing deficiency
>ENSF00000000671	3	2.2928	0.178	0	52.279
>ENSF00000000389	5	2.4549	0.22	0	53.107
>ENSF00000002053	2	1.8579	0.411	0	58.107
>ENSF00000001405	2	2.2754	0.042	0	58.055
>ENSF00000002395	4	2.5819	0.365	0	57.152
>ENSF00000000402	5	2.2446	0.561	0.056	57.012
>ENSF00000001931	5	2.3206	0.035	0.091	45.743
>ENSF00000003072	2	2.0413	0.093	0	54.973
>ENSF00000000492	6	1.9765	0.195	0.141	44.787
>ENSF00000002120	2	2.6622	0.02	0	54.427
>ENSF00000004883	4	2.7168	0.14	0	53.174
>ENSF00000002772	4	1.7219	0.132	0.094	51.132
>ENSF00000001313	3	2.5443	0.099	0.064	50.351
>ENSF00000001227	3	2.1405	0.285	0.17	33.99
>ENSF00000001199	2	2.9308	0.411	0.098	38.351
>ENSF00000001760	2	1.8274	0.123	0.088	37.322
>ENSF00000001365	3	1.5327	0.112	0.162	37.295
>ENSF00000000850	3	1.6986	0.193	0.335	22.644
>ENSF00000001242	3	1.8311	0.58	0.204	36.633
>ENSF00000002009	3	2.1064	0.339	0.267	31.05
>ENSF00000003693	2	2.8605	0.132	0.256	34.582
>ENSF00000000931	3	1.9106	0.07	0.35	24.055
>ENSF00000001181	3	2.5267	0.093	0.279	28.222
>ENSF00000000463	4	1.9925	0.134	0.152	32.358
>ENSF00000004286	2	1.869	0.564	0.385	29.439
>ENSF00000001127	2	2.7223	0.688	0.367	29.419
>ENSF00000000265	14	2.0125	0.699	0.213	28.91
>ENSF00000001157	4	2.3618	0.064	0.169	27.24
>ENSF00000002286	2	2.4737	0.046	0.41	17.284
>ENSF00000000715	9	2.4495	0.237	0.707	24.718
Class III. The 6 human families with $1.48 > K_s > 1.11$					
>ENSF00000001699	2	1.4313	0.223	0.408	21.703
>ENSF00000001755	4	1.4269	5.00E-001	0.136	31.305
>ENSF00000001091	4	1.4047	0.112	0.333	21.279
>ENSF00000000239	5	1.3547	0.442	0.298	34.019
>ENSF00000001198	3	1.3243	0.335	0	55.438
>ENSF00000000360	6	1.3127	0.18	0.343	27.938

(Continued)

Table 5.2. (*Continued*)

Ensembl ID	Size	max. K_s	Expression correlation	miRNA-target coincidence	Packing deficiency
Class IV. The 5 human families with 1.11 > K_s					
>ENSF00000000399	13	1.102	0.138	0	43.174
>ENSF00000002309	2	1.0081	0.551	0	49.846
>ENSF00000000530	19	0.615	0.23	0	49.235
>ENSF00000002885	2	0.4883	0.012	0	47.305
>ENSF00000000786	6	0.28	0.107	0	43.32

K_s (speciation) implies that orthologs of the paralog human genes are likely to be found in the diverging species [22]. Thus, paralogs for families in class I are likely to have orthologs in orangutan, gorilla and chimpanzee, those in class II, only in gorilla and chimpanzee, etc.

Human families with paralog coexpression and the most reliable miRNA site inference (class I) exhibit a tight anticorrelation ($R^2 = 0.697$) between packing deficiency and miRNA-target coincidence (Fig. 5.4): *paralogs with deficient packing are more likely to be localized separated from each other as dictated by their dissimilar miRNA-target patterns of post-transcriptional regulation:* $<\tau> \rightarrow 0$ *as* $<v> \rightarrow$ *maximum* $\approx$ *58%*. These disjoint localization patterns reduce paralog competition for binding partners, thereby buffering the evolution-related dosage imbalance. This result highlights the role of miRNA regulation as a capacitor for dosage imbalance.

An even tighter anticorrelation between packing deficiency and miRNA target coincidence is found for family class II ($R^2 = 0.792$, Fig. 5.4). The slope of the linear fit obtained by the least squares linear regression is now significantly larger in magnitude (−69.34 versus −57.54 for class I). This implies that for a fixed level of packing deficiency, a more effective buffer (lower miRNA target coincidence) is needed for the newer families (K_s-class II) than for the older ones (K_s-class I). This result is expected since a longer exposure of surviving paralogs to the selection pressure promoted by dosage imbalance is likely to promote higher level of adaptation

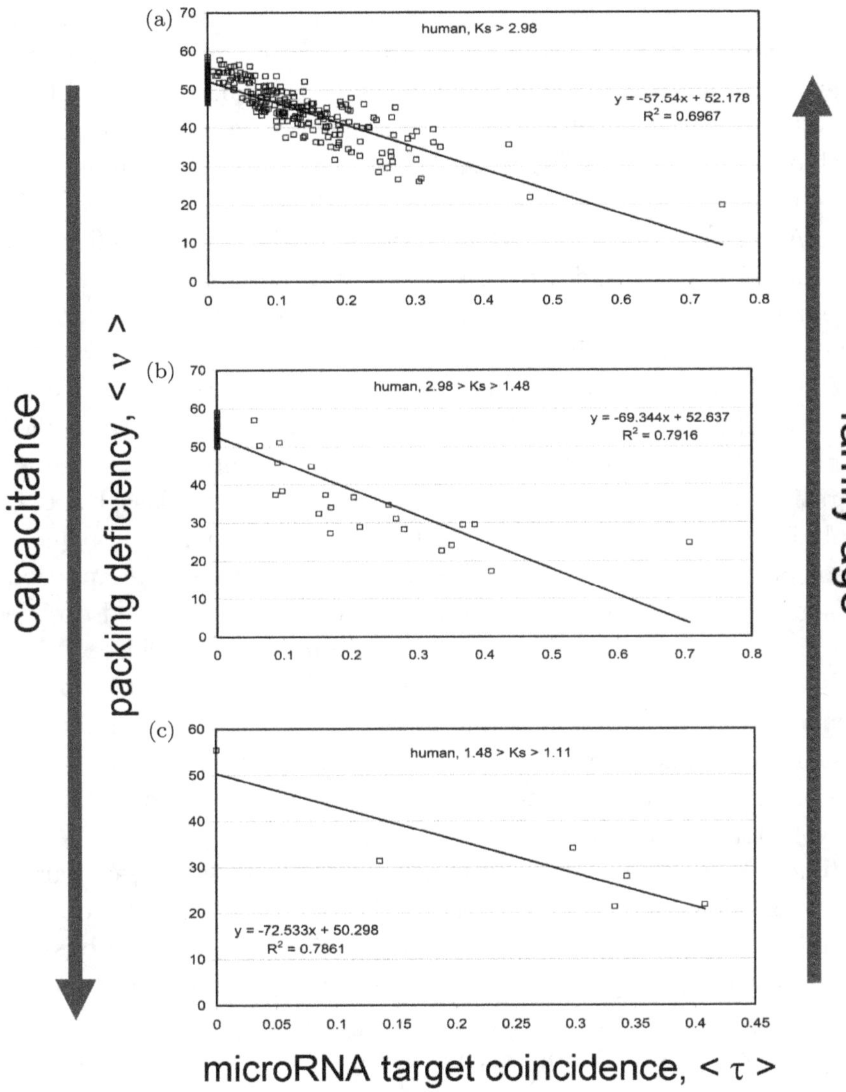

Figure 5.4. Negative correlation between under-wrapping or packing deficiency (ν) and miRNA target coincidence (τ) for human families in K_s-classes I (**A**), II (**B**), III (**C**). The linear fits were obtained by least-squares linear regression.

through functional divergence, and hence, as older paralogs become more differentiated, a capacitance to dosage imbalance becomes less necessary. The same trend is apparent as we examine class III (slope -72.53, $R^2 = 0.786$), although the scarcity of the data precludes a reliable statistical analysis. Class IV consists of only 5 families and hence no trend can be established, except that all families have zero miRNA target coincidence irrespective of their packing deficiency. This fact is clearly indicative of a pressing need to buffer dosage imbalances arising from duplicates that have not yet undergone sufficient functional differentiation.

The trends in terms of tighter $\nu - \tau$-anticorrelation and steeper slope as classes with lower K_s are considered (Fig. 5.4) implies that a miRNA-based capacitance to dosage imbalance is more operative for younger families (classes II–IV versus class I). This result is compatible with the fact that selection pressure on more recent paralogs has had comparably less time to promote adaptation through functional divergence and hence duplication-related dosage imbalances are more significant than those in older families.

These results reveal that the human capacitance to dosage imbalance is in part required due to the inefficiency of the selection pressure on duplicate genes, precluding sufficient differentiation over the evolutionary times of the latest speciations, thereby maintaining an evolutionarily related dosage imbalance.

The results of Fig. 5.4 imply that miRNA target dissimilarity across paralogs may be assimilated to a capacitance to dosage imbalance effects arising from gene duplication. The severity of such effects is in turn quantified by packing deficiency: Dosage imbalances are less tolerated for deficiently packed proteins forcing paralogs to be localized separately from each other.

5.6 Human capacitance to cope with the impact of dosage imbalances

In this section we examined dosage imbalances that have an evolutionary origin. Thus, gene duplication events generate dosage imbalances that impose selection pressure on paralogs, and the magnitude of the effects of this pressure depend on the extent of under-wrapping or packing deficiency of the gene product. However, this dependence varies widely from unicellular to higher eukaryotes, with human being particularly insensitive to dosage imbalances. In human, there is a significant amount of genes with packing deficiency which are nevertheless extensively duplicated. This suggests that humans are resilient to evolution-related dosage imbalances, a capacitance that may be rationalized in terms of escape routes available to human but not to unicellular organisms, where dosage imbalances have clear deleterious effects.

In the absence of expression dissimilarity, the initially identical paralogs of deficiently packed proteins are subject to high selection pressure because they compete for binding partners needed to maintain structural integrity. Conversely, tight protein packing reduces dosage sensitivity, thereby curbing selection pressure. Cross examination of genetic and structural data reveals that humans have a built-in resilience or capacitance to dosage imbalances. The determinant of this human capacitance is traced in this chapter to the paralog-discriminatory power of miRNA regulatory patterns. In this way, dissimilar paralog localization governed by post-transcriptional regulation of protein levels mitigates the competition of paralogs for common binding partners that become obligatory for proteins of low packing quality. In other words, dissimilarity in paralog localization operative through miRNA control offers an escape route to dosage imbalances created by gene duplication, and this escape route becomes more necessary as protein packing deficiency makes these dosage imbalances less tolerable.

If selection is indeed inefficient in human as Lynch and coworkers proposed [3], one may wonder how miRNA-based capacitance could be achieved through random genetic drift. The removal of a miRNA binding site is readily achievable through a single deleterious mutation in one paralog and is unlikely to occur at the same binding site in another paralog. For instance, if M non-overlapping miRNA-binding sites are present in the 3'UTR of two paralogs ($1 \ll M < 156$), the probability that a pair of mutations (one in each paralog) will discriminate paralogs is $(M - 1)/M$, while the probability that they both occur at the same site in the two paralogs and hence do not contribute to increase the capacitance is 1/M. Thus, dissimilarity and even orthogonality in post-transcriptional repressive patterns is readily achievable through widespread random mutation and hence may be the result of the nonadaptive forces prevalent in human.

5.7 Due to low population, humans are exposed to fitness catastrophes

Human biological functions are exquisitely regulated and resilient to external variations, owing to complicated webs of interactions. Yet, we may be doomed as a species precisely because of the way in which our complexity arose [24]. Paraphrasing science writer Philip Ball, nature seems to have activated a time bomb, and our complexity is only a short-term fix [25, 26].

To grasp the nature of the problem, we need to examine orthologous proteins across vastly different species [24].

As previously said, it has been generally recognized that the basic "fold" of a protein is conserved across species, because there is a tight correspondence between structure and function. Proteins that retain the same function across different species — generally the case with orthologs — are expected to keep the same fold. But the sequence of amino acids that make up the protein chains in these orthologs can vary significantly. Sometimes the extent of sequence identity between two orthologs can be as low as 25%, and yet their folds remain strikingly similar, attesting to the robustness of function to evolutionary change.

This conservation of the protein fold across species makes the origin of our complexity even more puzzling, as it is well known that the number of human genes is deceptively small, merely one order of magnitude larger than that of, say, rice. If the structure of the proteins is conserved across species, where is our complexity coming from? Better still, in what sense are we more complex?

We have discovered subtle structural variations occurring in orthologs from species that diverged from each other billions of years ago. In these structures, a feature subtler than overall topology changes across orthologs [24]. The structure in some seems "looser" than in others — less well wrapped, with surface regions that enable surrounding water to penetrate and disrupt the structure by interacting favorably with the protein backbone. These structural vulnerabilities known as *dehydrons* have been extensively studied in the preceding chapters.

As we examine orthologs, the proteins become more structurally degraded, or richer in dehydrons, in species with a lower effective population — a somewhat elusive indicator inversely related to the size and reproductive complexity of the organism (Fig. 5.2(a–c)). Thus, humans have significantly smaller (ten or more orders of magnitude) population than bacteria [24].

The observation that structural degradation is a reflection of decreasing species population (Fig. 5.2(a–c)) resonates in the field of evolution, because natural selection is known to be more inefficient as the population gets smaller [24–26]. Structural degradation is thus an indicator of the species' exposure to random genetic drift: mildly deleterious mutations that would typically degrade the protein structure are more likely to be selected against in bacteria before they can become fixed in the entire population (estimated in trillions of individuals), whereas such a mutation has a far better chance of prevailing in humans.

A protein that is richer in dehydrons than its ortholog is more vulnerable to becoming disrupted by surrounding water. Precisely for this reason, it becomes more reliant on binding partners to maintain its structural integrity. Furthermore, dehydrons are known to be sticky (chapter 2), so structurally degraded proteins are more likely to promote protein-protein associations than orthologs with a lower dehydron content. Thus, *protein-protein interactions, a hallmark of organismic complexity, are actually promoted by random genetic drift, the evolutionary force behind the protein degradation process.*

So, it seems, complexity is not really naturally selected, but instead arises as a short-term fix to the effects of selection inefficiency. At first reading, this assertion seems counterintuitive, but the root of the paradox is simply our dogmatic way of thinking, where complex traits are expected to be an outcome of natural selection.

And where is nature's gambit taking us? As shown in Chapter 4, the proteins with the largest accumulation of uncompensated structural defects are the prions, soluble proteins so poorly wrapped that they relinquish their functionally competent fold and form aberrant aggregates that may cause degenerative neuropathies.

This extreme case of an "aberrantly needy protein" illustrates the high level of genetic risk to which we are exposed as a species due to our small population. The prion is a "fitness" catastrophe that gives us clues as to where nature's gambit might take the human species. Perhaps the long-term evolutionary cost of our complexity is simply too high. Our survival as a species will ultimately depend on our ability to mitigate the fitness cost of our complexity through increasingly arduous therapeutic solutions.

Other fitness catastrophes seem to be in the horizon for the human species as dehydron enrichment caused by random genetic drift creates significant deviations from the architectural constraints required to maintain the structural integrity of soluble proteins (Chapter 4). If we monitor over species within established orthologies [24] the deviation $\Delta(\mathrm{X}, \mathrm{Y}) = \mathrm{Y} - (5\mathrm{X} + 20)$ from the $\mathrm{Y} = 5\mathrm{X} + 20$ rule (Y = number of dehydrons per 100 backbone hydrogen bonds; X = number of disulfide bonds per 100 aminoacids) averaged over proteins for each species, we can see that the human species is ostensible more vulnerable to fitness catastrophes than species with significantly larger population (Fig. 5.5).

5.8 Evolutionary insights for the drug designer

As discussed, in spite of the striking structural similarity arising from common ancestry, both ortholog and paralog proteins exhibit vast differences in their wrapping or dehydron patterns. However, the root of these variations is very different depending on whether orthologs or paralogs are considered. As indicated in the previous sections, differences in selection efficiency across species appear to be responsible for wrapping differences across orthologs. On the other hand, in the case of paralogs, significant dosage imbalances would arise if paralogs were identical, simply because paralogs coexist

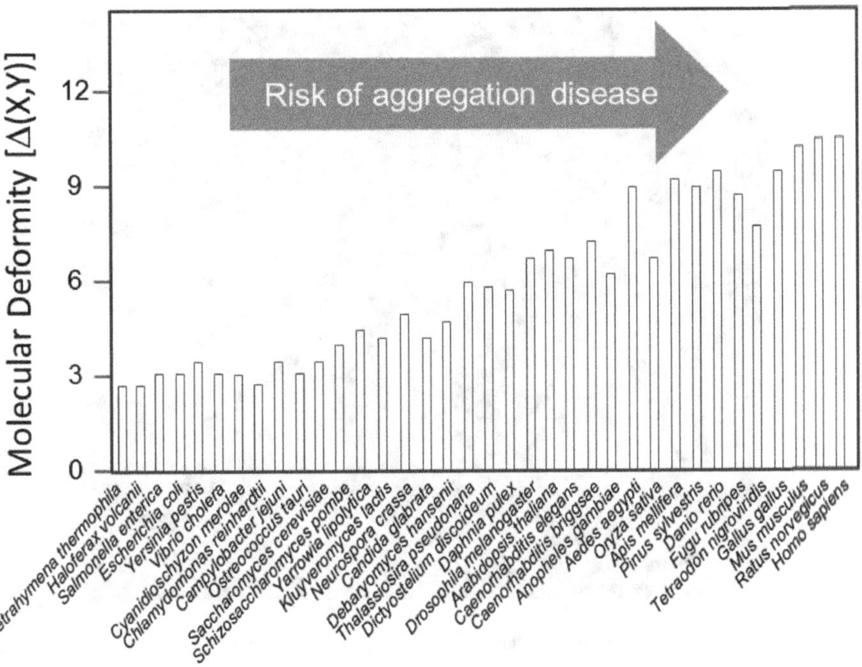

Figure 5.5. Averaged deviation $\Delta(X,Y)$, named molecular deformity, for 36 species with established protein orthologies [24].

in the same individual. To avert such imbalances and their fitness consequences, sufficient divergence of the original duplicate genes must take place through dissimilar expression regulation. Thus, in the previous sections we showed how paralog segregation is evolutionarily achieved.

An alternative evolutionary route to differentiate paralogs as needed to buffer the dosage imbalances they create is through dissimilar wrapping of their otherwise highly similar 3D-structures (Fig. 5.6). *This phenomenon has profound consequences for drug design because it enables designers to discriminate paralogs guided by their different dehydron patterns, exploiting the idea that a drug may function as an external wrapper of the packing defects in the target protein.*

Differences in wrapping patterns may be significant even for close paralogs with high levels (~88%) of sequence identity, such as the

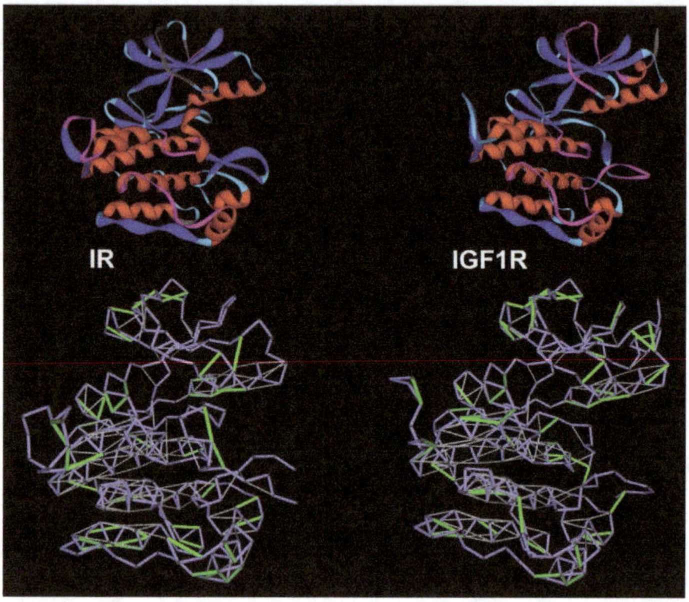

Figure 5.6. Comparison of structures (ribbon representation) and wrapping patterns of the human paralog kinases for the IR (insulin receptor) and the IGF1R (insulin-like growth factor 1 receptor).

kinase domains of the insulin receptor (IR) and that of the insulin-like growth factor receptor (IGF1R), as shown in Fig. 5.6. From the perspective of molecular targeted cancer therapy, there is a vested interest in engineering drugs able to discriminate between these two paralogs: IGF1R is probably a major target in the treatment of breast cancer [23], while inhibition of the IR kinase is likely to have devastating consequences, even the risk of inducing a diabetic coma in the patient. Yet, harnessing on the wrapping design concept, it should be possible to target differences in the wrapping patterns of both kinases (Fig. 5.6) to enhance therapeutic efficacy against breast cancer.

On the other hand, the observation that there are wrapping differences across orthologous proteins should also have a significant impact for the drug designer. *For example, the therapeutic efficacy of drugs is routinely tested in animal models through xenografts and other assays, always under the unwarranted assumption that the affinity and specificity of the drug for its target in human would be the same or very close to its affinity and specificity for the animal ortholog of the targeted protein. In light of the wrapping differences across orthologs, there is simply no assurance that this scenario is indeed valid. This observation could potentially undermine the very foundation on which animal testing is predicated.*

Yet, there is a positive implication of the observed wrapping differences across orthologs, and it relates to the drug-based treatment of infectious diseases such as AIDS. It is indeed highly advantageous for the drug designer to detect wrapping differences between the target protein in the infecting species and its human ortholog, if any: *A drug purposely designed to wrap specific dehydrons in the protein of the infecting species that are not present in the human ortholog is likely to be far less toxic than a drug that cannot tell apart the two orthologs.* Species selectivity is hardly a concern in an AIDS treatment geared at targeting the reverse transcriptase of the HIV-1 retrovirus, simply because this protein is not encoded in the human genome. On the other hand, a molecular design rooted in wrapping differences would be very helpful if the goal is to target a retroviral protein that is also represented in the human proteome. Species selectivity matters in this last context.

5.9 Drug designer's take-home message from epistructural evolution

In spite of the promises of the post-genomic era, structure-based drug design did not live up to the expectations, becoming a sort of hit-and-miss endeavor. Drug discovery and development remain serendipitous and deeply rooted in high-throughput screening methodologies. The methods of epistructural biology are intended to put rational drug design back on its feet, and thus, need to address the main hurdle that marred most structure-based design efforts: *the control of drug specificity*. The results of this chapter suggest that this goal may indeed be within reach, as schematically shown in Fig. 5.7. The crux of the argument is that protein homologies are the culprit for the

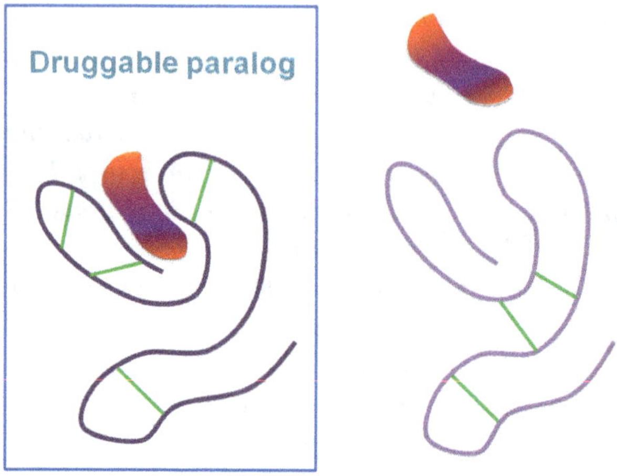

Figure 5.7. Differences in dehydron patterns across paralogous proteins sharing the same fold topology may be targeted by dehydron-wrapping ligands to achieve specificity, thus telling apart proteins with common ancestry in the human species.

lack of control of specificity in structure-based designs because of the structural similarity between target and off-target homologs, while variations in dehydron patterns across homologs may be targeted by dehydron-wrapping drugs to achieve the desired specificity.

References

1. Fernández A, Scott R, Berry RS (2004) The nonconserved wrapping of conserved folds reveals a trend towards increasing connectivity in proteomic networks. *Proc Natl Acad Sci USA* 101:2823–2827.
2. Fernández A, Berry RS (2004) Molecular dimension explored in evolution to promote proteomic complexity. *Proc Natl Acad Sci USA* 101:13460–13465.
3. Lynch M, Conery JS (2003) The origins of genome complexity. *Science* 302:1401–1404.
4. Kondrashov FA, Koonin EV (2004) A common framework for understanding the origin of genetic dominance and evolutionary fates of gene duplications. *Trends Genet* 20:287–290.
5. Liang H, Rogale-Plazonic K, Chen J, Li WH, Fernández A (2008) Protein under-wrapping causes dosage sensitivity and decreases gene duplicability. *PLoS Genetics* 4:e11.
6. Papp B, Pal C, Hurst LD (2003) Dosage sensitivity and the evolution of gene families in yeast. *Nature* 424:194–197.

7. Fernández A, Scheraga H (2003) Insufficiently dehydrated hydrogen bonds as determinants for protein interactions. *Proc Natl Acad Sci USA* 100:113–118.
8. Bartel D (2009) MicroRNAs: Target recognition and regulatory functions. *Cell* 136:215–233.
9. Fernández A (2004) Keeping dry and crossing membranes. *Nature Biotech* 22:1081–1084.
10. Veitia RA (2002) Exploring the etiology of haploinsufficiency. *Bioessays* 24:175–184.
11. Veitia RA (2004) Gene dosage balance: Deletions, duplications and dominance. *Trends Genet* 21:33–35.
12. Su AI, Wiltshire T, Batalov S, *et al.* (2004) A gene atlas of the mouse and human protein-encoding transcriptomes. *Proc Natl Acad Sci USA* 101:6062–6067.
13. Birney E, Andrews D, Caccamo M, *et al.* (2006) Ensembl 2006. *Nucl Acids Res* 34:D556–D561.
14. Yang Z, Nielsen R (2000) Estimating synonymous and nonsynonymous substitution rates under realistic evolutionary models. *Mol Biol Evol* 17:32–43.
15. Friedman RC, Farth KK, Burge CB, Bartel DP (2009) Most mammalian mRNAs are conserved targets of microRNAs. *Genome Res* 19:92–105.
16. Lewis B, Burge C, Bartel D (2005) Conserved seed pairing, often flanked by adenosines, indicates that thousands of human genes are microRNA targets. *Cell* 120:15–20.
17. Fernández A, Chen J (2009) Human capacitance to dosage imbalance: Coping with inefficient selection. *Genome Res* 19:2185–2192.
18. Grimson A, Farth KK, Johnston WK, *et al.* (2007) MicroRNA target specificity in mammals: Determinants beyond seed pairing. *Molecular Cell* 27:91–105.
19. Aloy P, Ceulemans H, Stark A, Russell RB (2003) The relationship between sequence and interaction divergence in proteins. *J Mol Biol* 332:989–998.
20. Gu Z, Nicolae D, Lu HH, Li W-H (2002) Rapid divergence in expression between duplicate genes inferred from microarray data. *Trends Genet* 18:609–613.
21. Chen F, Li W-H (2001) Genomic divergences between humans and other hominoids and the effective population size of the common ancestor of humans and chimpanzees. *Am J Hum Genet* 68:444–456.
22. Gao L, Innan H (2004) Very low gene duplication rate in the yeast genome. *Science* 306:1367–1370.
23. Surmacz E, Bartucci M (2005) Role of estrogen receptor alpha in modulating IGF-I receptor signaling and function in breast cancer. *J Exp Clin Cancer Res* 23:385–94.
24. Fernández A, Lynch M (2011) Nonadaptive origins of interactome complexity. *Nature* 474:502–505.

25. Ball P (2011) The Achilles' heel of biological complexity. Nature:Published online 18 May 2011 doi:10.1038/news.2011.294
26. Ball P (2011) Why Are You So Complex? Complicated Protein Interactions Evolved to Stave Off Mutations. Scientific American:Published online 18 May 2011 (http://www.scientificamerican.com/article/complicated-protein-interactions-evolved-to-stave-off-mutations/)

Chapter 6

Epistructural biochemistry

This chapter unravels the catalytic role of dehydrons in biological chemistry. It prompts a significant revision of the field to encompass the chemical functionality of frustrated interfacial water. Through the induced functionalization of vicinal water, the dehydron is shown to be an enabler and a promoter of enzymatic activity.

Interfacial water molecules around dehydrons become proton acceptors, an observation likely to revolutionize mechanistic aspects of biological chemistry. Most if not all transesterification reactions requiring the prior functionalization of nucleophilic groups will need to be revised to incorporate the catalytic enablement promoted by nearby dehydrons. Thus, a novel reactant ubiquitous in biological chemistry has been discovered and a frustration-based chemistry has been invented.

6.1 Catalytic dehydrons

This chapter is concerned with the biochemical role of dehydrons in protein enzymes. Our goal is to prove that dehydrons are not only stimulants but also enablers of enzymatic activity, hence prompting a substantial revision of the mechanistic aspects of biological chemistry. This general result has crucial consequences for drug design as it points to dehydrons as key targetable elements to block protein functions for therapeutic effect.

To assess the biochemical function of dehydrons, particular attention will be paid to what is likely to be the most ubiquitous mechanistic motif in biological chemistry: the functionalization of a nucleophile followed by nucleophilic attack leading to group substitution and displacement. Most biochemical transformations subsume this ubiquitous mechanistic motif in their underlying enzymatic function. However, the functionalization of the nucleophile itself is problematic and the extant explanations are befuddling. Let us generically denote the nucleophilic group as "-NucH", and the nearby proton acceptor as "AcH". The nucleophile functionalization is mechanistically described typically with a single elementary step: $\mathrm{AcH} + -\mathrm{NucH} \rightarrow [\mathrm{AcH_2}]^+ + [-\mathrm{Nuc}:]^-$. Yet, the species $[\mathrm{AcH_2}]^+$ is typically more acidic (lower pKa) than −NucH, hence the elementary step becomes unfeasible unless the enzymatic nanoenvironmental conditions enable the proton transfer, with effective pKa's satisfying: $\mathrm{pKa}([\mathrm{AcH_2}]^+) > \mathrm{pKa}(-\mathrm{NucH})$, which is the reverse of the relation that holds in bulk solvent: $\mathrm{pKa}([\mathrm{AcH_2}]^+) < \mathrm{pKa}(-\mathrm{NucH})$. The most common realization of this scheme is obtained when $\mathrm{AcH} = \mathrm{H_2O}$ and $-\mathrm{NucH} = -\mathrm{NH_2}$. In this realization, the paradox arises because the hydronium ion ($\mathrm{H_3O^+}$) is certainly more acidic than the ammonium group ($-\mathrm{NH_3^+}$) in the bulk phase, so it is unlikely or at least befuddling to postulate that the ammonium would get functionalized by handing a proton over to a water molecule.

Usually, through a cumbersome and uncertain quantum mechanical computation plagued with adjustable parameters and an arbitrary QM/MM (quantum mechanics/molecular mechanics) frontier, researchers have been able to assert the relative acidities that enable the functionalizing proton transfer in the quasi-condensed phase. This type of QM/MM computation provides no insightful justification other than the fact that the enzyme molecule furnishes a "special solvent environment" that is often distortive of bulk-phase affinities.

The quantum mechanical computation becomes greatly facilitated and insightful when we consider the fact that dehydrons shape the active sites of protein enzymes, as demonstrated in this chapter. In fact, the water molecule vicinal to a dehydron becomes functionalized into a proton acceptor, a chemical role that is directly related to the extent of frustration induced by the dehydron on the surrounding solvent. Thus, the dehydron may be regarded as a biochemical quasi-reactant. As such it would need to be broadly incorporated into the mechanisms of biological chemistry. Furthermore, because of its enabling role in protein function, coupled with its inherent stickiness demonstrated in chapter 2, the dehydron becomes a decisive targetable feature in the therapeutic quest to impair specific biochemical pathways.

The dielectric behavior of epistructural water in soluble proteins and other solutes endowed with nanometer-level detail is a subject of intense scrutiny [1–4]. The understanding and manipulation of such interfaces require a multiscale approach to water dielectrics, as described in the previous chapters. Such an approach demands a conceptual departure from the so-called "Debye *ansatz*" [1] intensely advocated by Arieh Warshel and coworkers [5] in their extrapolation from macroscopic behavior. The Debye ansatz has been incorrectly taken to mean that water polarization $\vec{P}$ at the protein-water interface must align with the internal electrostatic field $\vec{E}$ of the solute: $\vec{P} = \overrightarrow{P^{\parallel}}$, where $\overrightarrow{P^{\parallel}}$ is the Debye polarization component. In contrast with the bulk hydrogen-bond pattern, water molecules under nanoscale confinement are forced to relinquish hydrogen bonding opportunities to fit in the nanometer cavity, generating a net polarization component $\overrightarrow{P^{\#}}$ orthogonal and statistically independent of $\vec{E}$. While the Debye polarization introduces the well-known rescaling (screening) of the inherent solute charge [5], a consequence of the resilience of water structure to variations in the electrostatic field, the orthogonal polarization component induces an $\vec{E}$-independent net charge $\gamma^{\#} = -\vec{\nabla}\cdot\overrightarrow{P^{\#}}$. This charge contribution is of paramount importance in assessing chemical functionalities related to topographical features of protein interfaces as it generates charges that are not accounted for by the protein chemical composition. As shown in this chapter, this induced charge endows nano-confined water with a chemical functionality in accord with the sign of $\gamma^{\#}$, i.e. proton donor if $\gamma^{\#} > 0$ and proton acceptor if $\gamma^{\#} < 0$. Thus, the inequality $\gamma^{\#} > 0$ indicates that at least one water hydroxyl proton is on average forced by the interface geometry to relinquish its hydrogen-bonding capability, while $\gamma^{\#} < 0$ implies that at least one water oxygen atom remains on average unpaired to a hydroxyl proton (its orbital-localized lone electron pair is unutilized).

Building on the non-Debye treatment of the water interface, we identify the episteric chemical functionalities arising from nanoscale structural defects in soluble proteins, establishing their role as promoters or enhancers of catalytic activity [6]. To identify the chemical role of interfacial water subject to partial nanoscale confinement, we resort to the non-Debye treatment described in Chapter 2.

Within this framework, the interfacial energy, ΔU_ϕ, associated with spanning the solute-water interface is given by the elastic integral

$$\Delta U_\phi = \int \frac{1}{2}\lambda \parallel \vec{\nabla}\phi \parallel^2 d\vec{r} \tag{1}$$

where the integration is carried over a spatial domain Ω large enough so that its border $\partial\Omega$ is fully contained in bulk water. Thus, Ω is subject to the boundary condition

$$\{\phi(\vec{r}) = 0, \nabla\phi(\vec{r}) = 0\}\, \forall \vec{r} \in \partial\Omega \tag{2}$$

Integration of (1) by parts yields

$$0 \leq \Delta U_\phi = -\frac{1}{2}\lambda \int \phi\nabla^2\phi d\vec{r} = -\frac{1}{2}(\lambda/\varepsilon_0)^{1/2} \int \gamma^{\#}\phi d\vec{r} \tag{3}$$

since $\gamma^{\#} \propto \nabla^2\phi$ (cf. Chapter 2) and

$$\oiint \phi\vec{\nabla}\phi \cdot d\vec{\sigma} = 0 \text{ on } \partial\Omega \tag{4}$$

Since $\phi(\vec{r}) = 4 - g(\vec{r}) \geq 0$, the mean value theorem of integral calculus applied to (3) yields:

$$\gamma^{\#}_{\mathrm{MV}} = -\frac{(\lambda\varepsilon_0)^{\frac{1}{2}} \int ||\vec{\nabla}\phi||^2 d\vec{r}}{\int \phi d\vec{r}} \leq 0 \tag{5}$$

where $\gamma^{\#}_{\mathrm{MV}}$ is the mean-value constant yielding:

$$\gamma^{\#}_{\mathrm{MV}} \int \phi d\vec{r} = \int \gamma^{\#}\phi d\vec{r}. \tag{6}$$

We have then proven the following

Theorem 1: *Interfacial water under local nanoscale confinement with* $\phi \geq 0$ *yields a non-Debye polarization-induced charge* $\gamma^{\#}_{\mathrm{MV}} \leq 0$. *The net negative charge begets a proton-acceptor role compatible with unfulfilled hydrogen-bond coordination of water oxygen (where partial negative charge is located), turning the local interfacial water into a chemical base.*

As noted in Chapter 2, the interfacial tension is generated by dehydrons. While the physico-chemical properties of dehydrons have been characterized in previous work [1, 3] their chemical role has not been assessed so far. To determine the chemical functionality of *individual* dehydrons in the protein structure we consider a covering of the spatial domain Ω made up of M closed convex subsets $\Omega_j\, j = 0, 1, 2, \ldots, M$ fulfilling the following conditions (cf. Fig. 6.1(a)):

1) $\Omega = \bigcup_{j=1}^{M} \Omega_j$
2) For $i \neq j$, $\Omega_i \cap \Omega_j = \partial\Omega_i \cap \partial\Omega_j$ (closed subsets only overlap along their borders).
3) Let the dummy index $j = 1,\ldots$,M label the dehydrons in the protein structure, then the subset $\Omega_j\, j = 0, 1, 2, \ldots$,M contains dehydron j and also satisfies $\Lambda_j = \Lambda_j(\xi_j) \subseteq \Omega_j$, where the set Λ_j is the osculating (first-order contact) sphere of the water-smeared envelope of the protein surface at dehydron j with local curvature ξ_j [7].
4) $\forall j = 0, 1, \ldots;\ \forall \vec{r} \epsilon \Omega_j$ one of the two conditions holds:

   4a) $\{\phi(\vec{r}) = 0,\ \vec{\nabla}\phi(\vec{r}) = 0\}$
   4b) if $\{\phi(\vec{r}) \neq 0$ or $\vec{\nabla}\phi(\vec{r}) \neq 0\}$, $\exists \Omega_j : \vec{r} \epsilon \partial\Omega_i \cap \partial\Omega_j$, and the respective differential area normal vectors $d\vec{\sigma}(\vec{r})$ for $\vec{r}$ on the two subsets cancel each other out (cf. Fig. 6.1(a)).

Given conditions 1–4, the vanishing integral $\oiint \phi\vec{\nabla}\phi \cdot d\vec{\sigma} = 0$ over $\partial\Omega$ may be written as

$$0 = \oiint \phi\vec{\nabla}\phi \cdot d\vec{\sigma} = \sum_{j=1}^{M} \oiint \phi\vec{\nabla}\phi \cdot d\vec{\sigma}_j \tag{7}$$

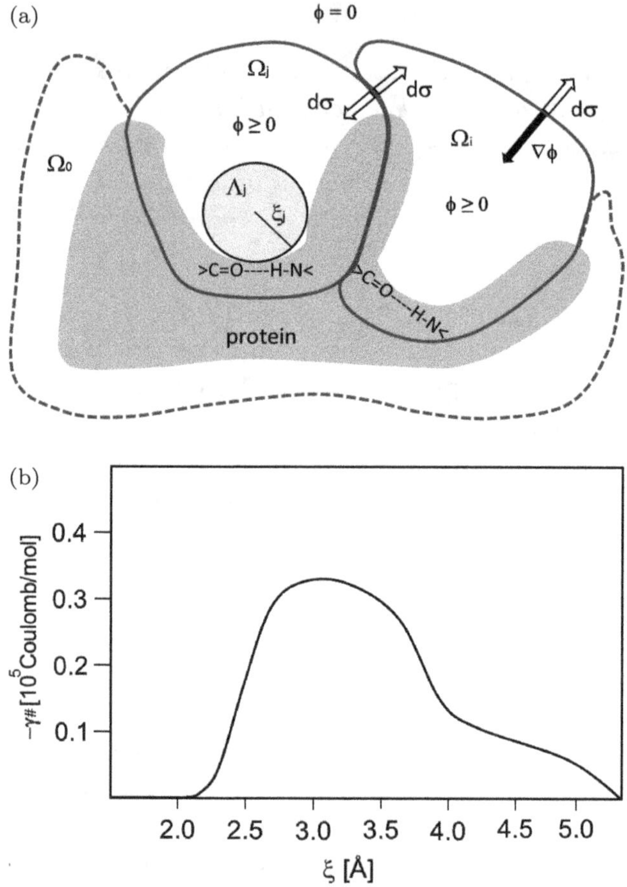

Figure 6.1. **(a)** Schematic representation of the partition of domain Ω into subdomains Ω_n $n = 0, 1, 2, \ldots, M$, where a single subdomain with $n > 0$ is required to contain each ($\phi > 0$)-dehydron in the protein structure and $\Omega_0 = \overline{\Omega \backslash \bigcup_{n=1}^{M} \Omega_n}$ where the over-bar denotes closure. The generic subdomain Ω_j contains the amide-carbonyl dehydron j and the first-order contact (osculating) sphere of the water-smeared envelope of the protein surface at dehydron j. **(b)** Net non-Debye polarization-induced charge $\gamma^{\#}$ as a function of the local curvature radius at a dehydron site. The charge units for $\gamma^{\#}$ are scaled by the proton charge 1.6×10^{-19} Coulomb or $\sim 10^5$Coulomb/mol. Reprinted from [6], copyright 2014 with permission from AIP Publishing LLC.

Where $\oiint \phi\vec{\nabla}\phi \cdot d\vec{\sigma}_j$ denotes the surface integral extended over $\partial\Omega_j$. Thus, we obtain:

$$0 \leq \Delta U_\phi = \frac{1}{2}\sum_{j=1}^{M}\left\{\lambda \oiint \phi\vec{\nabla}\phi \cdot d\vec{\sigma}_j - \left(\frac{\lambda}{\varepsilon_0}\right)^{\frac{1}{2}} \gamma_{\mathrm{MV}}^{\#}(j)\int \phi d\vec{r}_j\right\} \quad (8)$$

where the integral $\int \phi d\vec{r}_j \geq 0$ extends over Ω_j and the mean value constant $\gamma_{\mathrm{MV}}^{\#}(j)$ satisfies the relation: $\gamma_{\mathrm{MV}}^{\#}(j)\int \phi d\vec{r}_j = \int \gamma^{\#}\phi d\vec{r}_j$. Thus, the individual contribution of dehydron j to the protein interfacial tension is

$$0 \leq \frac{1}{2}\oiint \phi\vec{\nabla}\phi \cdot d\vec{\sigma}_j - \frac{1}{2}\left(\frac{\lambda}{\varepsilon_0}\right)^{\frac{1}{2}} \gamma_{\mathrm{MV}}^{\#}(j)\int \phi d\vec{r}_j \quad (9)$$

Since either $\vec{\nabla}\phi(\vec{r}) = 0$ or the vectors $\vec{\nabla}\phi(\vec{r})$ and $d\vec{\sigma}_j(\vec{r})$ point in opposite directions for $\vec{r}\epsilon\partial\Omega_j$ (cf. Fig. 6.1(a)), the following inequality holds for all j's:

$$\frac{1}{2}\oiint \phi\vec{\nabla}\phi \cdot d\vec{\sigma}_j \leq 0 \quad (10)$$

Combining (9) and (10), it follows that $\gamma_{\mathrm{MV}}^{\#}(j) \leq 0$. Thus we have proven the following

Theorem 2: *As a generator of interfacial tension, a dehydron yields a negative non-Debye polarization-induced charge. Thus, interfacial water enveloping a dehydron constitutes a chemical base.*

The proton-acceptor role of dehydrons, or rather, of interfacial water enveloping dehydrons, will probably revolutionize our understanding of biochemical mechanism. It is likely that many if not all intermolecular transesterification reactions in biochemistry requiring the activation of a nucleophilic group will need to be rewritten to incorporate the catalytic enablement provided by nearby dehydrons. In plain terms, *dehydrons have been the missing reactants in the chemical equations of biological catalysis.*

The net contribution to interfacial energy from dehydron j is:

$$\Delta U_\phi(j) = \int \frac{1}{2}\lambda \|\vec{\nabla}\phi\|^2 d\vec{r}_j = -\left(\frac{\lambda}{\varepsilon_0}\right)^{\frac{1}{2}} \gamma^{\#}_{\mathrm{MV}}(j) \int \phi d\vec{r}_j \tag{11}$$

yielding the net non-Debye polarization-induced charge

$$\gamma^{\#}_{\mathrm{MV}}(j) = -\frac{(\lambda\varepsilon_0)^{\frac{1}{2}} \int \|\vec{\nabla}\phi\|^2 d\vec{r}_j}{\int \phi d\vec{r}_j} \tag{12}$$

The disruption of bulk water structure quantified by the field $\phi(\vec{r})$ is computed using the molecular dynamics protocol previously described for dehydron cavities of variable curvature radius 1–6 Å [7]. The results are integrated according to (12) to yield a net non-Debye polarization-induced charge $\gamma^{\#}_{\mathrm{MV}}(j)$ shown in Fig. 6.1(b).

The basicity of dehydrons is in consonance with their abundance near catalytically active side chains involved in nucleophilic attacks in enzymatic reactions, as hereby shown. We may assert that the concentration of ($\phi > 0$)-dehydrons in the vicinity of side chains involved in intermolecular transesterification attests to their proton-acceptor role as promoters of active-site nucleophilicity. Dehydrons vicinal to the catalytic site stabilize the polarized deprotonated state that empowers nucleophilic activity. The paramount importance of this finding will likely invite a major revisiting of biochemical mechanism, as we have already emphasized.

6.2 The dehydron is a reactant in biochemical mechanism

To illustrate the chemical functionality of dehydrons we first examine the dehydron distribution of the aspartic (Asp) protease from HIV-1 virus (PDB.4DJP) [8], a functionally competent homodimer. Each monomer within the complex has two dehydrons located in the vicinity of the active site (Asp25) and at the highly flexible flap (Fig. 6.2), with a single ($\phi > 0$)-dehydron involving the pair Asp25-Ala28. "Vicinal" is hereby defined as being within 6 Å of the α-carbon

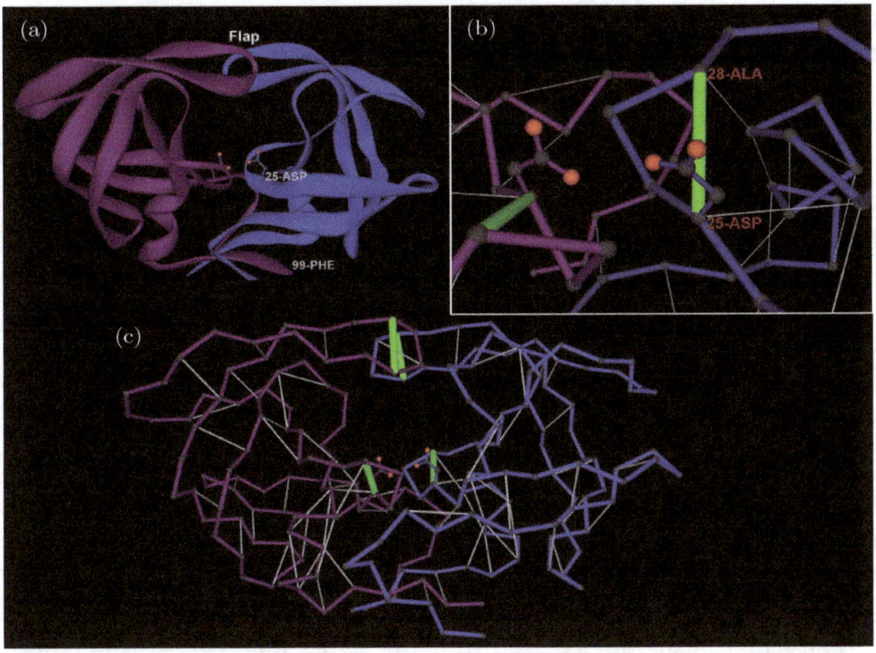

Figure 6.2. **(a)** Ribbon representation of the functional homodimeric HIV-1 protease (PDB.4DJP), with active site Asp25 with displayed side chain. The monomeric chains in the complex are depicted in magenta and blue, respectively. **(b)** Dehydron distribution in HIV-protease. Dehydrons are shown as green segments joining the α-carbons of the paired residues, while solvent-shielded (well wrapped) backbone hydrogen bonds are shown in grey. **(c)** The ($\phi > 0$)-dehydron Asp25-Ala28 flanking the active site Asp25 in the dimeric HIV-1 protease. Reprinted from [6], copyright 2014 with permission from AIP Publishing LLC.

(desolvation domain of a dehydron-paired residue) of the catalytically active residue. Examination of an exhaustive nonredundant set of 198 Asp proteases with PDB representation at resolution better than 1.5 Å and relational Uniprot [9] sequence annotation reveals the same localization pattern of ($\phi > 0$)-dehydrons found exclusively in the vicinity of the active site.

A similar localized concentration of ($\phi > 0$)-dehydrons is identified at phosphorylation sites that involve the participation of a nucleophilic group (usually hydroxyl and less frequently histidine amide) from a side chain (Ser, Thr, Tyr, His) in a transphosphoesterification of the ligand ATP [10]. The reaction promotes the cleavage of the terminal (gamma) phosphoryl group from ATP and its covalent attachment to the protein through a phospho-ester linkage. The net non-Debye polarization-induced charge at such sites is significantly larger in magnitude than that for a control residue of the same type but not susceptible to phosphorylation (Fig. 6.3(a, b)). This assertion has been validated by examining phosphorylation sites with reported local structure [11] in exhaustive nonredundant sets of PDB-reported kinases at resolution better than 1.5 Å with relevant sequence annotation on phosphorylation sites obtained from Uniprot. Thus, we examined 507 Ser/Thr kinases, 214 Tyr kinases and 19 His kinases. The tight correlation ($R^2 = 0.82$) between $\gamma^{\#}$ and bulk pK_a of the phosphorylation-susceptible residue is indicative of the de-protonation requirements of the side-chain group to enhance its nucleophilicity and thereby its susceptibility to phosphorylation. The basicity of the vicinal ($\phi > 0$)-dehydrons as measured by net non-Debye polarization-induced charge functionalizes the residue group implicated in the nucleophilic attack on the ATP terminal phosphoester linkage (Fig. 6.3(c)).

Due to the extremely high pK_a ($\approx$13), the functionalization of Ser/Thr as nucleophile requires a very large vicinal $\gamma^{\#}$-value, which in turn requires a substantial dehydron concentration. This situation is illustrated in the active Ser195 of the serine protease trypsin (PDB.4I8G [12]) that contains 5 vicinal dehydrons (Fig. 6.3(d)), the maximum concentration found in PDB [13]. Since dehydron clusters are unstable and expose the backbone to hydration, they become disruptors of protein structure and so an extreme concentration (>5) of vicinal dehydrons yields a natively disordered region [13], as shown in Chapter 4. Such disordered regions are often found around nucleophilically functional and extreme base-demanding Ser/Thr and may be regarded as "ephemerally basic" since they visit conformations so rich in dehydrons that can only be temporarily

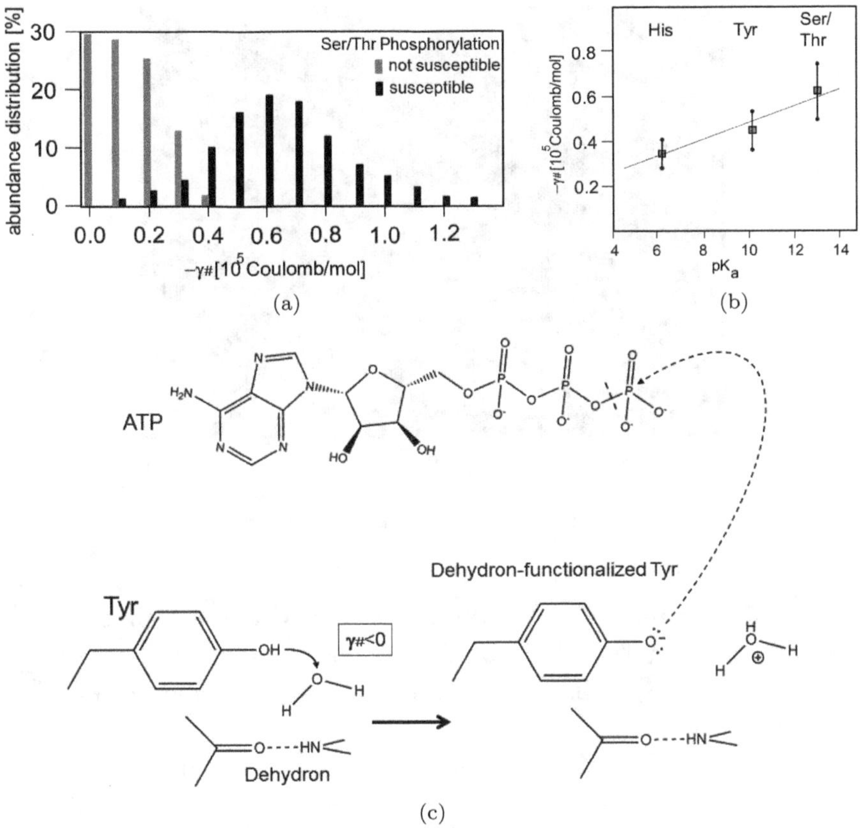

Figure 6.3. **(a)** Abundance distribution of phosphorylation-susceptible Ser/Thr residues according to their vicinal non-Debye polarization-induced charge $\gamma^{\#}$. The $\gamma^{\#}$-distribution for phosphorylation-impervious Ser/Thr residues is displayed as control. **(b)** Dispersion ranges (error bars) of $\gamma^{\#}$-values as a function of bulk pK_a of the phosphorylation-susceptible side-chain group. **(c)** Chemical reaction of trans-phosphoesterification involving a nucleophilic attack on the terminal phosphoester linkage of ATP by a dehydron-functionalized Tyr (the phosphorylation-susceptible residue). The nucleophilicity of the Tyr phenolic hydroxyl is significantly enhanced through polarization induced by the proton-acceptor water molecule that envelops the vicinal dehydron with $\gamma^{\#} < 0$. **(d)** Cluster of five ($\phi > 0$)-dehydrons (maximum concentration) vicinal to the catalytic residue Ser195 in bovine trypsin (PDB.4I8G). The structure is rendered following the convention in Fig. 6.2 with backbone in magenta. The chemical basicity of these structural defects enables the proton relay mechanism from Ser to His in the Ser-His-Asp catalytic triad of this enzyme, which would otherwise be impaired due to the significant gap in pK_a value (~7 log units) between adjacent side chains Ser and His. Reprinted from [6], copyright 2014 with permission from AIP Publishing LLC.

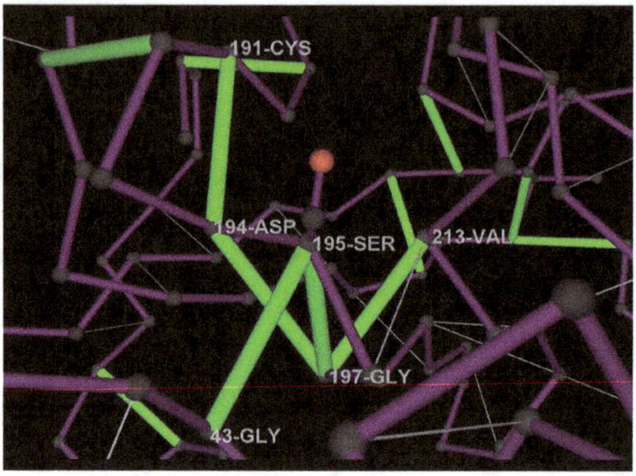

(d)

Figure 6.3. (*Continued*)

sustained in water [13]. Yet, while the dehydrons are present in a transient conformation they act as proton acceptors and functionalize the Ser/Thr by stabilizing the polarized state, switching on their nucleophilic nature.

In the case of serine proteases [14], the high concentration of serine-vicinal ($\phi > 0$)-dehydrons becomes adjuvant to the inherent Ser-His-Asp proton-relay mechanism of such enzymes, facilitating proton transfer from serine to the nearby histidine. It should be noted that such transference is unlikely to occur without the assistance of vicinal basic dehydrons due to the large gap in pK_a (approximately 7 log units) between serine and the nearby histidine in the catalytic triad.

This section reveals the chemical functionality of interfacial water enveloping nanoscale structural defects in soluble proteins or other nano-materials and asserts its role as a quasi-reactant in biochemical reactions. Many such reactions require the activation of protein groups that perform or promote a nucleophilic attack leading to transesterification. This section shows that interfacial water enveloping a dehydron under nanoscale confinement acts as a chemical-base effector, enhancing the nucleophilicity of the adjacent active site. The concept of functionalized episteric water is introduced in this chapter and the results invite a substantive revision of the purported elementary steps in biochemical reactions. On the other hand, novel biomolecular engineering is also likely to emerge from the physico-chemical foundations delineated, as dehydron-based enzymatic effectors may be created or removed though site-directed mutation altering side-chain packing.

6.3 Dehydron-based catalytic engines

The hereby established biochemical role of dehydrons as promoters of basicity actually complements their dehydration propensity [1,3,7] in the context of enzymatic mechanisms. Thus, water enveloping a dehydron becomes a better leaving molecule (hydronium seeking full hydration) as it functionalizes the nucleophilic moiety of the enzyme, while the dehydration propensity of the packing defect induces the expulsion of the hydronium as it promotes the binding of the substrate to the enzyme. This migration of the dehydron-enveloping hydronium is entropically favored due to a gain in translational and conformational freedom as the hydronium is transferred to the bulk, and is also enthalpically favored, as the transference enables the fulfillment of the hydration demands of the hydronium. Thus, the thermodynamic cost of transferring the proton from the pro-catalytic group to the dehydron-functionalized water molecule is defrayed by the subsequent stabilization of the dehydron that results from its wrapping or shielding upon substrate-protein association and by the free-energy gain associated with the transferring of confined ionized water to the bulk region. This established role of the dehydron as a two-step catalytic engine (Fig. 6.4) will surely prompt further research effort, as its impact in biotechnology is predicted to be of vast proportions.

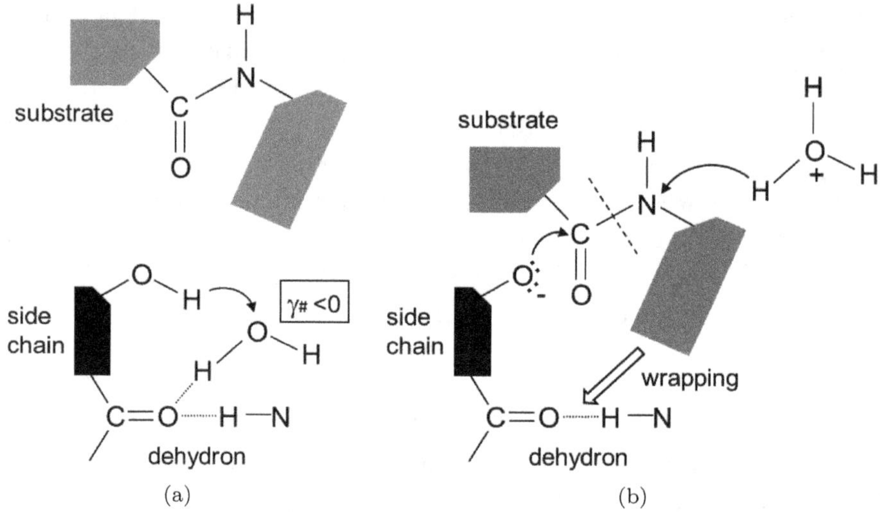

Figure 6.4. The dehydron as a two-step catalytic engine. **(a)** The dehydron functionalizes the nucleophilic group by inducing basicity in vicinal water. **(b)** The dehydron promotes substrate binding and concurrent hydronium expulsion to enable intermolecular trans-esterification.

6.4 Quantum dehydron chemistry

The following sections explore the participation of dehydrons in biochemical events through quantum mechanical (QM) calculations. We delineate the enabling role of dehydrons as activators of nucleophilic groups or enablers of proton transference. As previously shown, this functionality results from the induction of chemical basicity in interfacial water molecules, an event that triggers deprotonation of adjacent nucleophiles. Through multiple steering molecular dynamics with pulling along the proton-displacement coordinate, we now show that nucleophilic groups are functionally enabled by nearby dehydrons that promote proton transference. The computations are validated against experimentally determined pKa decreases at functional sites and biochemical probes of deregulated catalytic activity arising from dehydron-generating mutations.

Dehydrons are markers for protein associations [15] and have been conjectured in the previous sections to induce chemical reactivity in interfacial water [16]. These two properties are interrelated, and a chain of reasoning starting by assuming the validity of one property takes us to assert the validity of the other, as rigorously shown in section 6.1. Thus, dehydrons are known introduce structure-destabilizing nanoscale cavities on the protein surface. This interfacial tension is released upon protein associations that in effect displace the restricted interfacial water, turning dehydrons into promoters of protein interactions [17]. A simple computation of the interfacial tension leads us to the conclusion that water molecules enveloping dehydrons may act effectively as proton acceptors, as shown in section 6.1. This chemical behavior arises from a non-Debye polarization-induced negative charge arising as nanoscale confinement hampers the alignment of water dipoles with the electric field.

Here we unravel the mechanism of functional enablement promoted by dehydrons in their role as inducers of chemical basicity of the aqueous interface. To that effect, we investigate the chemical event of proton transference prompted by water molecules at dehydron interfaces. Specifically, we compute the shifts towards lower values in pKa [18] of groups functionalized through dehydron-promoted deprotonation. To assess this activity we need to consider chemically active dehydrons in the proximity of the functional site, i.e. those for which the water oxygen in the dehydron cavity is within 6 Å of the α-carbon of the functional residue. The method of choice to investigate the chemical event of dehydron-induced proton transference is multiple steering molecular dynamics computation [19]. The nucleophilic group and nearby proton-receptive water molecules at the dehydron interface are treated within a quantum mechanical (QM) scheme while the rest of the molecule and explicit solvent are treated using a classical molecular mechanics (MM) package, in accord with a QM-MM hybrid approach [20, 21]. The results are validated against experimentally determined pKa shifts [18] and functional studies of constitutively active mutant enzymes [22] whose aberrant deregulation is shown to arise from the creation of dehydrons not present in the wild type.

The study cases are selected so that the dehydron-promoted lowering of pKa value is significant and cannot be properly captured by current estimators of pKa shift. The latter are typically based on an empirical evaluation of pairwise interactions within a protein environment that favors a particular ionization state. Such estimators do not incorporate the unique electrostatic effects of structural or confined interfacial water molecules [16] into the empirical environmental field [18].

6.5 Quantum chemistry at the epistructural interface

To determine the functional stimulation caused by dehydrons, we compute the pKa decrease for nucleophilic side-chain groups with dehydrons in their proximity relative to the free residue in solution. As usual, the pKa shift, ΔpKa, estimates the difference in free energy increment, $\frac{\Delta\Delta G}{RT} = \frac{[\Delta G(p)-\Delta G(w)]}{RT}$, of the proton abstraction process in the protein environment $(\Delta G(p))$ relative to the bulk aqueous environment $(\Delta G(w))$. The results are contrasted against experimental data on ΔpKa. The free energy computation follows the multiple steering ansatz [19], where the molecular dynamics (MD) trajectories are generated by treating classically all groups except for those implicated in the chemical step of proton transference. The latter are treated in the quantum-mechanics (QM) density functional theory (DFT) setting [20]. The QM treatment is thus restricted to the side chain of the catalytic residues containing the weak-acid pro-nucleophilic group and to the reactive dehydron-associated water molecule. The reactive water molecule is defined as having its oxygen within 2.5 Å of the transitional proton that is initially covalently attached to a heavy atom (O, S or N) in the pro-nucleophilic group. The latter is generically denoted AH (or AH^+) and the neighboring distance cutoff is set so that the covalent bond A-H (or $[A\text{-}H]^+$ if protonation bestows charge) turns into hydrogen bond in the deprotonated state A^-—$H(H_2O)^+$ (or A—$H(H_2O)^+$) that results as the proton is transferred to the nearby dehydron-functionalized water molecule.

We denote by X the proton transference coordinate indicating the distance of the proton to the heavy atom initially covalently attached to it in the weakly acidic pro-nucleophile. Thus, $X(t = 0) = X_0$ is the bond length corresponding to covalent bonding to the heavy atom in the nucleophile and $X - X_0$ measures departure from covalent bond length. We denote by $\vec{R}$ the structural-coordinate vector for protein chain and water. In accord with Jarzynski's identity [19] conveniently written as

$$\frac{\Delta G(p)}{RT} = -\log\langle e^{-[\frac{W(X,\vec{R}(X))}{RT}]}\rangle \tag{13}$$

where the average $\langle e^{-[\frac{W(X,\vec{R}(X))}{RT}]}\rangle$ (W = computed work) extends over all trajectories $\vec{R}(X(t))$ with structural conformations steered by the pulling $X = X_0 \rightarrow X = X_0 + vt_f$ at constant speed v along the harmonic proton-transference linear coordinate. The pathway ensemble $\{\vec{R}(X(t))\}$ is generated by choosing a set of initial conformations $\{\overrightarrow{R_0} = \vec{R}(X_0)\}$ within an isothermal/isobaric equilibrated ensemble (T = 298K). This ensemble realizes the condition $X = X_0$ and is generated by a set of 20 classical thermalization trajectories, each lasting 1ns, with the PDB-reported structure fixed at the initial condition. The trajectory multiplicity arising from X-pulling is provided by the conformational dispersion in the initial ensemble $\{\overrightarrow{R_0} = \vec{R}(X_0)\}$, with each initial conformation responding differently to the X-pulling.

The QM region is treated using flexible basis sets of linear combinations of finite atomic orbitals in a real space grid optimized to N-scaling. The basis functions enable the matching of the radial wave function to the core region described by pseudopotentials by using pseudoatomic orbitals (PAOs) [23]. Split valence bases are generated by combining numerical Gaussian orbitals with the minimal basis described. The nuclei and core electrons are represented by norm-conserving pseudopotentials to avoid the computation of core states, a procedure that smoothens out the valence charge density in accord with grid requirements. Within the nonlocal pseudopotential approximation, a Kohn-Sham Hamiltonian is adopted incorporating the Hartree and exchange-correlation potentials, and a pseudopotential with additive contributions to account for local effects, long-range interactions and operation on valence electrons [24]. Calculations are performed on contracted Gaussian basis sets of double-zeta valence polarized (DZVP) quality (pseudoatomic orbital energy shift = 30 meV, grid cutoff = 135 Ry) [25].

The MM region is treated as detailed in Chapter 3 [17,26], where torsional degrees of freedom of backbone and side chains are coarse grained modulo basins of attraction in the potential energy surface in accord with Ramachandran (energetically allowed) regions in local conformation space. Interfacial water dipoles confined to dehydron cavities are subject to a torque resulting from the hindrance to alignment with the electrostatic field [17]. To equilibrate the PDB-reported structures with the solvent, we generated MD trajectories driven by the coarse-grained stochastic process, incorporating the potential energy associated with solvent orientation steering as the reversible work needed to align polarization-induced dipoles due to interfacial water confinement with the Debye electrostatic field [26]. To cover relevant timescales ($\sim$10ns), the dynamics are entrained by the metadynamics (Chapter 3), where the backbone dihedral torsions are specified "modulo basins of attraction" in the potential energy surface. Coarse moves are defined as transitions between basins of attraction (R-basins) in the Ramachandran torsional map for each residue. Thus, each residue is assigned an R-basin after a coarse move, and the coarse state of the chain becomes a conformational ensemble, with each conformation generated by selecting individual backbone torsional coordinates within the assigned R-basins [17].

The hybrid Hamiltonian incorporated includes QM-MM coupling comprised of three contributions: 1) electrostatic interaction between electrons and classical charges, 2) electrostatic interactions between nuclei in the QM subsystem and the classical point charges, and 3) a Lennard-Jones 6–12 potential to account for the van der Waals interactions between the atoms in MM and QM regions constructed using the force-field parametrization of Wang *et al.* [27]. The forces on the QM nuclei are obtained by taking the gradient with respect to atomic positions, and include derivation of the QM-MM coupling energy.

6.6 Dehydron quantum chemistry computations

The quasi-equilibrated work plots harvested in the free-energy computation associated with the dehydron-induced proton transfer event do not portend and are not required to reproduce the actual kinetics, which occurs on much faster timescales. The work performed by the system to reach the point $X = X_0 + vt$ along the proton transference coordinate is shown in Fig. 6.5(a) for the imidazole >NH group in His149 of xylanase (PDB.1XNB) for ten realizations $\{\overrightarrow{R_0} = \vec{R}(X_0)\}$ of the initial condition $X = X_0$ with harmonic force constant 48 kJ/mol. The thin lines indicate the work performed on the system at each point $X = X_0 + vt$ along the X-pulling steering trajectory with $v = 0.2$ Å/ns and $t_f = 6$ns. The thick lines correspond to slower pulling at $v = 0.1$ Å/ns with $t_f = 12$ns. The work histories for proton transference from imidazole in a free His amino acid in bulk water are shown in Fig. 6.5(b). The dehydronic environment of His149 in xylanase structure is displayed in Fig. 6.5(c). The His149 residue is required to be deprotonated in its structure-stabilizing function exerted by hydrogen bonding Ser130, internal water and by engaging in a putative aromatic-aromatic interaction with Tyr105 [28]. The case illustrated represents a dramatic pKa shift, with $\Delta pKa < -3.8$, from the pKa value ~6.1 for free protonated imidazole in bulk water to <2.3 in the xylanase environment [18]. The dehydron-functionalized water molecule around vicinal dehydron Ser100-Gly103 in the initial conformation picked from the set $\{\overrightarrow{R_0} = \vec{R}(X_0)\}$ shown in Fig. 6.5(d) serves as acceptor of the imidazole proton in His149, with the associated chemical event schematized in Fig. 6.5(e). Other conformations use the environment around the other vicinal dehydron Thr145-Asn148 for proton acceptance. A computed value of $\Delta pKa = -3.77$ is obtained for 20 trajectories generated by X-pulling at $v = 0.2$ Å/ns, while $\Delta pKa = -3.64$ obtained by collecting 20 trajectories at slower velocity $v = 0.1$ Å/ns, with both pKa shifts in good agreement with the experimental measurement [18].

A second computation of extreme pKa shifting, shown here to be due to dehydronic stimulation involves Asp70 in RNase H

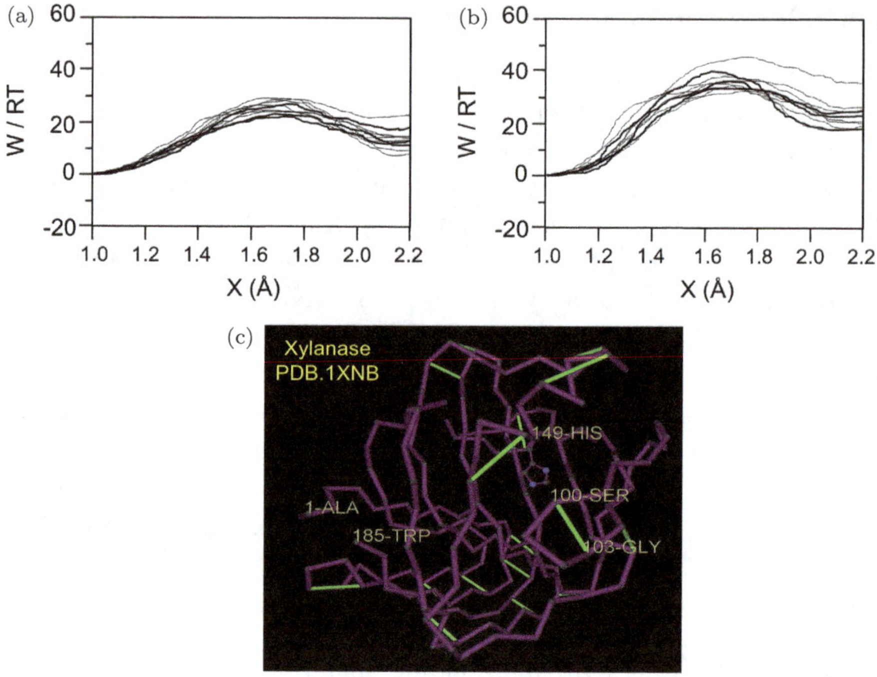

Figure 6.5. **(a)** Work performed by the xylanase-solvent system to reach the point $X = X_0 + vt$ along the proton transference coordinate X for the imidazole >NH group in His149. The histories displayed correspond to 10 initial conformations satisfying $X = X_0$. Thin lines were obtained at pulling speed $v = 0.2$ Å/ns and total pulling time $t_f = 6$ns. The thick lines correspond to $v = 0.1$ Å/ns, with $t_f = 12$ns. **(b)** Work associated with proton transference from a free His imidazole in bulk water, with pulling speeds along the X coordinate represented as in (a). **(c)** Dehydron pattern of an equilibrated xylanase structure at $X = X_0$, with dehydrons Ser100-Gly103 and Thr145-His149 flanking His 149 (side chain displayed). The backbone is schematically represented as virtual bonds joining alpha-carbons and dehydrons are displayed as sticks joining the non-adjacent alpha-carbons of the hydrogen bonded residues. **(d)** Dehydronic environment for His149 in xylanase at $X = X_0$ with the same structural representation as in **(c)**. The oxygen atoms of interfacial water molecules are displayed and the interfacial water molecule with proton-accepting capability induced by dehydron Ser100-Gly103 is indicated by the arrow. **(e)** Chemical event along proton transference coordinate X. Reprinted from [34] with permission from John Wiley and Sons.

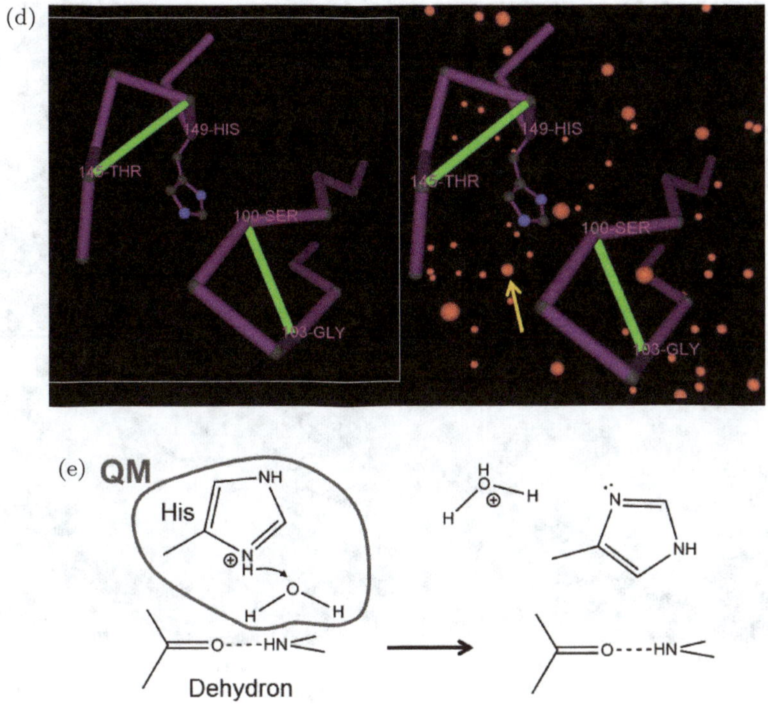

Figure 6.5. (*Continued*)

(PDB.2RN2), flanked by dehydrons Asn44-Glu48, Thr69-Val121, Lys122-Ala125 and His127-Glu131 (Fig. 6.6(a)). The carboxyl in Asp70 must remain highly nucleophilic since it is implicated in enzyme activation by ion coordination through lone electron-pair donation to Mn^{2+} [29]. In this case, the proton transference from the carboxyl group in Asp70 to proton-receptive vicinal water involves the water molecule associated with dehydron Asn44-Glu48 (Fig. 6.6(b)). The multiple steering QM-MM computation yields a shift $\Delta pKa = -1.3$ in coincidence with the experimental value [18] and in sharp contrast with other computations ($\Delta pKa = +0.3$ [18]) that ignored dehydronic effects.

A third study case revealing dehydronic effects in group functionalization is furnished by the pKa shift due to protein environment at His114 in RNase H. This residue in its deprotonated state is

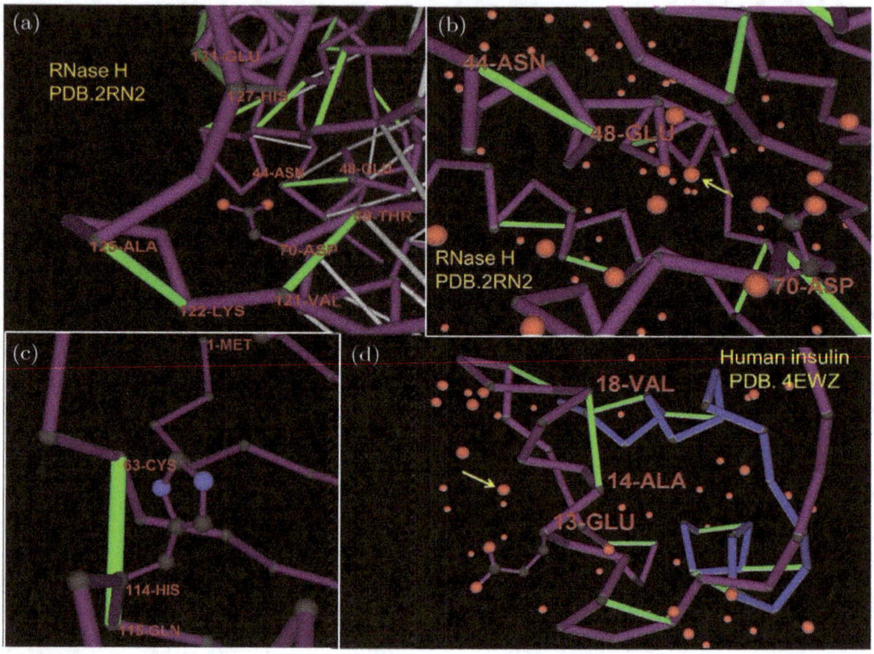

Figure 6.6. **(a)** Dehydronic environment for Asp70 in RNase H. The surrounding dehydrons are Asn44-Glu48, Thr69-Val121, Lys122-Ala125 and His127-Glu131. The representation convention is as described for Fig. 6.5(c). **(b)** Interfacial water around Asp70 in RNase H. The proton-receptive vicinal water marked by the arrow is associated with dehydron Asn44-Glu48 and promotes the proton transference from carboxyl group in Asp70. **(c)** Dehydron environment for His114 in RNase H with imidazole deprotonation induced by dehydron Cys63-Gln115. **(d)** Dehydronic environment for Glu13 in chain B of human insulin. The water molecule marked by the arrow hydrates dehydron Ala14-Val18 and behaves as a proton acceptor for the side chain of Glu13. Reprinted from [34] with permission from John Wiley and Sons.

implicated in structural stabilization [30]. A shift $\Delta pKa \approx -1.6$ is calculated by defining the reaction coordinate X through the imidazole deprotonation induced by dehydron Cys63-Gln115 (Fig. 6.6(c)). The pKa shift obtained is identical to the experimental value and at a variance with other computations ($\Delta pKa = +1.2$ [18]) that do not incorporate dehydronic effects.

Finally, residue Glu13 on chain B of human insulin is known to play a crucial role in oligomerization [31] and association with the islet amyloid polypeptide (IAPP) through an intermolecular salt bridge [32]. These structural roles require a functionalization evidenced in the shift $\Delta pKa = -1.9$. Current pKa computations that do not incorporate the dehydron influence yield the incorrect value $\Delta pKa = -0.3$ [18]. The shift is correctly estimated by taking into account the enabling role of vicinal dehydron Ala14-Val18 on chain B (Fig. 6.6(d)). The chemical event of deprotonation of Glu13 is captured by implicating the interfacial water molecule (marked by an arrow in Fig. 7.6(d)) turned into a proton acceptor by dehydron Ala14-Val18. The multiple steering MD computation pulling along the proton transference coordinate yields $\Delta pKa = -1.81$ is satisfactory agreement with experiment [18].

The biochemical consequences of dehydron-stimulated catalytic activity are probed by examining the effects of oncogenic mutations yielding constitutively active enzymes. We focus on cancer-related kinases altered by dehydron-generating mutation. As it is known, kinases get phosphorylated by performing a nucleophilic attack on the terminal ATP phosphoester linkage. Thus, our working hypothesis is that the nucleophilicity of the active side chain is enhanced in the mutant variant provided the mutation generates stimulating dehydrons nearby. With this rationale in mind, we investigate the oncogenic mutation D816V (Asp816Val) in the c-Kit kinase, found in mastocytosis [33] and other tumors, and known to induce a transforming capacity in c-Kit by turning it constitutively active [22]. The mutation D816V occurs in a floppy region of the kinase known as activation loop. A set of five 1.1μs MD trajectories were generated on the wild-type kinase and on the D816V substitution by equilibrating the PDB-reported conformation 1T46 following the coarse-graining protocol previously described [17, 26]. The hydrophobic replacement resulting from mutation D816V promotes water exclusion (wrapping) at backbone hydrogen bond Gly812-Arg815 that is retained as a dehydron (Fig. 6.7(a)). This hydrogen bond is disrupted in the wild type due to backbone hydration, as the activation loop becomes more solubilized by the presence of polar residue Asp816 (Fig. 6.7(b)). In turn, the presence of the Gly812-Arg815 dehydron in the vicinity of the phosphorylation site Tyr823 in the c-Kit mutant,

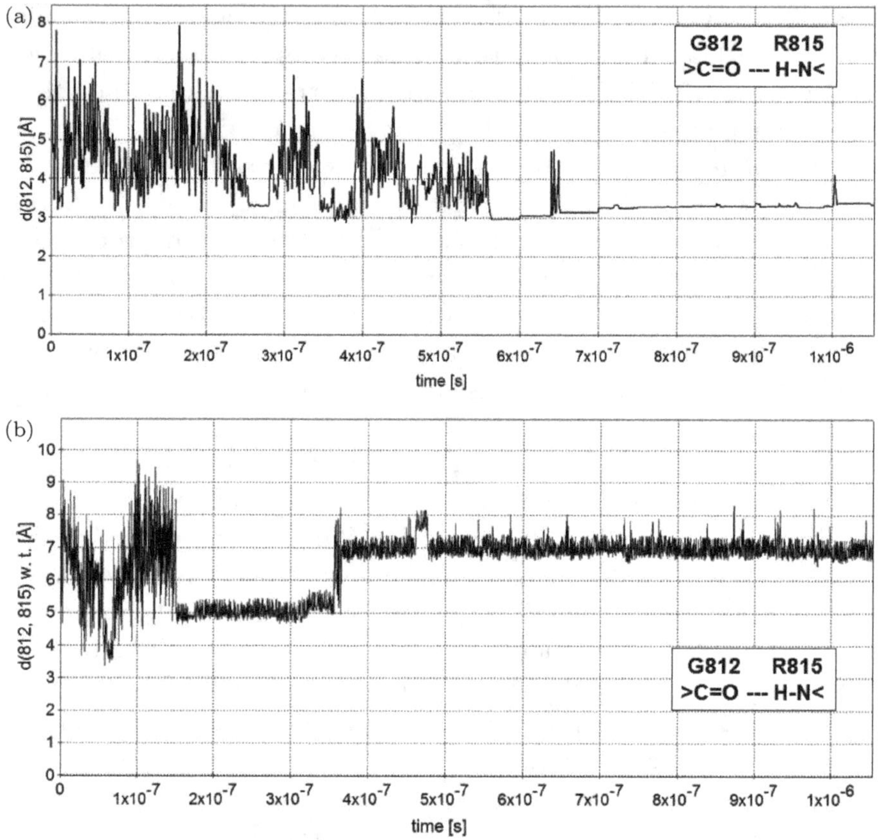

Figure 6.7. **(a)** Time-dependent O-N distance between backbone carbonyl of Gly812 and backbone amide of Arg815 in the activation loop of c-Kit D816V mutant along a typical MD trajectory generated as described in main text. The initial torsional state is the PDB-reported in entry 1T46. A stable Gly812-Arg815 backbone hydrogen bond emerges after 0.65 ± 0.20 microseconds in all 5 trajectories generated. **(b)** Time-dependent backbone O-N distance between Gly812 and Arg815 in wild type c-Kit along a typical MD trajectory. No stable backbone hydrogen bond is observed in any trajectory. **(c)** Snapshot of the activation loop of mutant D816V after 1.1 microsecond equilibration (cf. (a)) displaying dehydron Gly812-Arg815. The interfacial water molecule implicated in proton transference and functionalization of Tyr823 is marked by the arrow. **(d)** Chemical event of dehydron-based functionalization of a Tyr side chain as required for transesterification reaction with ATP. Reprinted from [34] with permission from John Wiley and Sons.

(c)

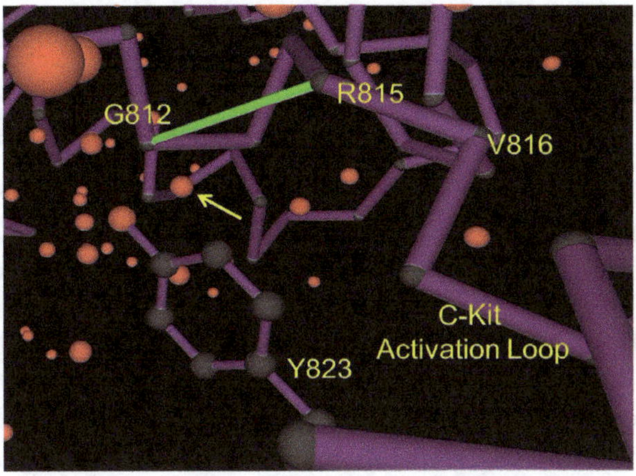

(d)

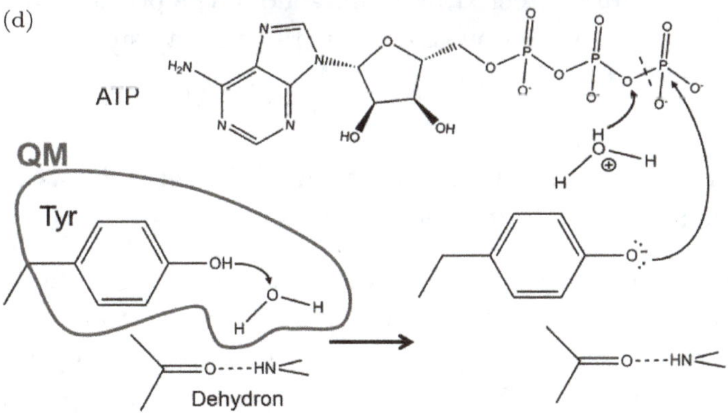

Figure 6.7. (*Continued*)

lowers significantly the pKa of the phenolic hydroxyl in Tyr823, as shown in the structural display for the mutant (Fig. 6.7(c)). The enhanced nucleophilicity of Tyr823 is the resultant of the proton acceptor activity of interfacial water (Fig. 6.7(d)) promoted by mutation-induced dehydron Gly812-Arg815. Multiple steering MD computations yield $\Delta pKa = -2.7$ as the mutation-generated dehydron functionalizes its adjacent water molecule into a proton acceptor (Fig. 6.7(c)) for the phenolic hydroxyl proton of Tyr823 (Fig. 6.7(d)). This enhancement in the nucleophilicity of the Tyr823 also enhances significantly its phosphorylation since the latter is contingent on nucleophilic attack on the ATP phosphoester linkage. Consequently, the mutation D816V turns the kinase constitutively active. It is now known that Tyr823 phosphorylation is essential to recruit anti-apoptotic pathways that bestow the transforming capability to c-Kit, leading to significantly longer tumor lifetime [22]. Thus, the oncogenic nature of the mutation may be now traced to its physico-chemical roots.

With these quantum mechanical computations we have mechanistically explored and validated the conjecture posed in sections 6.1, 6.2 that dehydrons participate as quasi-reactants in biochemical events. We focused on protein functions involving nucleophiles activated through deprotonation promoted by nearby dehydrons. Through molecular dynamics steered by pulling along the proton-transference coordinate, we have unraveled a general mechanism for dehydron-based chemical functionalization.

6.7 Why is dehydron-functionalized water a proton acceptor?: A heuristic approach

As indicated in chapter 2, interfacial water enveloping the structure of a soluble protein is often partially confined due to sub-nanoscale topographic detail in the protein surface [1, 34, 35]. When there is a dearth of coordination partners, this confinement brings about frustration of water molecules in regards to their hydrogen-bonding opportunities. Frustration makes water chemically reactive [34], a possibility that needs to be systematically explored. This picture is validated in this work focusing on uncompensated anticontacts or mismatches that classical electrostatics would deem untenable and classical molecular dynamics would treat as unstable. To delineate the frustration-related functionality, we need to focus on the physico-chemical properties of interfacial water that arise from the emergence of interfacial tension, known to be a consequence of frustration [35]. Such properties are not enshrined in a permittivity coefficient stemming from the "classical" Debye dielectric picture [36]. Due to subnanoscale confinement, the water dipoles are often precluded from aligning with the electrostatic field ($\mathbf{E}$), signaling a breakdown in the Debye *ansatz*. This breakdown is marked by the presence of an **E**-orthogonal polarization contribution $\mathbf{P}^{\#}$ that generates a net charge $\gamma^{\#} = -\nabla \cdot \mathbf{P}^{\#}$. The non-Debye term $\mathbf{P}^{\#}$ stores electrostatic energy that may be alternatively computed as interfacial tension [1]. In accord with the charge asymmetry with respect to hydration [37], we provide crystallographic evidence supporting the fact that hydrogen-bond frustration due to nanoscale confinement functionalizes interfacial water as a general base [6], thus determining a *frustration-related chemistry*. The consequences of this chemical role become apparent as we examine conformations featuring same-charge uncompensated anticontacts reported in crystallographic data [38] deemed "unstable" by classical molecular dynamics (MD) due the absence of nearby counterions. The stabilization of such configurations emerges in a quantum-mechanical treatment [34, 39], a suitable framework to incorporate frustration-based chemistry. As shown, the basicity of frustrated water enables titration of ammonium and guanidinium, both weaker acids than hydronium, implying that this effect cannot be accounted for in classical terms. This novel functionality of frustrated water is supported by the crystallographic record and by detailed information on water molecules in intramolecular proton transfer obtained by FTIR difference spectroscopy [40]. The results reveal a functionality of biomolecular interfaces intractable by mean-field dielectrics.

As previously described, the Debye polarization accounts for the screening of the solute charge, the $\mathbf{P}^{\#}$-component is responsible for chemical functionality associated with induced charge, hence not accounted for by protein chemical composition. The functionality is in accord with the sign of $\gamma^{\#}$, i.e. proton donor if $\gamma^{\#} > 0$ and proton acceptor if $\gamma^{\#} < 0$. Only one alternative becomes feasible, however. The consequences of such asymmetry will be the object of this study.

To describe the local dielectric distortion of interfacial water, we introduce a "frustration scalar field" $\phi = \phi(\mathbf{r}) = 4 - g(\mathbf{r})$ that quantifies the level of unrealized water hydrogen bonding at spatial location $\mathbf{r}$ relative to the bulk hydrogen-bond pattern [6].

As expected, the non-Debye field $\mathbf{P}^{\#}$ is proportional to the distortion gradient [6]: $\mathbf{P}^{\#} = -\xi\nabla\phi$. The net charge $\gamma^{\#}$ induced by $\mathbf{P}^{\#}$ is then $\gamma^{\#} = -\nabla\cdot\mathbf{P}^{\#} = \xi\nabla^2\phi$, and the interfacial energy ΔU_ϕ associated with spanning the solute-water interface becomes $\Delta U_\phi = (1/2)\lambda\int||\nabla\phi||^2 d\mathbf{r}$, where integration is carried over a spatial domain Ω containing the interface, so that its border $\partial\Omega$ is fully contained in bulk water, that is, subject to the condition: $\{\phi(\mathbf{r}) = 0\,\text{and}\,\nabla\phi(\mathbf{r}) = 0\}\,\forall\mathbf{r} \in \partial\Omega$. As previously shown in this Chapter, the mean value theorem (MV) of integral calculus yields $\gamma^{\#}_{\text{MV}} = -(\lambda\varepsilon_o)^{-1/2}\int||\nabla\phi||^2 d\mathbf{r}/\int\phi d\mathbf{r} \leq 0$. Thus, frustrated interfacial water resulting from nanoscale confinement yields negatively induced charge $\gamma^{\#}_{\text{MV}} \leq 0$, consistent with a proton-acceptor role resulting from frustrated hydrogen-bond coordination to water oxygen.

This result has important methodological consequences, explaining the acid-base interfacial chemistry explored in this section and may be also obtained based on the hydration differences between positive and negative charges [37]. Such differences arise because the water dipole center differs from the center of its van der Waals sphere, implying that the positive charges on the water protons are closer to the surface of the van-der-Waals sphere than the negative charge distributed on the lone electron pairs of the oxygen atom. Thus, a solute with negative charge may be more favorably hydrated than one with positive charge since the electrostatic interaction with water protons is facilitated relative to an electrostatic interaction involving the more internalized negative charge in the water molecule. This preferential hydration of negative over positive charges is in accord with the charge asymmetry ($\gamma^{\#}_{\text{MV}} \leq 0$, but not $\gamma^{\#}_{\text{MV}} > 0$) resulting from non-Debye polarization. A more detailed analysis requires that we consider dehydrons, water-exposed backbone hydrogen bonds that cause sub-nanoscale confinement and thereby frustration in surrounding water [1,34–36]. Such dehydrons are primarily hydrated by water molecules interacting with the dehydron carbonyl, rather than with the amide (cf. Fig. 6.8(a, b)). Since the water molecule is presented in the dehydron cavity as a carbonyl solvator, the question remains as to whether it becomes frustrated as proton

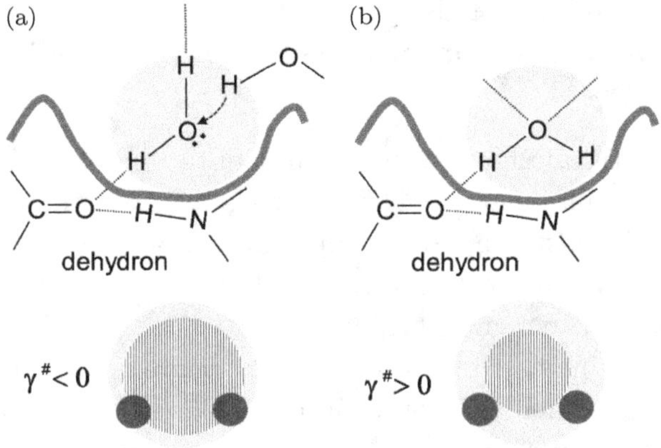

Figure 6.8. Dehydrons functionalize interfacial water by frustrating water hydrogen-bonding opportunities. **(a)** Schematic representation of the favored presentation of an interfacial water molecule within the dehydron cavity, featuring a proton acceptor role resulting from hydrogen bond frustration due to subnanoscale confinement. The van-der-Waals sphere is represented in light grey, positive charges are shown in dark grey, and the net negative charge ($\gamma^{\#} < 0$) resulting from unsatisfied lone electron pairs within the oxygen orbitals (patterned disk, lower panel) is expanded due to electronic repulsion, approaching the van-der-Waals border of the water molecule. **(b)** Disfavored water presentation within the dehydron cavity, yielding $\gamma^{\#} > 0$. The positive polarization-induced charge ($\gamma^{\#} > 0$) favors weaker electrostatic interactions with another water molecule because the latter's negative charge is far from the molecule's van-der-Waals border when compared with the positive charges on the protons.

acceptor (Fig. 6.8(a)), by developing a frustration-related negative charge $\gamma^{\#}_{\mathrm{MV}} < 0$, or a proton donor ($\gamma^{\#}_{\mathrm{MV}} > 0$), with a frustrated dangling hydroxyl (Fig. 6.8(b)). The option $\gamma^{\#}_{\mathrm{MV}} < 0$ is favored since the negative charge expands due to electronic repulsion within the oxygen shell, bringing the charge closer to the water van der Waals surface. This makes it susceptible to better electrostatic interaction with vicinal water protons, located close to the van der Waals surface [37]. This picture has been corroborated in molecular dynamics computations of water-filling dehydron cavities (Fig. 6.8(b), [6]) revealing a negative induced charge with maximum magnitude 3.31×10^4Coulomb/mol at curvature radius $\xi = 2.95\,\text{Å}$.

6.8 The discovery of dehydron-based catalysis prompts a revision of mechanism in biological chemistry

The mechanistic interpretation of enzymatic reactions in biological chemistry is still a matter of vigorous contention, shrouded in paradoxes. The latter arise as bulk-phase reactions are contrasted against their enzymatic counterparts. Perhaps the single most perplexing aspect of enzymatic mechanism is the functionalization of nucleophilic groups involved in transesterification reactions, with intervention of water as proton acceptor. In the bulk phase, water is hardly ever a proton acceptor because of the extreme acidity of hydronium. Proton acceptance would be typically regarded as an anomaly in bulk-phase chemistry, with the proposed underlying elementary step treated with skepticism. To reconcile this discrepancy between bulk-phase chemistry and enzymatic chemistry, we have been told that the enzymatic environment is "special" since it is able to alter significantly the pKa of the intervening groups. However, upon closer scrutiny, nothing is actually said about the way in which the enzyme protein structure shapes the dielectric environment at the active site, so as to alter the pKa of the active groups. This matter clearly pertains to the field of epistructural biology put forth in the first chapters of this book. As shown in this chapter, the protein-water interface of the enzyme is actually functionalized by the packing defects of the protein in ways that enable and stimulate the enzymatic activity. Specifically, the water molecule that behaves as proton acceptor in the enzymatic reaction is not within a bulk-like tetrahedral coordination lattice but is a frustrated molecule confined by the adjacent packing defect of the protein enzyme. *Dehydrons are strategically located along the protein surface to enable and stimulate the enzymatic activity.* This is a crucial matter pertaining to the field of epistructural biology and its unraveling in this chapter prompts a thorough mechanistic revision of the entire biological chemistry.

6.9 Dehydrons as enablers of conductance and determinants of pharmacological affinity in the M2 proton channel from influenza virus

The M2 proton channel from influenza virus offers a superb illustration of the dual role of dehydrons as promoters of water functionality and determinants of pharmacological affinity [41]. The helical tetrameric transmembrane domain M2(22-46)TM from the M2 channel is shown in ribbon rendering in Fig. 6.9(a) in complex with amantadine (PDB.6BKK). Calculations along the lines described in this chapter revealed unambiguously [41] that 1) the dehydron Ala30-Gly34 tetrad determines the high-affinity binding site for amantadine in the complex (Fig. 6.9(b)) and 2) the induced basicity of water molecules adjacent to the tetrad dehydron Ala30-Gly34 is the enabler for the elementary steps of proton transfer in the channel, marked by arrows in Fig. 6.10(a).

Strikingly enough, the two roles of dehydrons are intimately entwined: This is revealed by the positioning of the four water

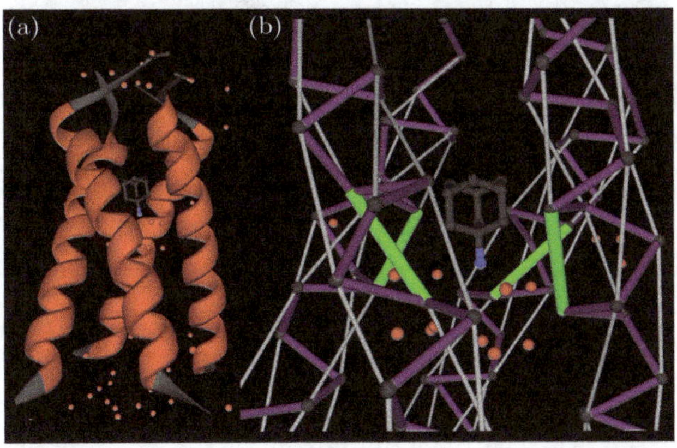

Figure 6.9. **(a)** Helical tetrameric transmembrane domain M2(22-46)TM from influenza virus M2 proton channel in complex with amantadine (PDB.6BKK) in ribbon display. **(b)** The dehydron Ala30-Gly34 tetrad determines the high-affinity binding site for amantadine in the complex from PDB entry 6BKK. Reprinted from [41] with permission from Elsevier.

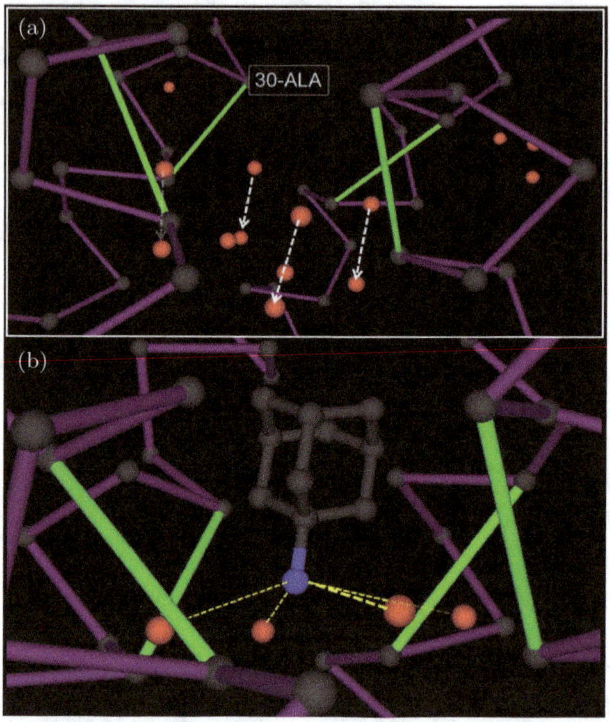

Figure 6.10. **(a)** Induced basicity of water molecules adjacent to the tetrad dehydron Ala30-Gly34. Elementary steps of proton transfer (arrows) from the water molecules functionalized by the adjacent Ala30-Gly34 dehydron tetrad. Spatial positions of water oxygens are indicated by red circles. **(b)** The four water molecules with higher proton affinity and negative net charge $\gamma^{\#}$ induced by the Ala30-Gly34 dehydron tetrad interact favorably (dashed lines) with the ammonium from the therapeutic salt formulation amantadine hydrochloride. Reprinted from [41] with permission from Elsevier.

molecules with higher proton affinity and negative net charge $\gamma^{\#}$ induced by the Ala30-Gly34 dehydron tetrad to interact favorably (dashed lines) with the ammonium from the amantadine ligand (Fig. 6.10(b)). Thus, the dehydrons that behave as enablers of proton transfer also contribute *in that same capacity* as enhancers of pharmacological affinity, exquisitely complementing their additional role as promoter of water exclusion, which is the typical determinant for binding affinity.

References

1. Fernández A (2013) The principle of minimal episteric distortion of the water matrix and its steering role in protein folding. *J Chem Phys* 139:085101.
2. Giovambattista N, Lopez CF, Rossky P, Debenedetti P (2008) Hydrophobicity of protein surfaces: Separating geometry from chemistry. *Proc Natl Acad Sci USA* 105:2274–2279.
3. Fernández A (2012) Epistructural tension promotes protein associations. *Phys Rev Lett* 108:188102.
4. Kumar P, Han S, Stanley HE (2009) Anomalies of water and hydrogen bond dynamics in hydrophobic nanoconfinement. *J Phys Condens Matter* 21:504108.
5. Schutz CN, Warshel A (2001) What are the dielectric "Constants" of proteins and how to validate electrostatic models? *Proteins-Struct Funct Gen* 44:400–408.
6. Fernández A (2014) Communication: Chemical functionality of interfacial water enveloping nanoscale structural defects in proteins. *J Chem Phys* 140:221102.
7. Fernández A (2010) Nanoscale thermodynamics of biological interfacial tension. *Pro Roy Soc A* 467:559–568.
8. Parai MK, Huggins DJ, Cao H, Nalam MN, Ali A, Schiffer CA, Tidor B, Rana TM (2012) Design, synthesis, and biological and structural evaluations of novel HIV-1 protease inhibitors to combat drug resistance. *J Med Chem* 55:6328–6341.
9. The *Uniprot* Consortium (2014) Activities at the Universal Protein Resource (UniProt) *Nuc Acids Res* 42:D191–D198.
10. Hardie DG ed (1999) Protein Phosphorylation: A Practical Approach. Oxford University Press, Oxford, New York.
11. Zanzoni A, Carbajo D, Diella F, Gherardini PF, Tramontano A, Helmer-Citterich M, Via A (2011) Phospho3D 2.0: An enhanced database of three-dimensional structures of phosphorylation sites. *Nuc Acids Res* 39:D268–D271.
12. Liebschner D, Dauter M, Brzuszkiewicz A, Dauter Z (2013) On the reproducibility of protein crystal structures: Five atomic resolution structures of trypsin. *Acta Crystall Sect D* 69:1447–1462.
13. Pietrosemoli N, Crespo A, Fernández A (2007) Dehydration propensity of order-disorder intermediate regions in soluble proteins. *J Proteome Res* 6:3519–3526.
14. Dodson G, Wlodawer A (1998) Catalytic triads and their relatives. *Trends Biochem Sci* 23:347–352.
15. Fernández A, Crespo A (2008) Protein wrapping: A molecular marker for association, aggregation and drug design. *Chem Soc Rev* 37:2373–2382.
16. Fernández A (2014) Protein Structural Defects Are Enablers and Stimulators of Enzyme Catalysis, Scientist Ariel Fernandez Finds. Market Watch (The Wall Street Journal):Published July 14, 2014 http://www.marketwatch.co

m/story/protein-structural-defects-are-enablers-and-stimulators-of-enzyme-catalysis-scientist-ariel-fernandez-finds-2014-07-14.
17. Fernández A, Lynch M (2011) Non-adaptive origins of interactome complexity. *Nature* 474:502–505.
18. Li H, Robertson AD, Jensen JH (2005) Very fast empirical prediction and rationalization of protein pKa values. *Proteins: Str Funct Bioinf* 61:704–721.
19. Jarzynski C (1997) Nonequilibrium equality for free energy differences. *Phys Rev Lett* 78:2690–2693.
20. van der Kamp MW, Mulholland AJ (2013) Combined Quantum Mechanics/Molecular Mechanics (QM/MM) Methods in computational enzymology. *Biochemistry (ACS)* 52:2708–2728.
21. Senn HM, Thiel W (2009) QM/MM methods for biomolecular systems. *Angew Chem Int Ed* 48:1198–1229.
22. Agarwal S, Kazi JU, Ronnstrand L (2013) Phosphorylation of the activation loop tyrosine 823 in c-Kit is crucial for cell survival and proliferation. *J Biol Chem* 288:22460–22468.
23. Sankey OF, Niklewski DJ (1989) Ab initio multicenter tight-binding model for molecular-dynamics simulations and other applications in covalent systems. *Phys Rev B* 40:3979–3995.
24. Kleinman L, Bylander DM (1982) Efficacious form for model pseudopotentials. *Phys Rev Lett* 48:1425–1428.
25. Chiodo S, Russo N, Sicilia E (2005) Newly developed basis sets for density functional calculations. *J Comput Chem* 26:175–184.
26. Fernández A (2014) Fast Track Communication: Water promotes the sealing of nanoscale packing defects in folding proteins. *J Phys Cond Matt* 26:202101.
27. Wang J, Cieplak P, Kollman PA (2000) How well does a restrained electrostatic potential (RESP) model perform in calculating conformational energies of organic and biological molecules? *J Comput Chem* 21:1049–1074.
28. Plesniak LA, Connelly GP, Wakarchuk WW, McIntosh LP (1996) Characterization of a buried neutral histidine residue in Bacillus circulans xylanase: NMR assignments, pH titration, and hydrogen exchange. *Protein Sci* 5: 2319–2328.
29. Goedken ER, Marqusee S (2001) Co-crystal of escherichia coli rnase hi with Mn2+ ions reveals two divalent metals bound in the active site. *J Biol Chem* 276:7266–7271.
30. Kanaya S, Katayanagi K, Morikawa K, Inoue H, Ohtsuka E, Ikehara M (1991) Effect of mutagenesis at each of five histidine residues on enzymatic activity and stability of ribonuclease H from Escherichia coli. *Eur J Biochem* 198:437–440.
31. Bentley GA, Brange J, Derewenda Z, Dodson EJ, Dodson GG, Markussen J, Wilkinson AJ, Wollmer A (1992) Role of B13 Glu in insulin assembly. The hexamer structure of recombinant mutant (B13 Glu–> Gln) insulin. *J Mol Biol* 228:1163–1176.
32. Wei L, Jiang P, Yau YH, Summer H, Shocha SG, Mu Y, Pervushin K (2009) Residual structure in islet amyloid polypeptide mediates its interactions with soluble insulin. *Biochemistry (ACS)* 48:2368–2376.

33. Piao X, Bernstein A (1996) A point mutation in the catalytic domain of c-kit induces growth factor independence, tumorigenicity, and differentiation of mast cells. *Blood* 87:3117–3123.
34. Fernández A (2015) Packing defects functionalize soluble proteins. *FEBS Lett* 589:967–973.
35. Fernández A (2012) Epistructural tension promotes protein associations. *Phys Rev Lett* 108:188102.
36. Fernández Stigliano A (2013) Breakdown of the Debye polarization ansatz at protein-water interfaces. *J Chem Phys* 138:225103.
37. Mobley DL, Barber AE, Fennell CJ, Dill KA *et al.* (2008) Charge asymmetries in hydration of polar solutes. *J Phys Chem B* 112:2405–2414.
38. Magalhaes A, Maigret B, Hoflack J, Gomes JN, Scheraga HA (1994) Contribution of unusual arginine-arginine short-range interactions to stabilization and recognition in proteins. *J Protein Chem* 13:195–215.
39. Fernández Stigliano A (2015) Biomolecular Interfaces: Interactions, Functions and Drug Design, Epilogue. Springer, Heidelberg.
40. Garczarek F, Gerwert K (2006) Functional waters in intraprotein proton transfer monitored by FTIR difference spectroscopy. *Nature* 439:109–112.
41. Fernández A (2019) Protein structural defects enable pharmaceutical targeting while functionalizing the M2 proton channel. *Biochem Biophys Res Comm* 514:86e91.

Chapter 7

Epistructural drug design: Next-generation targeted therapeutics

This chapter is devoted to the control of specificity for the next-generation targeted therapeutic agents. It is shown that epistructure-based molecular design enables a funneling of the drug inhibitory power towards targets of clinical relevance while suppressing off-target cross reactivity. Wrapping design is thus established as a paradigm in molecular engineering that broadens the technological base of the pharmaceutical industry.

7.1 Mastering specificity in rational drug design requires transcending the analysis of the target structure

Structure-based drug design is typically viewed as the mainstream rational approach to the engineering of ligands that bind to protein targets. This form of rational design is primarily geared at achieving a therapeutic blockade of specific functions which, in the context of oncotherapy, usually means interfering with pathways to which cancer cells are addicted. Yet, as argued extensively in chapter 2, the promising leads for new therapeutic agents are discovered in practice via a combination of high-throughput screening and serendipity, and are seldom if ever optimized through rational design. The rationale for a specific ligand design is almost invariably presented *a posteriori*, that is, pursuant on the availability of the structure of the drug-target complex. The rationale typically involves a physical description of pairwise interactions across the protein-ligand interface, including matched charge pairs, hydrophobic associations of nonpolar groups and van der Waals contributions.

When one carefully examines the lead optimization steps that turn the scaffold into a final therapeutic agent, one finds plenty of "counterintuitive" chemical modifications of the lead compound that cannot be rationalized based on a structural analysis of the protein-ligand interface. Thus, polar groups on the target protein surface appear to be matched up against nonpolar groups purposely incorporated to the drug scaffold during the lead-optimization phase. These mismatches are actually not what they *a priori* appear to be. In fact, the mismatches are not so when one examines protein interactions as many-body contributions. Thus, a nonpolar group in the ligand may be favorably placed within electrostatic proximity to a polar group in the target protein provided the latter is paired via a hydrogen bond with another polar of opposite charge. This is the basic physical description for the wrapping 3-body interaction, which in certain microenvironments constitutes a favorable interaction driven by the so-called dehydronic drag (chapter 2). This field, orthogonal to the underlying coulomb potential of the preformed hydrogen bond in the target protein, is the mechanical equivalent of the dehydration propensity of the hydrogen bond and serves as the guidance to epistructural design. From a solvent-centric perspective the removal of water from the surroundings of an under-wrapped hydrogen bond (dehydron) in the target protein is a thermodynamically favorable process. These dehydron properties encourage a lead-optimization design consisting on incorporating a nonpolar water-displacing moiety matched against the preformed hydrogen bond across the protein-ligand interface. This description highlights the stark contrast between epistructural and structural drug design. It makes apparent the essential differences arising as we regard the potential governing protein associations as a sum of many-body terms versus a sum of two-body contributions.

This chapter describes the operational steps required to actually implement epistructural drug design to control the specificity of an anticancer agent. The lead optimization steps are steered by the dehydron pattern of the target protein, that is, by an evolutionary meta-reading of structural information vis-à-vis the surrounding solvent. A striking aspect of epistructure-based optimization decisions is their counterintuitive nature when regarded from the perspective of structure-based design. Yet, the epistructural drug design is shown to enable the control of specificity to unprecedented levels that are definitely unfeasible when adopting structure-based design. These results are therefore expected to prompt a paradigm shift in rational drug design. According to the new paradigm, the drug favorably wraps the packing defects (dehydrons) of the target protein upon formation of the target-ligand complex.

In summary, epistructural drug design requires a meta-analysis of the target protein structure and is guided by a structure-encoded feature, namely, its dehydron pattern. Since dehydrons are computationally identified from structural coordinates, as indicated in Appendix 1, epistructural drug design becomes an open source bioengineering platform. This important feature sets apart epistructural design from other rational discovery platforms which pivotally rely on proprietary software. Thus, epistructural drug design is not only inherently accessible and physically more transparent than other approaches but its open-source nature also enables the possibility of progressively contributing to its improvement.

Proteins with common ancestry typically share a common fold. Thus, a protein target for a specific disease or malignancy may have off-target homologs that will likely be impacted by structure-based drug designs. This fact introduces a major hurdle in the quest to control specificity. On the other hand, the dehydron pattern of a protein is not conserved across homologs, as discussed in chapter 5. This fact argues for an epistructure-based rather than a structure-based approach to drug design, since the specificity filter appears to be enshrined in the aqueous interface and not in the protein structure.

Rational drug design remains essentially structure-based, therefore, the impact of drug-based inhibition often spreads to off-target members of the target protein family. This uncontrollable cross-reactivity leads to detrimental side effects that may be toxic or even health-threatening. The problem becomes particularly acute when attempting to interfere with signaling pathways involved in cell fate and cell proliferation, the type of molecular intervention often exploited in molecular anticancer therapy. In this context, the therapeutically relevant targets are the kinases, signal transducers with extensive homology in humans (and in most other species) thereby sharing significant structural similarity. However, as shown in Chapter 5, *dehydrons* are typically *not* conserved across proteins of common ancestry, in particular within kinase superfamilies. This evolutionary property combined with the fact that dehydrons promote their own dehydration, thereby triggering protein-ligand associations, implies that dehydrons constitute valuable *a-priori* targets to enhance specificity. Validating this assertion and exploring its ramifications and actual implementation is the thrust of this chapter.

The main rationale for this design strategy can be summarized as follows: If the packing defect is an enabler and stimulator of catalytic function (chapter 6), then its removal through intermolecular wrapping upon drug/target association should impair the function of the targeted protein and do so with high specificity, which is precisely the goal of molecular targeted therapy. Thus, the paradigmatic concept of "drug as dehydron wrapper" is established.

Engineering potent drug-based inhibitors of protein functions with controlled specificity and without harmful side effects remains a major goal in drug design. Drug-promoted inhibition of enzymatic activity may have at least two sources of side effects: a) the drug may interfere with pathways other than the one of therapeutic relevance because of the manifold roles of the target protein in off-target cellular contexts; b) paralogous proteins (homologs in the same species, i.e., humans), being structurally similar, may alternatively associate with the inhibitor, creating undesired cross-reactivities. Both sources of side effects have an evolutionary root that is traceable to the fate of duplicate genes, as shown in chapter 5. Building on the evolutionary knowledge acquired in chapter 5 and on the physical understanding of biomolecular interfaces acquired in Chapters 1–4, we introduce new and paradigmatic concepts to control selectivity and minimize drug interactions with toxicity-related targets.

In essence, the epistructure of the protein varies significantly across members of the protein family, while the structure remains topologically invariant across homologs [1–3]. The lesson that distills from this argument is that *mastering epistructural targeting of the protein is crucial to control drug specificity.*

The insights gained in the previous chapters prompt us to focus on a singular feature, the dehydron, a sticky packing defect shown to be of paramount importance in promoting protein associations [4–6]. Quantifiable features of these interactions allow us to introduce a target phylogeny that we can exploit to infer drug cross-reactivities and modulate the inhibitory impact of a drug, funneling it onto the realm of clinical relevance.

Considerable research has helped clarify many aspects of protein-ligand interaction [7]. Various methods enable one to predict such interactions, such as the assessment of packing defects [8], analysis of protein interface geometry [9], docking dynamics [10], modeling free energy [11], computational molecular probing [12], sequence threading [13], and learning-theory approaches [14]. The first four of these are based on properties of protein interfaces; the latter two are based only on sequences, and attempt to 'learn' features encoded in those sequences. Combined methodologies are also being developed [14]. Some of these techniques seek features of protein surfaces that promote protein-protein interactions. In this chapter we show how features with a quantifiable metric can be used to compare paralogs in a way that provides a guidance to develop more selective drugs.

To function, soluble proteins must retain relatively stable structures, a condition often requiring protein-protein associations [15–17]. Isolated structures with packing defects arising from poorly protected backbone hydrogen bonds typically do not prevail in water [3, 18]. On the other hand, such defects are inherently sticky, promoting removal of surrounding water through protein associations [8], as indicated in chapter 2. Accordingly, in this chapter we show that *dehydrons may be targeted in a new generation of highly selective drug-based inhibitors.* As shown in chapter 2, known structures of protein-inhibitor complexes [19–24] provide the blueprint to design inhibitors that in effect become wrappers or protectors of dehydrons.

Yet, the latter feature belongs to a meta-category, the *epistructure*, requiring an understanding of the dynamic relation between protein and solvent structure, as described in the previous chapters.

As shown in Chapter 5, while folds are typically conserved across homologous proteins, dehydron patterns are typically not conserved [3], and this property provides the main motivation for advocating a paradigmatic shift in drug design. While every targettable protein family may in principle be subject to the same analysis, we shall narrow down the scope of the discussion for the sake of clarity. Thus, we shall restrict ourselves to the goal of designing molecular therapeutic agents that selectively interfere with cell signaling. In this context, structure-based design becomes particularly daunting because the basic signal transducers in the cell, the kinases, share a common molecular ancestry and hence possess an uncanny structural similarity. This fact turns drug specificity into a major issue.

Kinase inhibitors are designed to impair the ATP-dependent signal transduction (Fig. 7.1). Hence they should be capable of

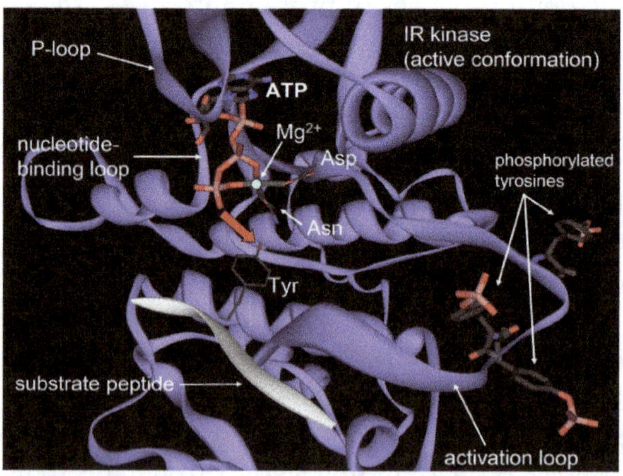

Figure 7.1. Generic structural features of a ternary complex involving a phosphorylated (active) kinase, its natural ligand ATP, and its phosphorylation substrate peptide (white). The phosphorylation event (red arrow) involves trans-phosphoesterification of the substrate tyrosine with transference of the γ-phosphate from ATP to the substrate, concurrent dismantling of the anchoring Mg(II)-coordination complex, and finally, release of ADP.

binding to the target competitively or noncompetitively vis-à-vis the natural kinase ligand ATP. The main structural features of the binding of ATP to a kinase are illustrated in Fig. 7.1, where an active (phosphorylated) tyrosine kinase, that of the insulin receptor (IR), is shown bound to ATP and to a substrate peptide. The kinase substrate becomes phosphorylated at a tyrosine residue through a trans-esterification reaction involving transference of the γ-phosphate of ATP (Fig. 7.1). Thus, a major challenge to design ATP-competitive inhibitors is the fact that the ATP-binding regions of most kinases are structurally very similar (with a RMSD <1.2Å in backbone coordinates) and have a very high level of amino acid conservation.

Contrasting with this troublesome aspect, the lack of conservation of the wrapping (dehydron) pattern across kinases has paramount potential to promote drug specificity, as illustrated in Fig. 7.2(a, b). Thus, the structural alignment of the focal adhesion kinase (FAK, PDB.2J0L) and the insulin receptor kinase (PDB.1GAG) reveal a significant similarity, with RMSD (root mean square displacement) <1.3Å (Fig. 7.2(a)). Yet, there are crucial differences in the dehydron patterns of both proteins (Fig. 7.2(b)), particularly in their ATP-binding pockets, where the ATP-competitive inhibitors bind [18]. These differences can be exploited with considerable therapeutic advantage: FAK is a target of major clinical relevance to treat cancer metastasis and yet the probably activity of a purported FAK inhibitor against the structurally related insulin receptor kinase is likely to have potentially devastating effects, arising mainly from the induction of a diabetic coma in the patient [18]. However, *there are dehydrons unique to FAK and not found in its paralog* (*arrows in Fig.* 7.2(*b*)) *which may be targeted to satisfy the therapeutic imperative of specificity*. This peculiar way of targeting a molecular feature materializes as inter-molecular wrapping, as illustrated in Fig. 7.2(c). The example shown in Fig. 8.2(a, b) dramatically reveals the difficulty in telling apart targets of clinical relevance from toxicity-related targets in molecular targeted therapy and unravels a possible avenue to solve this problem.

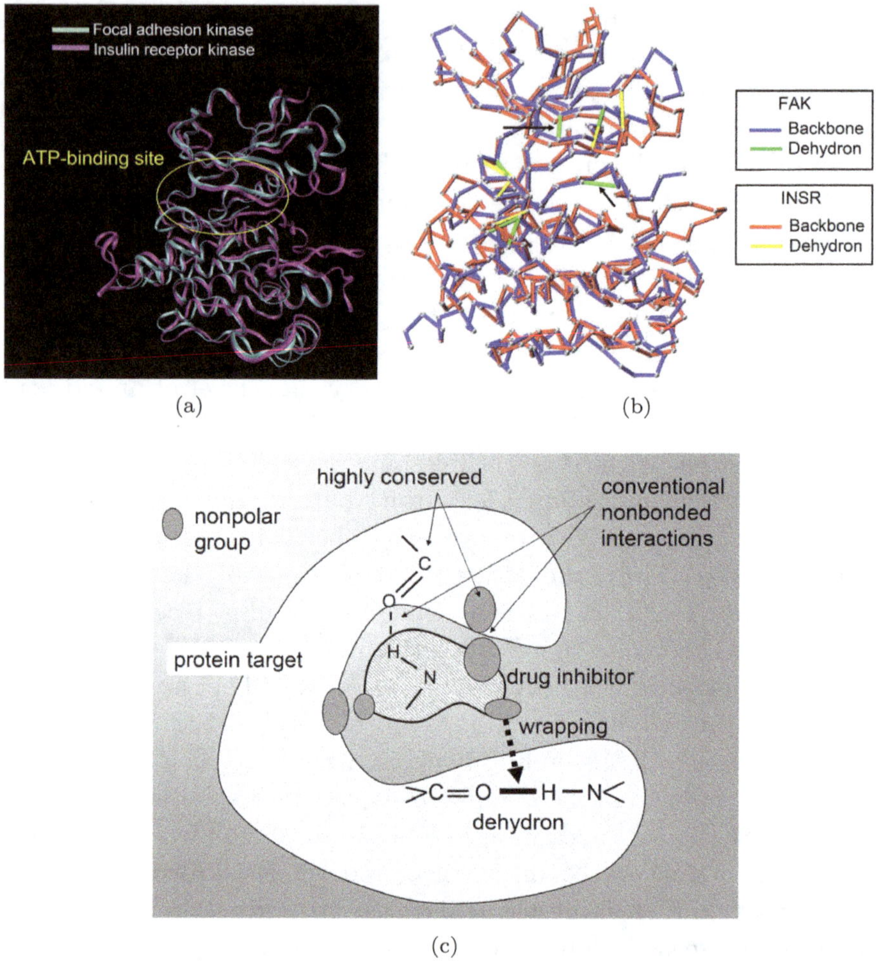

Figure 7.2. Structural **(a)** and wrapping **(b)** comparison between the focal adhesion kinase (FAK, PDB.2J0L) and the insulin receptor kinase (INRK, PDB.1GAG). The dehydrons in the ATP-binding region that are unique to FAK are marked by arrows. **(c)** Drug paradigmatically represented as a wrapper of pre-formed dehydrons in the target protein. Conventional nonbonded interactions between drug and target such as hydrophobic contacts and intermolecular hydrogen bonds typically foster drug promiscuity as they involve conserved features in the target protein.

Thus, in principle, side effects resulting from off-target ligand binding may be minimized by selectively targeting nonconserved dehydrons unique to the desired target protein with the guidance of a measure of wrapping proximity between structures. In this regard, this chapter reveals that packing defects may act not only as selectivity filters operative across homolog proteins, but also as selectivity switches, to re-engineer a protein inhibitor to redirect its impact towards another target. This latter role requires taking advantage of the spatial displacement of packing defects across aligned homologous structures.

Functional differences across homolog proteins sharing a common fold are very frequent in biology. Previous studies revealed that the wrapping constitutes a molecular dimension explored when evolution is constrained to preserve the fold for functional reasons. Thus, it is likely that wrapping differences across paralogs are indicative of the functional fine tuning needed to avoid dosage imbalances (chapter 5). It is precisely this fine tuning that needs to be discriminated in drug-based molecular therapy. *As this chapter reveals, such wrapping differences offer a new control in constructing the selectivity filters and selectivity switches that may endow the wrapping technology with a high therapeutic value.*

Structural descriptors of protein binding sites, such as hydrophobicity [25], curvature [26] and accessibility [27] are routinely used to guide inhibitor design. However, examination of the 814 non-redundant protein-inhibitor PDB complexes reveals that 488 of them have binding cavities with only average hydrophobicity [25], not significantly higher than the rest of the surface. In such cases, ligand affinity is attributed to the intermolecular hydrogen-bonding propensities of the inhibitor, inferred from protein-substrate transition-state mimetics [21–24]. However charge screening in water renders putative intermolecular hydrogen bonds unlikely promoters of protein-ligand association, unless water removal is favored at the interface by some pre-existing feature on the surface of the protein [8].

One obvious such feature is the solvent-exposed nonpolar moiety, except that, as stated above, such features occur infrequently on binding sites and if they do, they are highly conserved across homologs. A more common and less troublesome water-excluding feature has been recently identified. We have reported [3,8,18,28,29] that dehydrons constitute sticky sites with a propensity to become dehydrated as a result of protein associations.

To explore the potential of dehydrons as promoters of drug selectivity, we start by noting that *in most PDB protein-inhibitor complexes, the ligand is in effect a wrapper of protein dehydrons, although it was not purposely designed to fulfill this role.* In this way, the available bioinformatics data support the novel design concept. Ultimately, we shall develop a wrapping technology and provide evidence supporting the idea that targeting dehydrons that are not conserved across paralogs constitutes a useful strategy to enhance the selectivity of the inhibitor. Thus, the notion of wrapping (packing) similarity will be rigorously introduced and used selectively to modify a multiple-target inhibitor to achieve a higher specificity towards a particular target and subsequently to redirect its impact towards an alternative target.

7.2 Epistructure-based drug design

If the protein dehydron is a catalytic stimulator (chapter 6), then its removal through intermolecular wrapping upon drug/target association should impair the function of the targeted protein. This line of thought marks the genesis of the paradigmatic concept of "drugs as dehydron wrappers". This leads to pose a simple question: Is intermolecular wrapping a hitherto undetected factor contributing to ligand affinity and selectivity? To answer this question, the interfaces of the 814 protein-inhibitor PDB complexes were re-examined to determine whether inhibitors were "dehydron wrappers", that is, whether nonpolar groups of inhibitors penetrated the desolvation domain of dehydrons. This feature was found in 631 complexes, and *invariably* found in the 488 complexes whose the binding cavities presented average or no surface hydrophobicity [25]. Figure 7.3 illustrates such wrapping for the HIV-1 protease [21, 31]. The inhibitor contribution to improve the protein packing is not fortuitous since the substrate must be anchored and water must be expelled from the

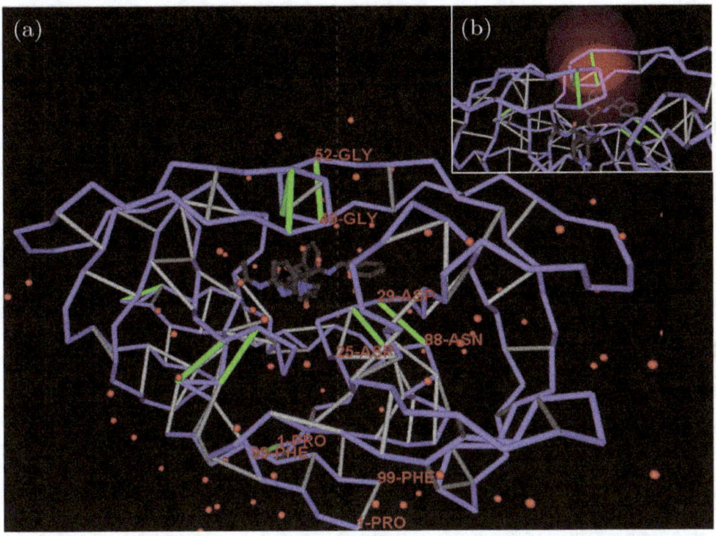

Figure 7.3. HIV-1 protease in complex with inhibitor that acts as dehydron wrapper. **(a)** Indinavir (Crixivan) inhibitor crystallized in complex with HIV-1 protease (PDB.2BPX). The packing defects in the dimeric HIV-1 protease are displayed jointly with their spatial relation to the inhibitor position. The chain backbone is represented by blue virtual bonds joining α-carbons, well wrapped backbone hydrogen bonds are shown as light grey segments joining the α-carbons of the paired residues, and dehydrons are shown as green segments. **(b)** Desolvation spheres for flap Gly49-Gly52 dehydron containing nonpolar groups of the wrapping inhibitor. Reprinted from [1], copyright 2005 with permission from Elsevier.

enzymatic site. *Strikingly, the wrapping of dehydrons is not purposely targeted in current drug design.*

The Merck inhibitor *Indinavir* (Crixivan) bound to the functionally dimeric HIV-1 protease (PDB.2BPX) is shown in Fig. 7.3 [21, 31]. The dehydrons in the protease are marked in green. On each monomer, these are backbone hydrogen bonds between these residue pairs: Ala28-Arg87; Asp29-Asn88; Gly49-Gly52 and Gly16-Gln18. The cavity associated with substrate binding contains the first three dehydrons, with dehydron 49-52 located in the flap and dehydrons 28-87 and 29-88 adjacent to the catalytic site (Asp25), to anchor the substrate. This "sticky track" determined by dehydrons 28-87 and 29-88 is required to align the substrate peptide across the cavity as needed for nucleophilic attack by the Asp25. The flap, on the other hand, needs an exposed and hence labile hydrogen bond to confer the flexibility associated with the gating mechanism. The lack of protection on the flap (49-52) hydrogen bond becomes the reason for its stickiness, as the bond can be strengthened by the exogenous removal of surrounding water (Fig. 7.3(b)). The positioning of all three dehydrons in the cavity (six in the dimer) promotes inhibitor association (Fig. 7.3(a)).

Indinavir is a wrapper of packing defects in the enzymatic cavity: it contributes 12 desolvating groups to the 49-52 hydrogen bond (Fig. 7.3(b)), 10 to the 28-87 hydrogen bond and 8 to the 29-88 hydrogen bond. All functionally relevant residues are either polar or expose the polarity of the peptide backbone (Asp25; Thr26; Gly27; Ala28; Asp29; Arg87; Asn88; Gly49; Gly52), and thus are not *themselves* promoters of association to hydrophobic groups of the ligand. The strategic position of dehydrons involving these residues in their microenvironments becomes a decisive factor to drive water removal or charge de-screening required in facilitating the enzymatic nucleophilic attack.

Central to drug design is the minimization of toxic side effects and the enhancement of safety. Achieving such goals is proving to be extremely challenging and yet a more modest yet crucially related aim, the control of specificity, seems clearly within reach, as advocated in this section and proved in the subsequent chapters. Because paralog proteins are likely to share a common structure [32], the possibility of multiple binding partners for a given protein inhibitor arises, unless the inhibitor specifically targets nonconserved features. Thus, the problem of controlling specificity may in principle be circumvented by targeting dehydrons because, in contrast to the fold, the wrapping is generally *not* conserved across homologs [3]. This evolutionary fact makes the dehydron pattern a possible selectivity filter for drug design. The usefulness of this filter of course depends on our ability to design drugs that may contribute intermolecularly to a better wrapping of the target.

To determine whether dehydron targeting is likely enable a control of specificity, we first investigated the extent of conservation of dehydrons across human paralogs in PDB. The paralogs for every crystallized protein-inhibitor complex were identified and dehydron patterns at binding cavities were compared. A 30% minimal sequence alignment was required for paralog identification. Packing defects were found to be a differentiating marker in paralogs of 527 of the investigated 631 proteins crystallized in complex with inhibitors. Protein chains are often reported in complexes with different inhibitors.

The PDB contains 440 redundancy-free pairs of human paralogs. Of these, 308 involve some of the 527 proteins containing binding dehydrons. In 269 pairs, the intramolecular wrapping at the binding cavity differs in the location or presence of at least one dehydron, and in 203 pairs, the difference extends to two or more dehydrons. Thus, *the probability of avoiding side effects by selectively wrapping packing defects is estimated at 88%* (269 pairs out of 308).

7.3 Dehydron targeting and promiscuity

The natural product *staurosporine* has been singled out as the ligand inhibitor most promiscuously interactive with the human kinome [33]. Its complexes are extensively reported in the PDB and high-throughput screening reveals nanomolar inhibitory impact over ∼80% of the screened kinases. In spite of this extremely high affinities, staurosporine has shown very limited therapeutic possibilities, and that is -we anticipate- because it is a poor wrapper of preformed dehydrons in the proteins to which it binds. We have examined all 96 staurosporine-protein PDB complexes and found no instance of the inhibitor acting as dehydron wrapper. All interactions were hydrophobic in nature, involving nonpolar groups on the protein surface. An illustration of such type of binding is given in Fig. 7.4, where the Syk tyrosine kinase-staurosporine complex (PDB.1XBC) is shown to hinge on three pivotal hydrophobic interactions engaging Phe382, Val385 and Leu377. It should be noticed that staurosporine does not wrap the single dehydron Gly380-Gly382 closest to the binding site. Thus, since surface hydrophobic residues tend to be conserved as markers for interactivity and staurosporine does not discriminate among packing differences in the kinome, its promiscuity

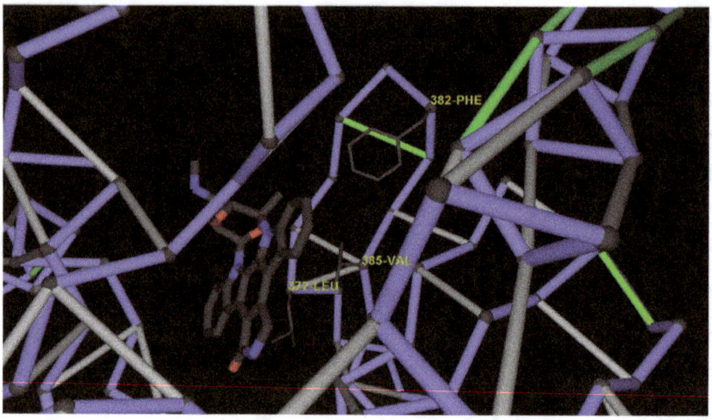

Figure 7.4. Staurosporine does not wrap dehydrons and thus, it does not discriminate proteins with different packing, which makes it highly promiscuous within the kinome. The staurosporine-Syk complex (PDB.1XBC) reveals a binding mode determined exclusively by hydrophobic interactions engaging residues Leu377, Phe382, Val385. The closest Gly380-Gly383 dehydron is not wrapped by staurosporine.

becomes entirely expected, and so is its uselessness as a therapeutic agent.

7.4 Exploiting the epistructural interface as a filter for drug selectivity

The subtle structural differences among paralogs of a kinase target may be quantified by introducing a "wrapping homology". Assessing wrapping similarity across paralogs requires comparing the microenvironments of backbone hydrogen bonds [8] that can be effectively carried out following the structural alignment [30]. This "wrapping homology" becomes a useful tool to control specificity by targeting a packing defect. For a protein chain of length N, a matrix of dehydrons $D_{ij}, i, j = 1, 2, \ldots, N$ may be constructed by choosing $D_{ij} = 1$ if residues i and j are paired by a dehydron and $D_{ij} = 0$, otherwise. This representation is illustrated in Fig. 7.5(a). When the dehydron matrices for two proteins m and n are aligned, they are trimmed by restricting them to those residues that have been structurally aligned in a one-to-one correspondence. Then a Hamming distance

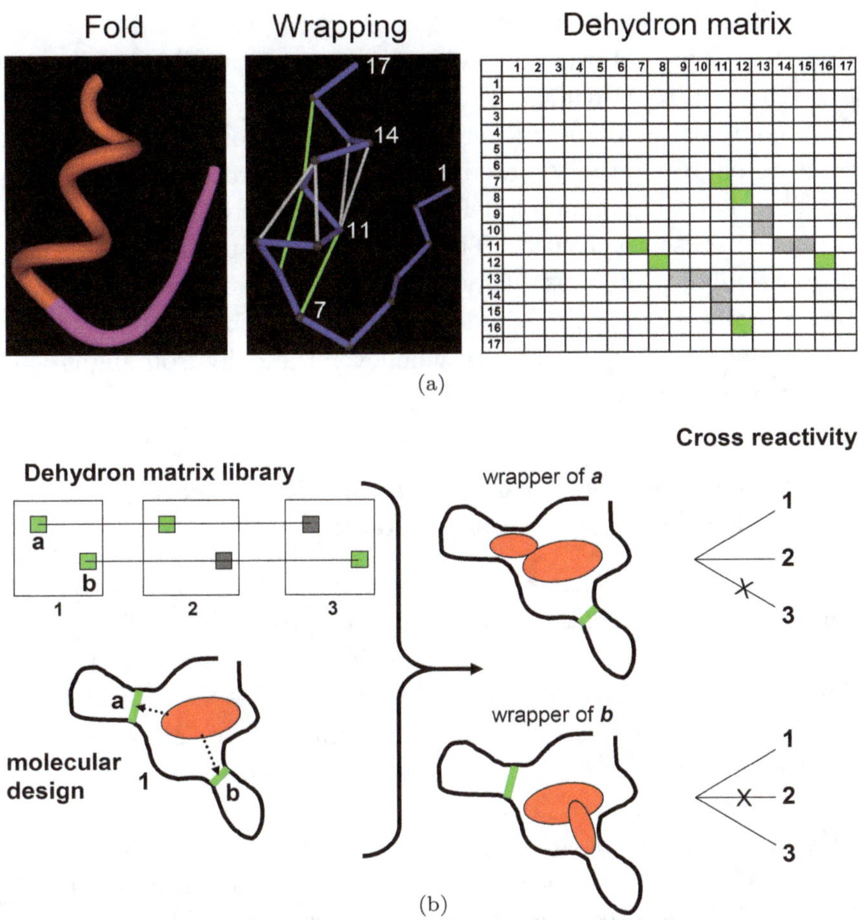

Figure 7.5. Dehydron matrices and *a-priori* cross reactivities derived from their alignment. **(a)** Three different representations of a folded peptide chain of length N = 17: fold, wrapping and dehydron matrix. The grey entries in the matrix indicate well-wrapped hydrogen bonds and the green entries represent dehydrons. **(b)** A-priori cross reactivities across three proteins (**1**, **2**, **3**) of drugs/ligands designed to wrap specific dehydrons (**a**, **b**) in protein **1**. The cross-reactivities are inferred from the alignment of the dehydron matrices.

$M_H(m, n) = \Sigma_{i<j}|D_{ij}(m) - D_{ij}(n)|$ may be computed to serve as indicator of the wrapping similarity between proteins m, n. Given a collection of paralogs $m, n = 1, \ldots, F$, and its corresponding packing-similarity matrix $\mathbf{M}_H = [M_H(m, n)]$, a wrapping-similarity tree

(WST) may be easily constructed by adopting the premise that the minimal pathway between protein-nodes m and n crosses a number of nodes equal to $\mathrm{M_H(m, n)}$.

A comparison of dehydron matrices for proteins with aligned structure enables an automated digitalization of the drug selectivity problem. The alignment of dehydron matrices reveals the pattern of *a-priori* cross reactivities: Thus, targeting a specific dehydron in one particular protein is likely to promote cross reactivities with other targets where this dehydron is found at the aligned position and preclude inhibitory activity whenever the dehydron aligns with a well-wrapped hydrogen bond (Fig. 7.5(b)).

7.5 Epistructural re-design of *imatinib* (*Gleevec*®) to eliminate adverse side effects

Molecular cancer treatments are often geared at interfering with signaling pathways that govern cell fate or proliferation. These therapeutic strategies target kinases, the signal transducers in the cell. This approach remains challenging because kinases are evolutionarily and therefore structurally related and thus kinase inhibitors often lack the required specificity, which may lead to toxic or health-threatening side effects. The next sections illustrate the power of the wrapping concept in engineering safer kinase inhibitors, thus unraveling a rational approach to fulfill this therapeutic imperative. The focus of these sections chapter is the redesign of the anticancer drug imatinib (Gleevec) used to treat chronic myeloid leukemia, where its primary target is the chimeric Bcr-Abl kinase, as well as certain solid tumors based on its impact on the C-Kit kinase. Imatinib also has potentially cardiotoxic effects traceable to its impact on the Abl kinase in off-target cells. These sections describes a wrapping modification of imatinib purposely designed to prevent inhibitory impact against Abl (and Bcr-Abl), to re-focus the impact towards C-Kit and to promote inhibition of an additional target, JNK, required to reinforce the prevention of cardiotoxicity and recognized as a target of significant therapeutic interest in its own right. The molecular blueprint for target discrimination, described in chapters 2 and 5, is now validated through assays that span a vast testing ground, from *in silico* assessment and test-tube probes to animal models. The findings surveyed identify the wrapping-based re-engineered imatinib as an agent to treat gastrointestinal stromal tumors and possibly ovarian cancer with reduced side effects, thereby illustrating the therapeutic impact of the wrapping technology.

7.6 Target blueprint for imatinib redesign

The possibility of molecular interference with signaling pathways that control cell fate and cell proliferation opened up many therapeutic opportunities for the treatment of malignancy. Thus, protein kinases, the signal transducers of the cell, have become paradigmatic targets for drug-based cancer therapy [34–46]. However, their evolutionary- and hence structural-relatedness often leads to unforeseen and uncontrollable cross-reactivities [46–49]. Although the relationship between specificity, anti-cancer activity and therapeutic efficacy remains opaque to our understanding, a lack of controlled specificity towards targets of therapeutic relevance typically underlies toxic side effects [38–47]. Undesired and even health-threatening side effects can even be traced to inhibitory impact on a primary molecular target in off-target (i.e. normal) cells. This scenario is superbly illustrated by the reported potential cardiotoxicity of imatinib (STI571, Gleevec) attributed to its impact on Bcr-Abl [48], the chimeric Abelson (Abl) kinase target in the treatment of CML (chronic myeloid leukemia) already introduced in the preceding chapter.

In this chapter we survey a rational drug-redesign strategy to control and re-focus the inhibitory impact adopting a blueprint that is strictly equivalent to dehydron pattern to guide molecular design [47]. Furthermore, for validation of the design strategy, we present a broader testing ground, from *in silico* assay to animal model.

While wrapping remains the epistructural target discriminator, we may exploit its link to the physically tangible hydration structure of the target protein (Chapter 2, [47]) to guide our molecular design. Thus, we first determine the target dehydration or de-wetting hot spots as a blueprint for drug design. Then, we modify imatinib to

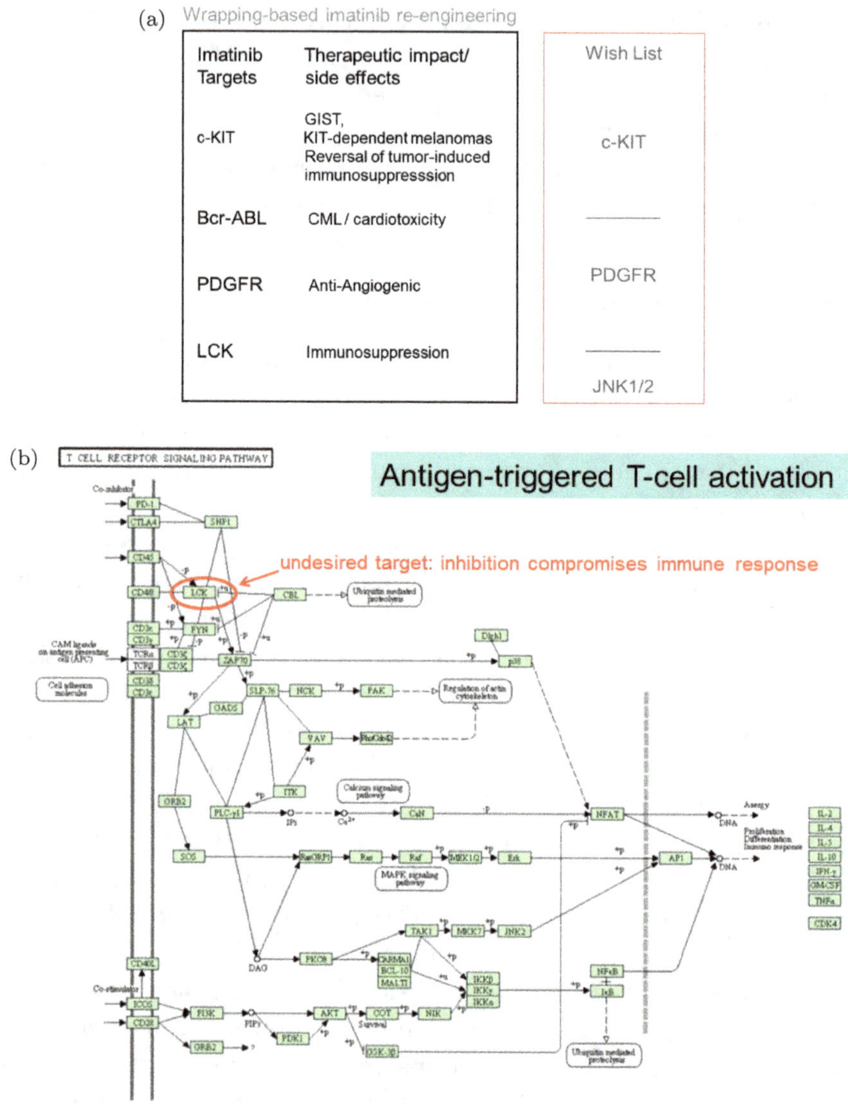

Figure 7.6. **(a)** Imatinib targets and specific plans for its epistructure-based re-engineering. **(b)** Role of undesired target LCK as signal transducer in antigen-triggered T-cell maturation. The signaling pathways for this immune response were reported in *KEGG*, the Kyoto Encyclopedia of Genes and Genomes.

significantly reduce its impact on Bcr-Abl (cf. [48, 49]), *prima facie* curbing its cardiotoxicity [49], while retaining the anticancer activity associated with its other primary targets.

In concrete terms, by sculpting into the ligand the de-wetting differences across imatinib targets, we are able to focus the inhibitory impact specifically on the C-Kit kinase, a target for GIST (gastrointestinal stromal tumor) [42–44] while suppressing Bcr-Abl inhibition (Fig. 7.6(a)). In addition, our wrapping-based redesign is expected to avoid binding LCK, because this kinase is implicated in antigen-triggered T-cell activation (Fig. 7.6(b)), and therefore LCK inhibition is likely to bring about immunosuppressive effects in a therapeutic context where they would be most unwelcomed, as argued in forthcoming chapters. Finally, we encourage JNK inhibition, as needed to reinforce the prevention of cardiotoxicity [48] and because of the importance of JNK as a target in the treatment of ovarian cancer [50]. The discriminating molecular design is reflected in selective anticancer activity on GIST cell lines and a GIST animal model, and a *prima facie* reduction of Abl-related cardiotoxicity. The program for imatinib redesign is sketched in Fig. 7.6(a).

7.7 Avoiding side effects by redesigning imatinib into a better dehydron wrapper

As indicated Chapter 2, dehydrons generate de-wetting hot spots, that is, defects in the hydration layer of the protein. This physical property clearly suggests a molecular design strategy where, upon association with the target, the drug/ligand contributes to the removal of the hydrating molecules at the de-wetting hot spot. This design strategy is often but not always equivalent to the dehydron-wrapping approach. The latter is based on an arithmetic counting of side-chain nonpolar groups in protein microenvironments disregarding their relative positions, while the former is rooted in the physical properties of interfacial biological water, providing a more rigorous approach.

To engineer an affinity discriminator for C-Kit following the de-wetting (see Chapter 2) blueprint, we compare the patterns of residence times of water molecules that solvate the aligned interfacial regions of PDB-reported imatinib targets Bcr-Abl (PDB.1FPU), C-Kit (PDB.1T46) and Lck (lymphocyte specific tyrosine kinase, PDB.3LCK) (Fig. 7.7(a–c)). The de-wetting patterns introduce a descriptor of hydration tightness to assess the functional role of dehydrons and are generated as follows:

Hydration tightness is defined by the extent of mobility of interfacial water molecules. Thus, the mean residence time of hydrating molecules within a domain around each residue on the protein surface serves as an adequate indicator of hydration tightness. Our results lead us to identify dehydrons as the structural feature causative of the most dramatic decrease in residence times (highest mobility) of hydrating molecules. Dehydrons promote local de-wetting because the Coulomb energy of the intramolecular hydrogen bonds becomes magnified upon water removal, and the net gain in stability upon dehydration offsets the work required to remove surrounding water (chapter 2).

To assess the local mobility of water molecules in the epistructural interface, the local mean residence time, $\langle\tau\rangle_i$ of hydrating molecules around residue i is defined with respect to a microenvironment in the form of a spherical domain $D(i)$ of 6Å-radius (~width of more than two water layers) centered at the α-carbon of residue i (Fig. 2.13). The computations are performed for a range of radii (see below). The residence time is obtained as follows:

$$\langle\tau\rangle_i = \int \tau f_i(\tau)d\tau \Big/ \left(\int f_i(\tau)d\tau\right);$$

$$\int_0^{\tau} f_i(\tau')d\tau' = P_i(0) - P_i(\tau); \qquad (1)$$

$$P_i(\tau) = \Theta^{-1}\int_0^{\Theta}\left[\sum_{\substack{v(t)\in U(i,t)\\ w(t+\tau)\in U(i,t+\tau)}} \delta(v(t), w(t+\tau))\right] dt;$$

Where $f_i(\tau)d\tau/\int f_i(\tau)d\tau$ is the expected fraction of water molecules that exit $D(i)$ within time interval $[\tau, \tau + d\tau]$; $P_i(\tau)$ is the expected

(a)

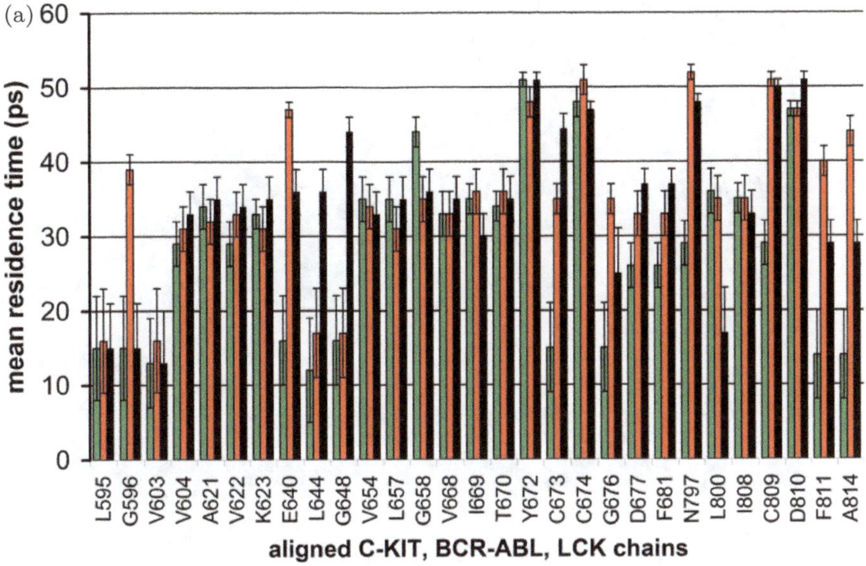

(b)

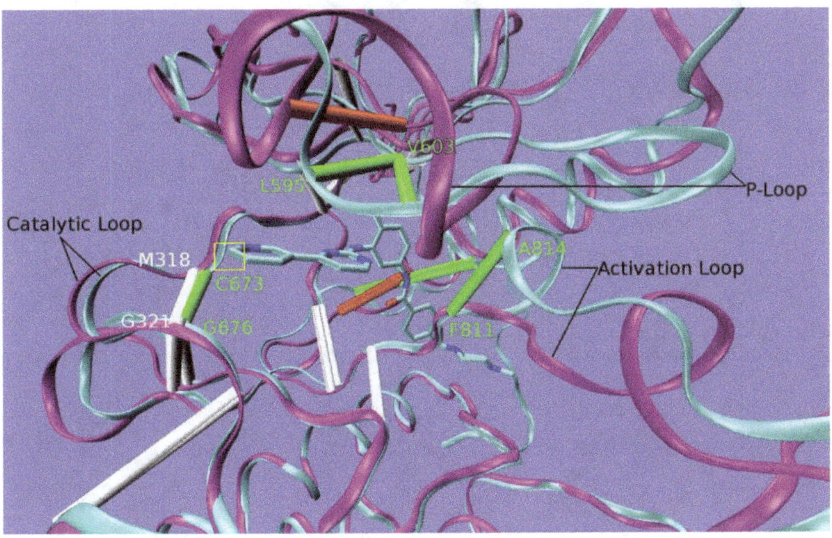

Figure 7.7. (*Continued*)

(c)

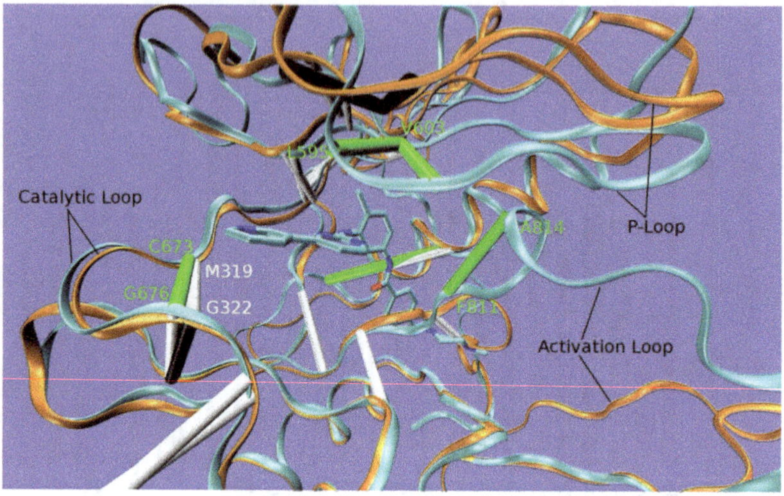

(d)

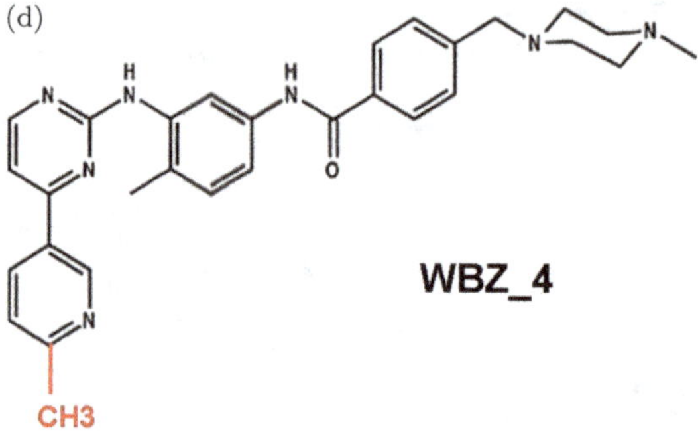

(e)

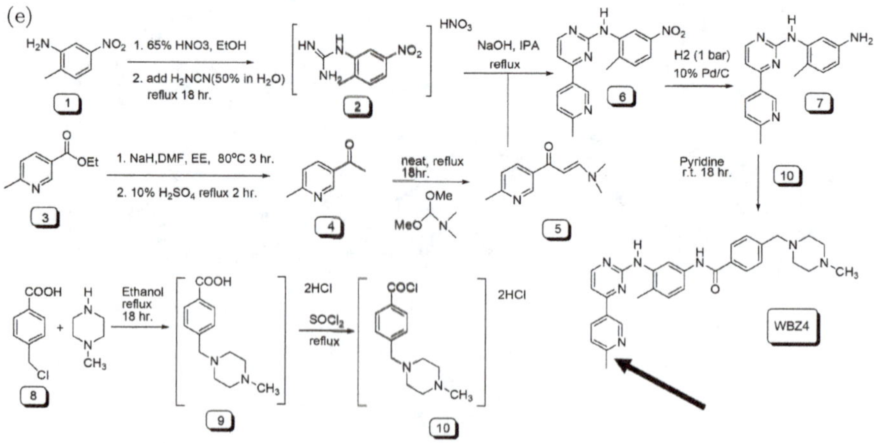

Figure 7.7. (*Continued*)

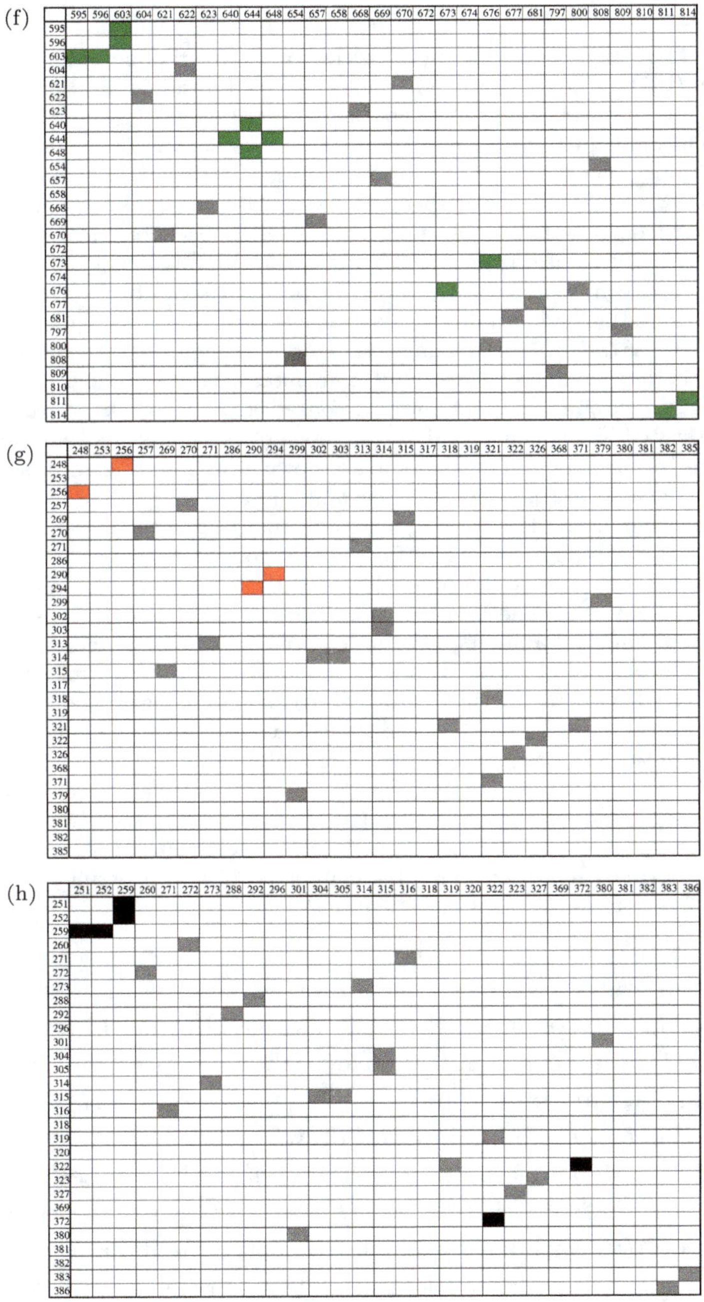

Figure 7.7. (*Continued*)

Figure 7.7. **(a)** Dewetting propensities of C-Kit residues in contact with imatinib (PDB.1T46, green bars) and of aligned residues in Bcr-Abl kinase (PDB.1FPU, red bars) and Lck (PDB.3LCK, black bars). Residue i is in contact with the ligand if an atom of the latter lies within its domain $D(i)$. The de-wetting propensity is quantified by the mean lifetime of solvating water molecules. Error bars denote Gaussian dispersion over 5 MD (molecular dynamics) runs. **(b)** Pattern of de-wetting hot spots that arise as backbone hydrogen-bonded residues in C-Kit kinase (ribbon backbone representation in light blue, de-wetting hot spots in green), aligned with Bcr-Abl kinase (magenta backbone, de-wetting hot spots in red). The imatinib methylation site leading to the expulsion of water from C-Kit C673-G676 de-wetting hot spot is highlighted (yellow rectangle). Imatinib is thus modified to favorably expel interfacial water molecules from the C-Kit microenvironment, a feature not conserved in Bcr-Abl. Hydrogen bonds are represented as segments joining α-carbons of the paired residues, and those lacking the propensity for dehydration are shown as light grey segments. Residues from C-Kit chain are labeled in green and those from Bcr-Abl are labeled in white. **(c)** Differences in de-wetting hot spots upon alignment of C-Kit (light blue backbone, hot spots in green) and Lck kinase (gold backbone, black hot spots). Labels for Lck residues are shown in white. **(d)** Prototype molecule WBZ_4 (N-{5-[4-(4-methyl piperazine methyl)-benzoylamido]-2-methylphenyl}-4-[3-(4-methyl)-pyridyl]-2-pyrimidine amine). The added methyl group is indicated in red. **(e)** Total synthesis of WBZ_4. The wrapping modification (methylation) of imatinib is indicated by the thick arrow. **(f–h)** Dehydron matrices of Kit, Abl and Lck kinases respectively, derived from PDB entries 1T46, 1FPU and 3LCK and restricted to the residues in contact with imatinib. Rows and columns are labeled by residue numbers, well-wrapped bonds are displayed in grey and dehydrons are shown in green, red and black for Kit, Abl and Lck, respectively. The entry denoting a selectivity-promoting feature for the wrapping design is circled in red. Fig. 7.7**(a–e)** reprinted from [47], copyright 2007 with permission from the American Society for Clinical Investigation.

number of water molecules remaining in $D(i)$ at time τ ($P_i(0) - P_i(\tau)$ = number of molecules that exited $D(i)$ in the time period $[0, \tau]$); $v(t), w(t + \tau)$ denote indexes labeling water molecules contained in $D(i)$ at times t and $t + \tau$, respectively; $U(i, t)$, $U(i, t + \tau)$ denote the collection of indexes of water molecules contained in $D(i)$ at times t and t + τ, respectively; δ is the Kronecker symbol ($\delta(v(t), w(t + \tau)) = 1$ if $v(t) = w(t + \tau)$ and 0, otherwise); and the integration over variable t is carried out over the interval of sampled times ($t = 0$ to $t = \Theta = 10$ns) after 5ns of prior equilibration (the sampling is considered exhaustive since $\langle\tau\rangle \ll \Theta$ for all residues).

The mean residence times are obtained from classical trajectories generated by molecular dynamics (MD) simulations starting from the PDB structure embedded in a pre-equilibrated cell of explicitly represented water molecules and counterions. Computations are performed by integration of Newton's equations of motion with time step 2fs in an NPT ensemble with box size $8 \times 8 \times 8\,\text{nm}^3$ and periodic boundary conditions maintained at 300K and 1atm. The box size is calibrated so that the solvation shell extended at least 12Å from the protein surface at all times. Specific details on the generation of these classical trajectories may be found in chapter 2.

In this way, we introduce a descriptor of hydration tightness for targeted soluble proteins defined as the mean residence time of hydrating molecules within a domain around each residue on the protein surface. Hydrating molecules with short residence times constitute our blueprint for ligand re-engineering since they signal a local propensity for water removal. *The crux of the redesign strategy is then the sculpting in the ligand of nonconserved local de-wetting propensities in the aligned targets: the ligand is engineered to remove interfacial water upon association according to weaknesses in the target hydration shell* (*chapter* 2). This blueprint is typically not conserved across drug targets (cf. Fig. 7.7(a)), enabling us to modulate the inhibitory impact of the drug and funnel it on the realm of therapeutic relevance. The key de-wetting hot spots correspond to amide-carbonyl backbone hydrogen bonds pairing backbone-exposed residues [46]. As noted in chapter 2, such bonds become energetically enhanced and stabilized upon removal of surrounding water and thus constitute de-wetting sites.

A de-wetting hot spot in C-Kit not conserved in the alternative targets corresponds to the residue pair C673-G676, which is mapped into the M318-G321 pair in Bcr-Abl and the M319-G322 pair in Lck (Fig. 7.7(a–c)). Thus, this local difference in de-wetting propensity, prompted us to conceive and synthesize a methylated variant of imatinib, named WBZ_4 [47] (Fig. 7.7(d, e)). To achieve a higher level of favorable and selective interactivity required an exogenous modulation of the target microenvironment, in turn, requiring a modification of the parental compound. As dictated by

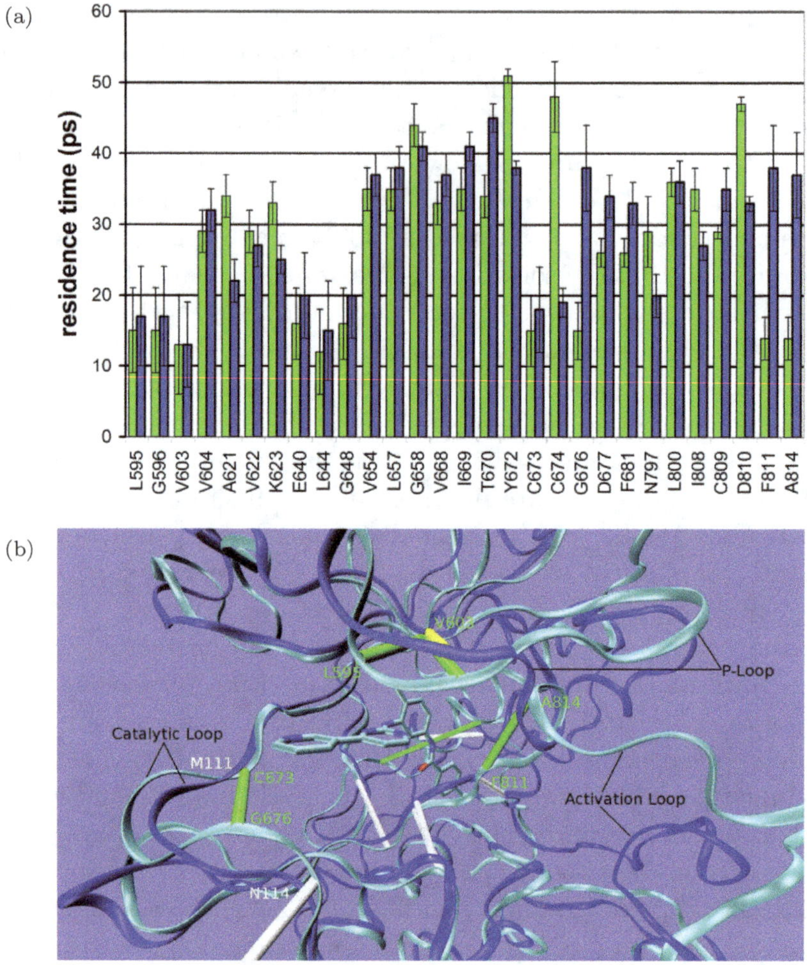

Figure 7.8. **(a)** Aligned de-wetting patterns for C-Kit kinase (green) and JNK1 (blue) restricted to the C-Kit residues in contact with imatinib. **(b)** De-wetting hot spots arising as backbone hydrogen-bonded residues in C-Kit kinase (backbone in light blue, de-wetting hot spots in green), aligned with JNK (blue backbone, de-wetting hot spots in yellow). The JNK residues M111 and N114, aligned with the de-wetting hot spot C673-G676 in C-Kit are not paired by a hydrogen bond. Yet, M111 is a de-wetting hot spot for JNK (Fig. 9.3(a)), hence a harnessing spot for the designed imatininb modification. Reprinted from [47], copyright 2007 with permission from the American Society for Clinical Investigation.

the de-wetting blueprint, the added methyl group would promote the favored dehydration of the pair C673-G676 upon binding to C-Kit, while it would hamper the association with Bcr-Abl and Lck, since the latter kinases favor hydration of the nucleotide-binding loop residues aligned with the targeted C-Kit residues C673-G676.

A comparison of the aligned dehydron matrices of the three imatinib-targeted kinases restricted to the imatinib-binding region single out the C673-C676 dehydron in C-Kit as the selectivity-promoting feature (red circles in Fig. 7.7(f–h)), in good agreement with the de-wetting analysis. The dehydron matrix is precisely the representational tool that enables the simplest and fastest *in silico* assessment of drug cross reactivity across the entire human kinome.

Reported assays on imatinib-promoted cardiomyocyte damage suggest that JNK (JNK1) inhibition may be beneficial to reduce the induced collapse of mitochondrial membrane potential and preserve sarcolemmal integrity [48]. For this reason, we tested the binding of WBZ_4 as it anchors on the de-wetting pattern of JNK1 (PDB.2G01). This analysis required alignment of JNK1 with the imatinib-C-Kit complex (PDB.1T46) (Fig. 7.8(a, b)). The high de-wetting propensity at JNK1 residue M111, the residue that aligns with C673 in C-Kit, instills confidence in the affinity of WBZ_4 for JNK.

7.8 Interfacial thermodynamics to assess efficacy of imatinib wrapping variant WBZ_4

The target-dewetting patterns or equivalently, the target dehydron patterns, constitute powerful tools to assess the efficacy of wrapping drugs or ligands in favourably displacing interfacial water from the target. In this regard, we tested WBZ_4 *in silico* by monitoring the spatio-temporal effect of the specific methylation on the kinase-inhibitor association through molecular dynamics (Fig. 7.9(a, b)). As C-Kit associates with imatinib, the loop facing the para-position on the terminal ring (Figs. 7.7(b), 7.9(a)) was found to be unstable. In all five simulation trajectories, the backbone hydrogen bond between Cys673 and Gly676 was irreversibly replaced by water-mediated interactions within 1ns (Fig. 7.9(a)). When WBZ_4 replaced imatinib

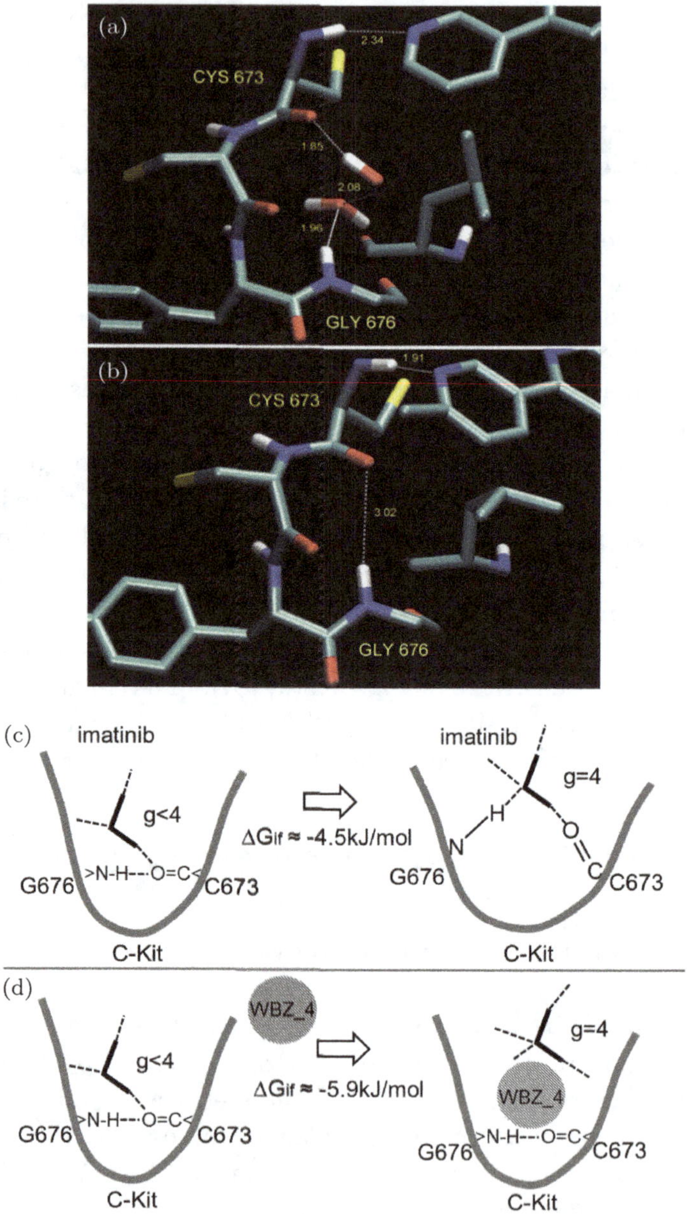

Figure 7.9. *(Continued)*

within the C-Kit complex, the same loop was found to be stabilized due to the improved dehydration of the hydrogen bond by the added methyl group on the ligand (Fig. 7.9(b)). Thus, for C-Kit, WBZ_4 introduces favorable interactions engaging the solvent-exposed preformed hydrogen bond and consequently stabilizes the inhibitor binding. The effect of WBZ_4 is the opposite on Bcr-Abl. The simulations demonstrate that in this case, the imatinib complex has a better stability in the same loop region, while WBZ_4 significantly destabilizes the loop. This is due to the fact that the Met318-Gly321 backbone hydrogen bond on the Bcr-Abl loop is well dehydrated intramolecularly and positioned closer to imatinib, thus this bond becomes well protected [51] by imatinib and the addition of the methyl group clashes sterically with the loop. Thus, molecular dynamics provides a rationale for the discriminatory power of WBZ_4 relative to the parent drug.

The solvent-centric physical understanding of the mechanism of action of the wrapping drug WBZ_4 requires evaluation of the change in epistructural free energy, ΔG_{if}, associated with interfacial water dynamics in the C-Kit/imatinib versus the C-Kit/WBZ_4 complex. The C673-G676 dehydron in the C-Kit/imatinib complex becomes irreversibly disrupted due to backbone hydration in ~5ns.

Figure 7.9. **(a)** Snapshot of the molecular dynamics simulation for C-Kit kinase bound to imatinib at 1ns. The main-chain hydrogen bond between Cys673 and Gly676 is competitively and irreversibly replaced by hydrogen bonding to a water molecule, revealing the instability of the intramolecular interaction. **(b)** Snapshot of the simulation of C-Kit kinase in complex with WBZ_4 at 1ns. The main-chain hydrogen bond between Cys673 and Gly676 is stabilized by the water expulsion promoted by the added methyl on the inhibitor. Reprinted from [47], copyright 2007 with permission from the American Society for Clinical Investigation. **(c)** Mechanism of mitigation of interfacial tension generated by the unique nonconserved C-Kit dehydron C673-G676 within the nucleotide-binding loop of the kinase. If the drug is unable to wrap the dehydron upon associating with the C-Kit target (as is the case with imatinib), the dehydron simply breaks apart to reduce water frustration ($g < 4 \rightarrow g = 4$) and thereby reduce interfacial tension. **(d)** Dehydron-wrapping drug WBZ_4 stabilizes the dehydron C673-G676, as it displaces interfacial frustrated water surrounding the dehydron upon associating with C-Kit.

The hydrogen-bond disruption is thermodynamically favored as the means of releasing the interfacial tension created by the C673-G676 dehydron. Based on the decrease in interfacial water frustration, from $\phi = 1$ (g = 3) around the dehydron-sustaining conformation to $\phi = 0$ (g = 4) in the conformation with the dehydron disrupted, and applying the thermodynamic functional methods described in chapter 1, we estimate the decrease in interfacial free energy associated with dehydron disruption in the C-Kit/imatinib complex at $\Delta G_{if} \approx -4.5$kJ/mol. On the other hand, the mitigation of interfacial tension generated by the C673-G676 dehydron upon formation of the C-Kit/WBZ_4 complex follows a completely different mechanism, as it befits the wrapping effect of WBZ_4 upon the C673-G676 dehydron. In this case the frustrated water molecule hydrating the C673-G676 dehydron becomes displaced to a bulk-like locus with $\phi = 0$ (g = 4) upon C-Kit binding to WBZ_4. The reduction in water frustration in this case yields $\Delta G_{if} \approx -5.9$kJ/mol, a figure obtained as the difference in association free energy between WBZ_4 and the parental drug imatinib, which only evaluates the extra dehydron wrapping.

Thus, as shown in Fig. 7.9(c, d), we observe a qualitative difference in the mechanism of mitigation of the interfacial tension generated by the unique nonconserved C-Kit dehydron C673-G676. If the drug is unable to wrap the dehydron upon associating with the target, the dehydron simply breaks apart to reduce water frustration (Fig. 7.9(c)), whereas, a dehydron-wrapping drug stabilizes the dehydron upon binding, as it displaces surrounding frustrated water (Fig. 7.9(d)). This dynamic aspect of epistructure-based drug design will be further developed in subsequent chapters, but it is important to highlight its importance at this early stage of conceptual maturation of the wrapping technology.

7.9 Experimental validation of enhanced specificity for epistructure-based imatinib redesign WBZ_4 (part I)

Screening methodologies for kinase inhibitors have been revolutionized in their breadth with the advent of bacteriophage libraries of kinase display [39], enabling a huge amplification of the affinity signal of the test compound. With panels now covering the majority of the 519 kinases that comprise the human kinome, this screening methodology has become the benchmark of high-throughput assays in the test tube. Thus, kinases are expressed on the capside of bacteriophages and this display construct is subject to a competitive binding assay. In the assay, the test compound and the kinase-display construct are in solution and the high-affinity and promiscuous ATP-mimicking ligand is in a fixed phase within a chromatographic column. Thus, the affinity of the test compound is measured relative to that of the fixed-phase ligand through its ability to displace the latter and hence enable the kinase-display bacteriophage to elute from the column.

To test whether wrapping-based design truly enables the control of specificity, WBZ_4 was screened for affinity against the T7-bacteriophage kinase-display library (Fig. 7.10), using imatinib screening as control [47]. The selective affinity of WBZ_4 for C-Kit kinase and JNK1 is noteworthy. Predictably, the affinity of WBZ_4 for ABL1 is reduced by 75% and by 95% or more on all other Abl variants, while, in contrast with imatinib, WBZ_4 shows no detectable affinity for Lck. The impact of WBZ_4 on all additional imatinib targets was comparable, while its controlled specificity is apparent.

7.10 Experimental validation of enhanced specificity for epistructure-based imatinib redesign WBZ_4 (part II)

As shown in [47], the specificity of WBZ_4 towards C-Kit was established first through *in vitro* assays that probes the phosphorylation kinetics of competitive inhibition. These spectrophotometric assays couple ADP production, the byproduct of phosphorylation activity, with oxidative steps following the glycolysis cycle [52,53], as described in [47]. The inhibitory impact of imatinib (triangles) and WBZ_4 (squares) on the rate of phosphorylation was determined by spectrophotometry, assaying for the activity of C-Kit and Bcr-Abl

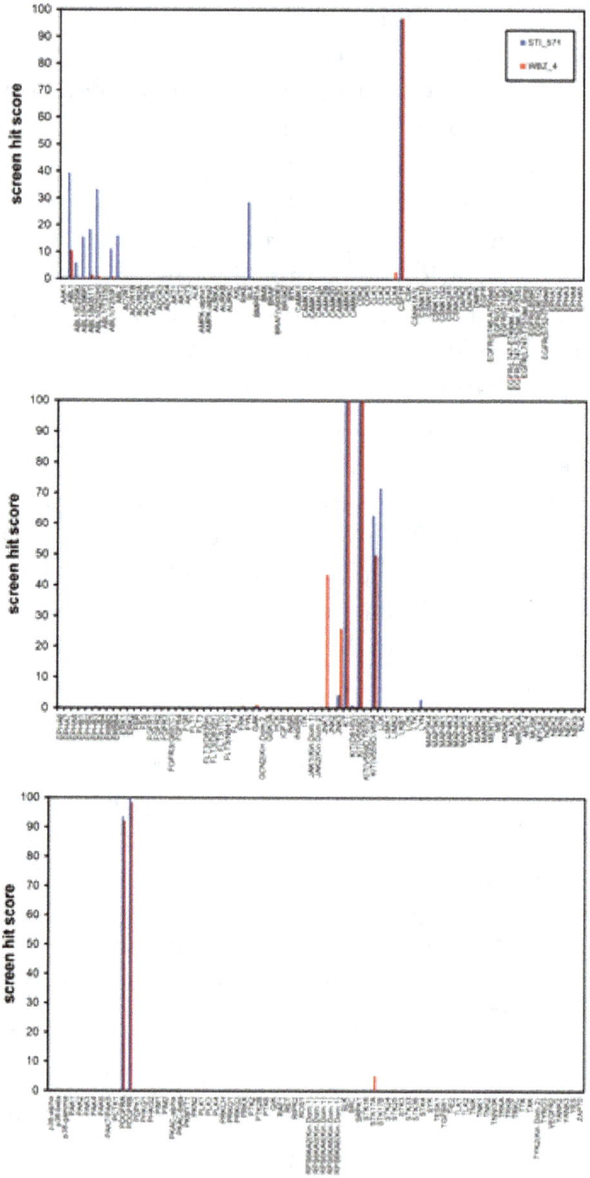

Figure 7.10. High-throughput screening at 10mM for WBZ_4 (red) and imatinib (STI_571, blue, control) over a battery of human kinases displayed in a T7-bacteriophage library (Ambit Biosciences, San Diego, CA). Hit values are reported as percentage bound kinase. Reprinted from [47], copyright 2007 with permission from the American Society for Clinical Investigation.

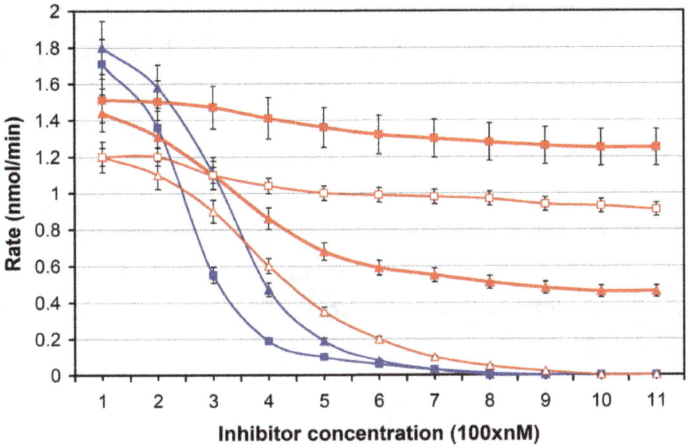

Figure 7.11. Kinetic inhibitory impact of compounds WBZ_4 and imatinib determined by measuring phosphorylation rates through spectrophotometric assays of C-Kit and Bcr-Abl kinase activity. The kinases are inhibited by WBZ_4 (squares), and by the parental compound (triangles). Phosphorylation rate plots are given for Bcr-Abl (red) and C-kit (blue). The open red symbols correspond to inhibition of unphosphorylated Bcr-Abl, while the full red symbols correspond to the Tyr412-phosphorylated form. Error bars represent dispersion over 5 runs for each kinetic assay. Reprinted from [47], copyright 2007 with permission from the American Society for Clinical Investigation.

(blue and red plots, respectively, Fig. 7.11). These kinetic assays revealed a high specificity of WBZ_4 for C-Kit, in contrast with imatinib. WBZ_4 enhances the inhibition of C-Kit activity even beyond imatinib levels, revealing a higher competitive affinity of the prototype compound for the adenosine tri phosphate (ATP)-binding pocket (K_I(imatinib) $\approx 55 \pm 7$nM; K_I(WBZ_4) $\approx 43 \pm 5$nM). On the other hand, the pattern of inhibition for Bcr-Abl is dependent on the phosphorylation state of this kinase [53, 54]. At 1μM concentration, imatinib reduces 66% of the activity of Tyr412-phosphorylated kinase [41] ($K_I \approx 5 \pm 1\mu$M) and ~100% of the activity of the unphosphorylated state ($K_I \approx 50 \pm 5$nM). By contrast, 1μM WBZ_4 reduces by less than 20% the activity of both states of Bcr-Abl. The prototype compound has reciprocal affinity constants $K_I \approx 18 \pm 3\mu$M and $K_I \approx 11 \pm 2\mu$M, for phosphorylated and unphosphorylated Bcr-Abl, respectively.

In vitro colorimetric assays were performed over a 1pM–100μM range in ligand concentration to assess the inhibition of phosphorylating activity by antibody recognition of phosphorylated peptide substrates [47]. The IC50 (50%-inhibition concentration) for imatinib/Abl is $\sim$1μM, while the WBZ_4/Abl value is above 100μM (Fig. 7.12(a)). The active recombinant Abl kinase and its substrate (Abl-tide) were incubated in the presence of various WBZ_4 or imatinib concentrations and ATP (100nM). Phosphorylation of Abl-tide peptide was detected by spectrophotometry following incubation with phospho-Abl-tide antibodies.

The specificity of the inhibitory impact on C-Kit is significantly enhanced as WBZ_4 substitutes imatinib (Fig. 7.12(a, b)), while C-Kit inhibition is 23 $\pm$ 12% greater for WBZ_4 (Fig. 7.12(b)). The impact of the wrapping prototype ligand on alternative imatinib targets, such as the platelet dependent growth factor receptor (PDGFR) kinase, could not be modulated since such proteins are not reported in PDB and thus, no de-wetting pattern can be reliably identified (cf. high-throughput screening of WBZ_4 versus imatinib in Fig. 7.10). On the other hand, the PDGFR kinase is a close paralog of the Kit kinase and hence it is largely expected that any Kit kinase inhibitor would be cross reactive with the PDGFR kinase.

7.11 Assaying the selective anticancer activity of the wrapping imatinib redesign

The controlled inhibitory impact of prototype WBZ_4 was further tested through assays on cancer cell lines representative of CML and GIST [47]. The initial tests entailed treating the GIST882 [45] cell line and the CML K562 [40] cell line with WBZ_4 and contrasting its inhibitory impact on cell proliferation and in-cell specificity with those associated with imatinib. Because of its relative insolubility, WBZ_4 was incorporated into liposomes to promote cellular delivery. The proliferation of C-Kit-expressing GIST882 cells treated with WBZ_4 was significantly inhibited in a quantitative dose-dependent manner similar to imatinib, with maximum impact at 1μM bulk concentration (Fig. 7.13(a)). By contrast, the inhibitory

(a)

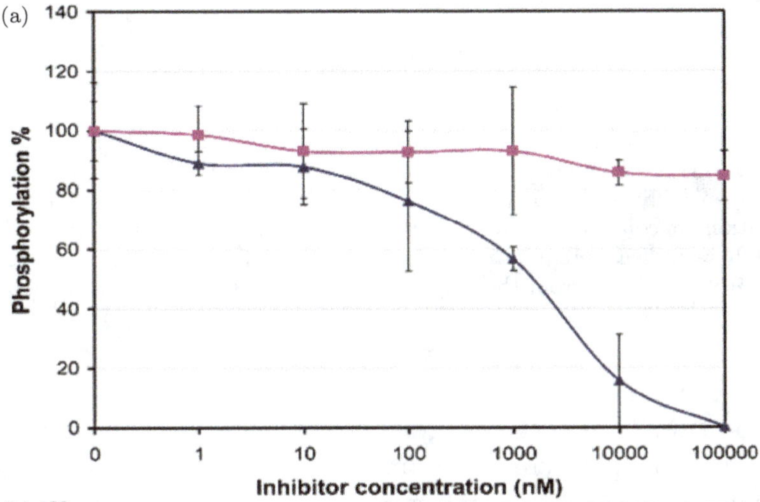

(b)

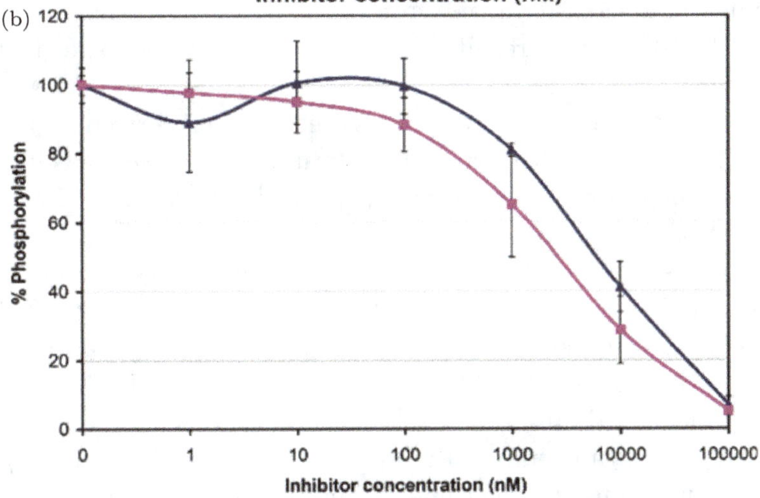

Figure 7.12. **(a)** *In vitro* phosphorylation inhibition assay for Abl enzyme in the presence of WBZ_4 (pink) or imatinib (blue). Active recombinant Abl enzyme (1μg/mL) and its substrate (Abl-tide, 1μg/ml) were incubated for 1h at 37°C in the presence of various WBZ_4 or imatinib concentrations. ATP (100nM) was added to the reaction mixture. Phosphorylation of Abl-tide peptide was detected by incubation in consecutive order with anti-rabbit phospho-Abl-tide antibody and anti-rabbit horseradish peroxidase (HRP) antibody. Phosphorylation of the substrate was quantified as absorbance units (AU) by spectrophotometry at 450nm. Values obtained with the enzyme without the inhibitors (WBZ_4 or imatinib) were assumed to be 100% phosphorylation and were compared to the

Figure 7.12. (*Continued*) values obtained with the addition of the inhibitors. **(b)** *In vitro* phosphorylation inhibition assay for C-Kit in the presence of WBZ_4 (pink) or imatinib (blue). Active recombinant C-Kit kinase (25ng/ml) and its substrate Poly (Glu4-Tyr, 150nM) were incubated for 1h at 37°C in the presence of various WBZ_4 or imatinib concentrations. ATP (100nM) was added to the reaction mixture. Phosphorylation of Poly (Glu4-Tyr) peptide was detected by incubation in consecutive order with anti-phosphotyrosine antibody and anti-rabbit horseradish peroxidase (HRP) antibody. Reprinted from [47], copyright 2007 with permission from the American Society for Clinical Investigation.

impact of WBZ_4 on CML K562 cells at the same bulk physiological dose of 1μM is almost negligible (cell proliferation less than 10% lower than the proliferation of untreated cells), while 1μM imatinib promotes a decrease in cell proliferation of approximately 66% (Fig. 7.13(b)). These results demonstrate the higher specificity in anti-cancer activity of WBZ_4.

A Western blot assay on treated cancer-derived cell lines (Fig. 7.14(a, b)) was performed to determine the *in-cell* specificity of WBZ_4. The immunoblots revealed specificity towards C-Kit consistent with the selective anticancer activity on the GIST882 cell line that expresses C-Kit. Thus, the activating phosphorylation of C-Kit at sites Tyr703 and Tyr721 in ST882 cells is inhibited by WBZ_4 in a dose-sensitive manner similar to imatinib (Fig. 7.14(a)). By contrast, phosphorylation of Bcr-Abl at Tyr 412 [55, 56] in K562 cells was not significantly inhibited (<15%) by WBZ_4, while densitometry revealed an imatinib-induced inhibition of ~85% (Fig. 7.14(b)).

Since imatinib is a micromolar inhibitor of phosphorylated Bcr-Abl (Fig. 7.11), the attack on CML cells at 1μM bulk concentration (growth decrease 63%, Fig. 7.13(b)) must be attributed to the inhibition of phosphorylated Bcr-Abl (Fig. 7.14(b)) combined with the effective nanomolar inhibition of the unphosphorylated form (Fig. 7.11). By contrast, WBZ_4 hinders the phosphorylation of Bcr-Abl only partially (Fig. 7.14(b)) and in any case, it is an ineffective (micromolar) inhibitor of *both* forms of Bcr-Abl (Fig. 7.11). Hence, its anti-tumor activity is predictably minimal on CML

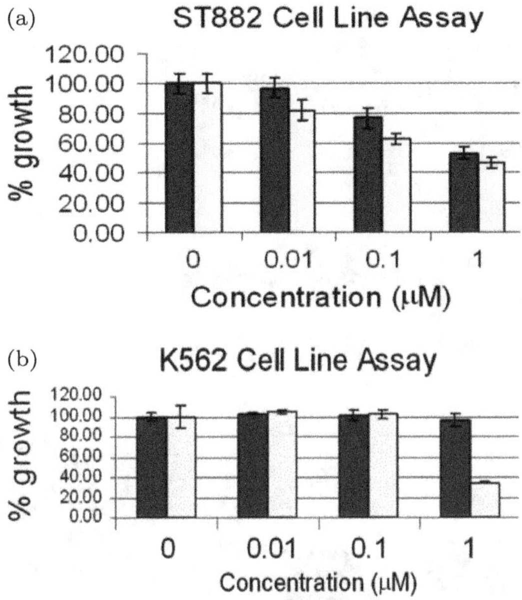

Figure 7.13. **(a)** Cell-proliferation assay for GIST 882 cells. WBZ_4 inhibits cell proliferation of C-Kit positive ST-882 cells. GIST cancer cells ST882 (GIST 882) were seeded in 96 wells plates at a density of 8×10^3 cells per well. The cells were treated with various concentrations of WBZ_4 (crimson) and imatinib (light blue) for an additional 48h. Cell proliferation is expressed as the percentage of proliferating cells relative to untreated cells. **(b)** Cell-proliferation assay for K562 cells. WBZ_4 does not significantly inhibit cell proliferation of Bcr-Abl-expressing K562 cells. K562 cells were seeded in 96 wells plates at a density of 1×10^4 cells per well in 50μl of medium. Two hours later, 50μl medium containing different concentrations 0.01, 0.1, 1μM of liposome-encapsulated WBZ_4 (crimson) or soluble imatinib (light blue) were added to the wells to reach a final volume of 100μl per well. Following 48h of exposure, the Alamar blue assay was performed. Plates were read at dual wavelength (570–595nm) in an Elisa plate reader. Reprinted from [47], copyright 2007 with permission from the American Society for Clinical Investigation.

cells (Fig. 7.13(b)). In the case of GIST cells, comparable anti-tumor activity of both compounds (Fig. 7.13(a)) is likely to arise from comparable inhibitory impact (~85%, Fig. 7.14(a)) on C-Kit phosphorylation, and the fact that both compounds are nanomolar-affinity inhibitors of C-Kit (Fig. 7.11).

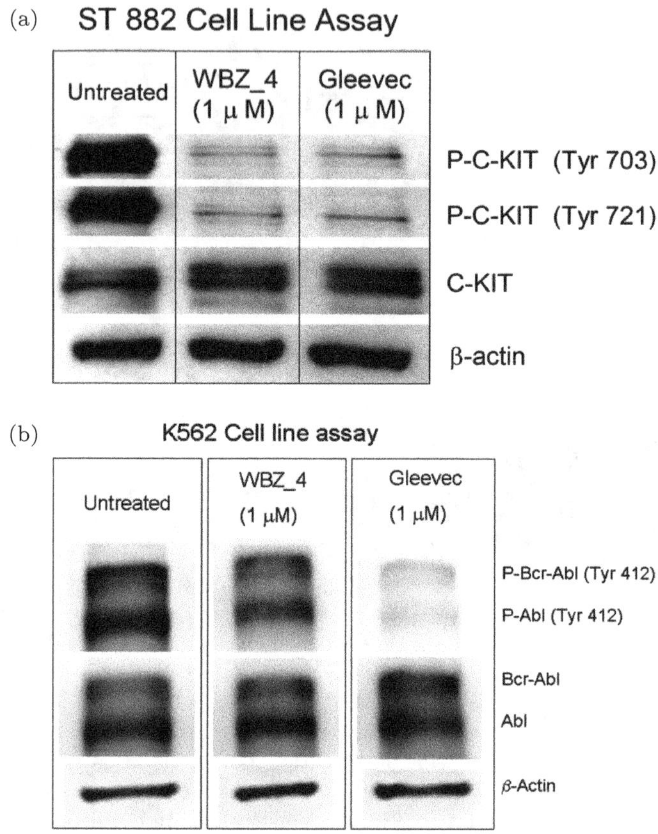

Figure 7.14. **(a)** Western blot of C-Kit inhibition. WBZ_4 inhibits phosphorylation of C-Kit kinase in ST-882 GIST cells. Gel bands from the Western blot assays of C-Kit and its phosphorylated (P-) form in GIST cells treated with WBZ_4 and imatinib. The β-actin assay was adopted as control. **(b)** Western blot of Bcr-Abl inhibition. Phosphorylation of Bcr-Abl kinase is not significantly inhibited by WBZ_4 in K562 CML cells. Electrophoretic gel bands for Western blots for Bcr-Abl kinase and its phosphorylated (P-) form in CML cells treated with WBZ_4 and imatinib. Reprinted from [47], copyright 2007 with permission from the American Society for Clinical Investigation.

7.12 Efficacy and safety of epistructural drug design tested in animal models

To assay the epistructural design WBZ_4 for anticancer activity *in vivo*, an animal model for GIST growth based on female

C.B-17/IcrHsd-*Prkdc*^{SCID} nude mice was developed *de novo* [47]. The model involved the subcutaneous injection of GIST882 cells [55]. The efficacy of WBZ_4 was found to be comparable to that of imatinib, as determined by the decrease in tumor volume and weight (Fig. 7.15(a, b)). No obvious toxicities were observed in the animals during treatment. Selectivity of WBZ_4 in the animal model was corroborated by assaying on the xenograft induced by CML cells K562 (Fig. 7.15(c)). While imatinib is shown to significantly impair tumor growth ($p < 0.01$), the prototype WBZ_4 has virtually no effect. This result is in perfect accordance with the engineered superior specificity of WBZ_4, reflected in a lack of inhibitory impact on the Bcr-Abl kinase.

Previous studies of imatinib-induced cardiotoxicity identified a protective JNK (JNK1) inhibition as a means to reduce the collapse of mitochondrial membrane potential [48]. Accordingly, WBZ_4 was engineered to also inhibit JNK, a feature preliminarily corroborated *in vitro* (Fig. 7.10). This protective role of WBZ_4 is also validated *in vivo*. Western blotting of cell extracts derived from the same imatinib- and WBZ_4-treated cardiomyocytes (Fig. 7.16(a)) revealed that both drugs increased the phosphorylation state of ERK1/2 and p38^{MAPK} as compared to untreated cultures. In contrast, cells treated with WBZ_4 showed reduced levels of JNK activation at each concentration tested, as compared to untreated cells, or cells treated with imatinib. These results confirm other observations [48] demonstrating that imatinib induces the endoplasmic reticulum (ER) stress response and activates JNKs in neonatal rat ventricular myocytes (NRVM). JNK activation has been clearly associated with cardiomyocyte apoptosis via collapse of the mitochondrial membrane potential and release of cytochrome C [55]. It was further confirmed that imatinib (and WBZ_4) had little effect on p38^{MAPK} activation at concentrations below 50μM, and actually increased ERK activation in these cultured cells. In contrast, WBZ_4 appeared to reduce levels of pJNK at each dose tested, suggesting that upstream activation of JNKs was inhibited by WBZ_4. Thus, a direct inhibitory effect on JNK activity would predict that WBZ_4 should have reduced cardiotoxicity *in vivo*.

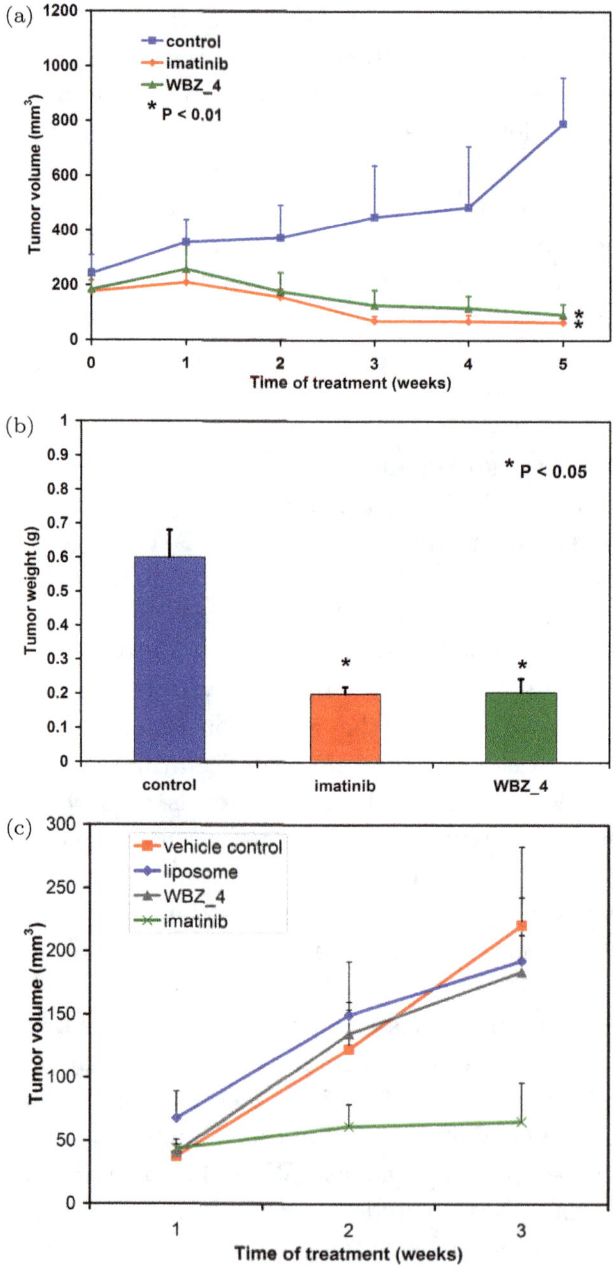

Figure 7.15. *(Continued)*

This expectation is supported by other observations using the surrogate marker brain natriuretic peptide (*BNP*), a most sensitive indicator of myocardial hypertrophy and cardiac impairment [57]. The expected curbing of cardiotoxity in WBZ_4 anticancer therapy was confirmed by examining the mRNA levels of BNP in the left ventricle of mice from the same groups assayed for anticancer activity. The *BNP* mRNA levels were about 58% higher in the ventricles from imatinib-treated animals (Fig. 7.16(b)), while no significant difference was detected in the WBZ_4-treated animals when compared with untreated mice. Finally, the reduced cardiotoxicity of WBZ_4 was directly tested in mice by determination of the percentage ejection fraction (EF) in the left ventricle by magnetic resonance (MR) imaging of treated mice subject to imatinib or WBZ_4 therapy (Fig. 7.16(c, d)). Following 6 weeks of therapy, the cardiac EF was significantly lower in the imatinib group compared to controls ($p = 0.02$), which is consistent with previous findings [48]. Remarkably, WBZ_4 treatment had no effect on cardiac EF despite prolonged therapy (Fig. 7.16(c, d)).

7.13 Epistructural design and drug safety

The top-down approach presented in this chapter is centered in a rational ligand re-design sculpting target-specific molecular features. The approach harnesses fundamental concepts pertaining to the

Figure 7.15. Xenograft models of anticancer activity. **(a)** Effect of WBZ_4 or imatibib therapy on *in vivo* GIST growth determined by longitudinal tumor volume measurements. Mice were randomized to treatment with either control (normal PBS and empty liposomes give indistinguishable results within experimental uncertainty), imatinib or liposome-formulated WBZ_4. **(b)** Effect of WBZ_4 or imatibib therapy on *in vivo* GIST growth determined by weight measurements. Animals from all groups were sacrificed after 6 weeks of therapy, tumors were excised, and the weight was recorded. **(c)** Effect of WBZ_4 or imatibib therapy on *in vivo* CML growth induced through a xenograft of K562 tumor cells, determined by longitudinal tumor volume measurement. The WBZ_4 selectivity is hereby corroborated *in vivo*. Reprinted from [47], copyright 2007 with permission from the American Society for Clinical Investigation.

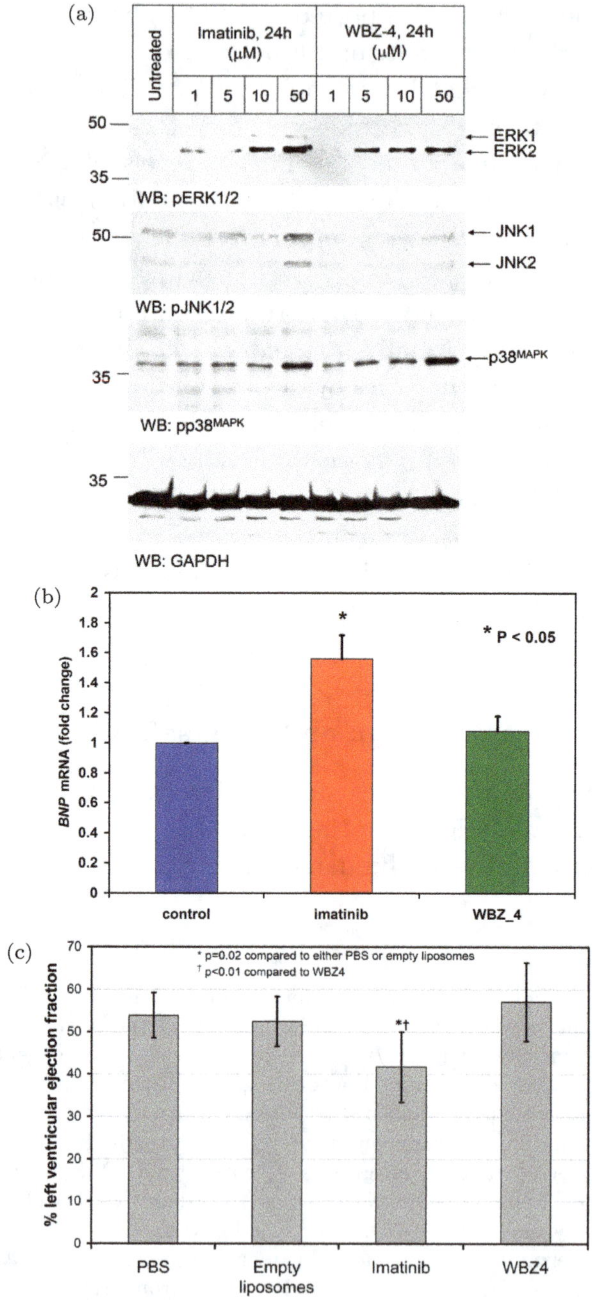

Figure 7.16. *(Continued)*

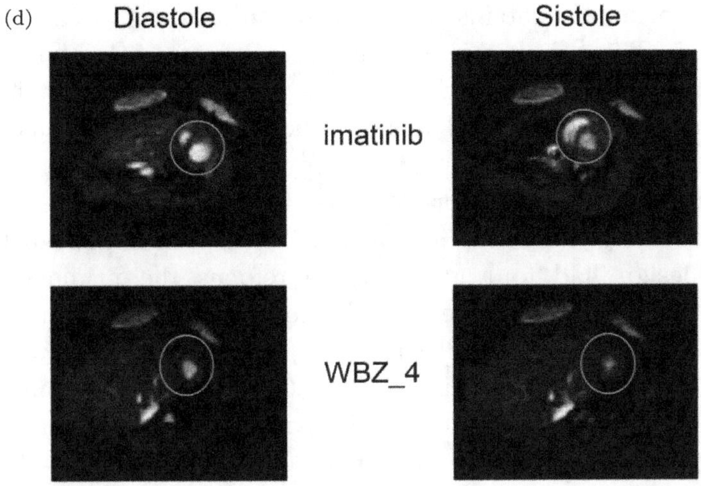

Figure 7.16. Cardiotoxicity assays. **(a)** Western blot of JNK inhibition in cardiomyocytes. Western blots were probed with primary antibodies specific for the phosphorylated forms of ERKs, JNKs, and $p38^{MAPK}$. The position of molecular weight standards is indicated to the left of each blot. **(b)** Effect of WBZ_4 or imatinib therapy on mouse heart brain natriuretic peptide (*BNP*). The mRNA levels of *BNP* (a sensitive marker of myocardial hypertrophy and cardiac impairment) were examined in the left ventricle of mice from the groups in Fig. 7.15(a). The *BNP* mRNA levels were about 58% higher in the ventricles from imatinib-treated animals ($p = 0.02$), but no significant difference was noted in the WBZ_4 treated animals. **(c)** Comparison of left ventricular ejection fraction after 6 weeks of control (groups treated with either PBS or empty liposomes), imatinib, or WBZ_4 therapy in mice. **(d)** Magnetic resonance imaging of cardiac function. Assessment of left ventricular function (red circle, lower cavity) was performed as follows: representative *in vivo* axial images of the left ventricle in diastole and systole of control and test mice were acquired in a 4.7T MR scanner cardiac gating using a magnetization-prepared spoiled gradient echo sequence. To assess cardiac function, short axis cardiac cine images were acquired using a magnetization-prepared, cardiac-gated spoiled gradient echo sequence (TE/TR 2.1 ms/$\sim$23.5 ms; 16 phases covering 1.5 R–R cycles; in-plane resolution $312\mu m \times 312\mu m$; 1.25 mm slice thickness). For assessing EF, regions of interest encompassing the cavity of the left ventricle were drawn. For each animal, the average region of interest of four central slices in systole was divided by the average region of interest of four central slices in diastole taken at the same location in the left ventricle to derive the EF. Fig. 7.16**(a–c)** reprinted from [47], copyright 2007 with permission from the American Society for Clinical Investigation.

discrimination of proteins with a common ancestry, as described in chapter 5. These discriminatory features are associated with unique dehydration or de-wetting hot spots found on the protein/water interface of the purported target. The de-wetting propensities are in turn promoted by dehydrons in the protein structure, and hence the hydration blueprint of the target becomes a design tool complementing the wrapping concept. In this particular illustration, the re-design had four goals: a) to refocus the primary impact on C-Kit kinase; b) to reduce the inhibitory impact on Bcr-Abl kinase; c) to reduce the inhibitory impact against LCK in order to prevent immunosuppression (cf. Fig. 7.6(b)); and d) to promote JNK inhibition in order to reduce cardiotoxic effects and because JNK is a recognized target in the treatment of ovarian cancer [50]. These three goals have been achieved [47], as attested by the *in vitro* and *in vivo* results described in this chapter, clearly revealing that *drug specificity can be rationally controlled.* The imatinib re-design turned the wrapping ligand into a selective proto-therapeutic agent to treat GIST with a *prima facie* reduction of cardiotoxicity.

7.14 Targeting catalytic dehydrons to block enzyme functions

This chapter already revealed how and why dehydrons may be exploited as selectivity filters in drug design. Yet, a more fundamental question has not been dealt with, at least explicitly: Why would targeting dehydrons by wrapping them with small-molecule drugs be effective at blocking specific protein functions, as required for therapeutic applications? One would argue that the dehydron wrappers discussed so far displace the natural ligand ATP of the target protein in a competitive manner, but this limits the discussion to dehydrons in the ATP-binding pocket, and we are interested in a more general answer. The answer may be found in chapter 6, where the chemical role of dehydrons as participants in biochemical reactions has been highlighted and their function as enablers and stimulators of catalytic activity has been unraveled. For the sake of the argument, let us say that we intend to block a signaling cascade that promotes cancer-related cellular activity. Then, our focus is to block the phosphorylation of a signal transducer, a kinase. Phosphorylation is an enzymatic activity whereby a kinase residue with a pro-nucleophilic side chain (tyrosine, serine, threonine and sometimes even histidine) performs a nucleophilic attack on the terminal phosphor-ester linkage of ATP triggering an intermolecular trans-esterification reaction which in effect amounts to phosphorylating the nucleophilic residue through covalent attachment of the terminal (gamma) phosphate group from ATP. If our intent is to block this chemical process, one way of doing it is to wrap and thereby annihilate the dehydron involved in stimulating the kinase catalytic activity. The dehydron-based enablement and stimulation of phosphorylation hinges upon the capacity of the dehydron to induce basicity in interfacial water, thereby triggering proton transference from the nucleophilic group assumed to undergo phosphorylation (Fig. 7.17(a)). Once deprotonated, the latter group is habilitated to

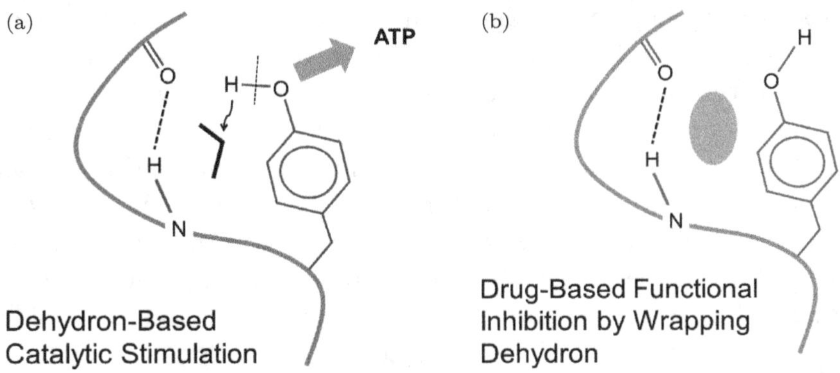

Figure 7.17. Drug-based dehydron wrapping impairs phosphorylation of a tyrosine kinase. The latter is schematically represented by the side chain susceptible to phosphorylation (Tyr) and the nearby dehydron that stimulates the enzymatic activity. **(a)** The dehydron-based enablement of phosphorylation depends on the capacity of the dehydron to induce basicity in nearby interfacial water (represented by thick sticks), thereby triggering proton transference (indicated by the arrow) from the nucleophilic group susceptible to phosphorylation. The latter group is now enabled to perform the nucleophilic attack on the ATP terminal ester linkage. **(b)** A drug that wraps the dehydron displaces the interfacial water that stimulates kinase catalytic activity, and thus the drug impairs phosphorylation upon binding.

perform the nucleophilic attack on the ATP terminal ester linkage. A drug that wraps the dehydron displaces the basic interfacial water molecule that enables and promotes the kinase catalytic activity (Fig. 7.17(b)), and thus a dehydron-wrapping drug impairs phosphorylation, which is the goal of the molecular targeted treatment.

7.15 Caveats with targeting dehydrons in floppy regions

The activation loop in a kinase is in some ways very well suited as a drug target. Its high amino acid variability relative to other regions makes it a good selectivity feature, since it is fairly unique to each kinase. In addition, dehydrons created by oncogenic mutation in the activation loop (such as D816V in c-Kit) are particularly dangerous, especially if they are close to side chains susceptible of phosphorylation (Ser, Thr, Tyr, His), as they functionalize such side chains for transesterification reactions. One such dehydron-creating mutation may in principle deregulate the kinase into a constitutively active signal transducer, with devastating consequences. As said, this is due to the catalysis-stimulating role of the dehydron (chapter 6). On the other hand, activation loops tend to be structurally disordered in their phosphorylated state, and highly fluctuating in their unphosphorylated state. Thus, targeting dehydrons in the activation loop may require a mastery of drug-induced folding that we currently do not fully possess. Be as it may, subsequent chapters describe a number of situations where such control of induced folding is possible, in particular when the latter is restricted to inducing dehydrons. This level of control of the drug target requires the participation of artificial intelligence, as demonstrated in Chapter 12.

7.16 Interfacial thermodynamics for drug design

The structure-based identification of dehydrons utilizes a geometric criterion to determine the wrapping of the backbone hydrogen bond. Dehydrons thus identified constitute a proxy for hot spots of protein-water interfacial tension, as shown in chapter 1. The latter represent more accurate indicators of the singularities of the aqueous interface that may be exploited as selectivity filters in ligand/drug design. Counting nonpolar groups surrounding the hydrogen bond may not yield the optimum indicator of solvent exposure: the spatial distribution of wrapping groups needs to be also factored in to assess the extent of water exclusion from the bond microenvironment. The latter criterion is ultimately captured by an interfacial thermodynamics filter, whereupon hot spots in interfacial tension not conserved across homologous proteins become the true targets for selectivity control. As shown in Fig. 7.18, the thermodynamic filter operates by evaluating the interfacial free energy difference $\Delta\Delta G_{\mathrm{if}}$ associated with mutating a poor wrapper residue (Gly in Fig. 7.18) paired by a backbone hydrogen bond (BHB) into a better wrapper residue (Val in Fig. 7.18). Thus, if the BHB happens to be a "thermodynamic dehydron" (a dehydron based on the thermodynamic criterion) that becomes a well-wrapped

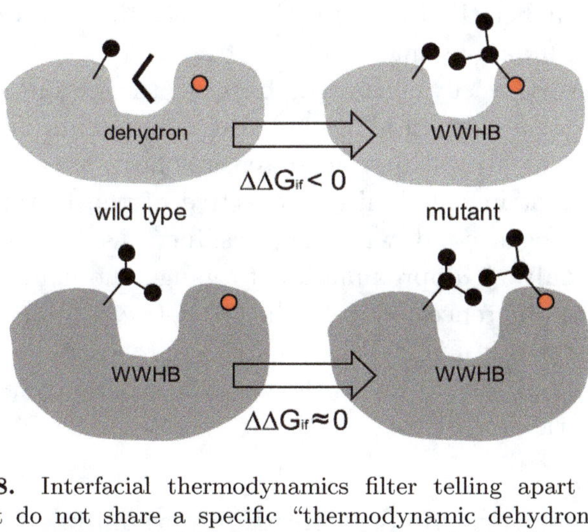

Figure 7.18. Interfacial thermodynamics filter telling apart two homolog proteins that do not share a specific "thermodynamic dehydron" ($\Delta\Delta G_{\mathrm{if}} \leq -2k_{\mathrm{B}}T$). A "thermodynamic dehydron" in one protein is identified by quantifying the interfacial free energy change associated with a mutation that improves the wrapping of the hydrogen bond (G $\rightarrow$ Val in the figure, with α-carbon of the mutation site in red). The thermodynamic dehydron aligns with a well-wrapped backbone hydrogen bond (BHB) in the homologous protein. This is evidenced by quantifying the negligible thermodynamic effect ($\Delta\Delta G_{\mathrm{if}} \approx 0$) of the mutation replacing a poor hydrogen-bond wrapper (G, red spot) for a good wrapper (Val) in the homolog protein.

BHB in the mutated version, then $\Delta\Delta G_{if} < 0$, since dehydrons generate interfacial tension and this tension is removed by the wrapping-enriching mutation. In fact, the thermodynamic criterion for identifying interface hot spots is more precisely formulated by the inequality $\Delta\Delta G_{if} \leq -2k_BT$, since the free energy decrease associated with removing a dehydron by improving its wrapping is of the order of $-2k_BT$, as shown in chapter 2. On the other hand, if the dehydron aligns with a well-wrapped hydrogen bond in a homologous protein, then in the latter protein the effect of the mutation replacing a poor wrapper for a good wrapper becomes negligible: $\Delta\Delta G_{if} \approx 0$. Thus, if two homologous proteins differ in a hot spot for interfacial tension so that $\Delta\Delta G_{if} \leq -2k_BT$ in one protein and $\Delta\Delta G_{if} \approx 0$ in the other, then the thermodynamic dehydron thus identified constitutes a filter for selectivity, meaning that if a ligand is designed to wrap it upon association, then the affinity of the ligand for the protein containing the dehydron will be significantly higher than that for the protein that does not contain the dehydron upon alignment.

As it can be easily surmised, because the geometric criterion ($\rho \leq 19$) is only a proxy for the thermodynamic criterion ($\Delta\Delta G_{if} \leq -2k_BT$) that identifies interfacial tension hot spots, the latter is actually more stringent. This is reflective of the fact that merely counting hydrogen-bond wrapping residues, as in the geometric criterion, is only an approximation to gauge the extent of solvent exposure. The differences between the geometric and thermodynamic filter is illustrated in Fig. 7.19(a, b) for the Src kinase, where the set of thermodynamic dehydrons is shown to be strictly contained in the set of geometric dehydrons.

7.17 Epistructural drug design for personalized medicine

Personalized molecular therapy is a major imperative of post-genomic medicine. This perception is reinforced with the frequent news that promising therapeutic agents are recalled because of idiosyncratic side effects detected in patient subpopulations. Rational

(a)

(b)

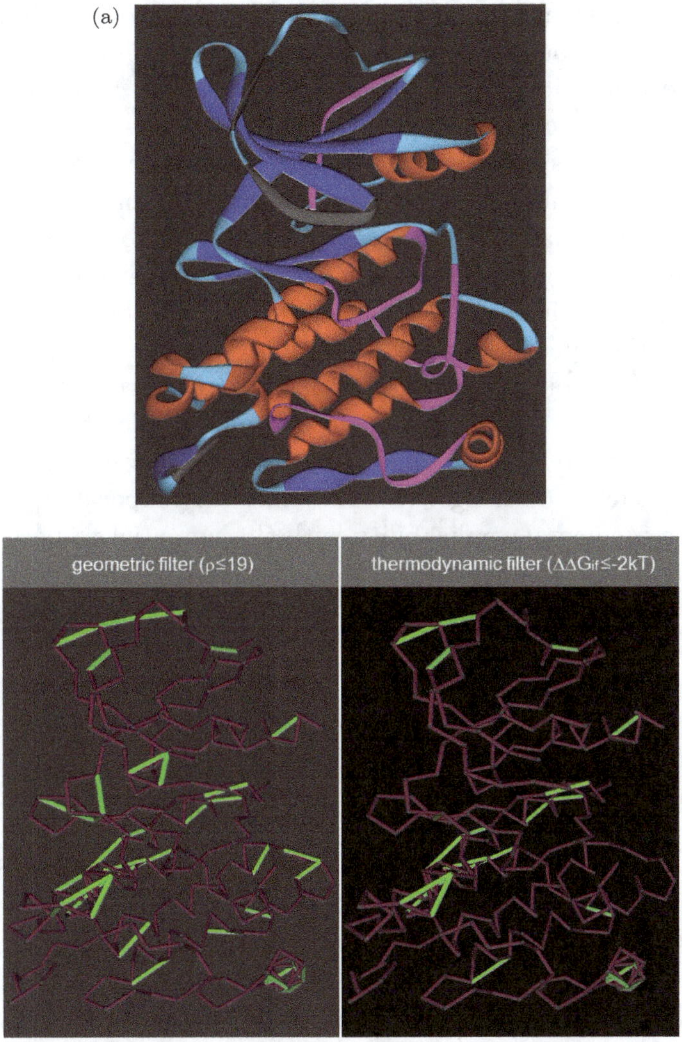

Figure 7.19. **(a)** Ribbon representation of Src kinase (PDB.3G5D) included as an aid to the eye. **(b)** Dehydron pattern of Src kinase identified by adopting a geometric (left panel) or a thermodynamic criterion (right panel).

approaches to personalized drug therapy will ultimately depend on our ability to translate genomic idiosyncratic variations into molecular biomarkers that can guide a patient-tailored design [58, 59]. This aspect is particularly challenging when the target proteins have no reported structure, and the molecular features promoting specificity need to be predicted from sequence, as shown subsequently. This section addresses this issue and describes how the wrapping design concept can be brought to fruition in this area. This section introduces plausible scenarios in which oncogenic idiosyncrasies may promote targetable differences in the wrapping patterns of the gene products. Ultimately an invitation is extended to adopt and exploit protein wrapping as a molecular biomarker for personalized medicine within an enabling platform to tailor drugs to patient idiosyncrasies.

The therapeutic imperative to make more efficacious and safer drugs by exploiting the enormous output of genomic forays has proven to be a daunting challenge, far more difficult than originally expected. No reliable rational approach has been identified so far to meet such a challenge. In addressing this imperative, the dearth of ideas of general applicability with the potential to become transformative and broaden the technological base of the pharmaceutical industry is quite evident. From the perspective of a rational drug designer, one can only speculate that a personalized approach would require an effective translation of genomic idiosyncrasies and disease-related variations into structural differences that may guide the molecular engineering of the therapeutic agent. While this conclusion may be inevitable, it has not been pursued beyond a limited number of anecdotal instances [47].

It is seldom the case that idiosyncratic or disease-related genomic differences would translate as significant structural changes in the gene products. The functional demands of the wild-type locus cannot generally be compromised without a serious fitness cost and misfolded proteins are generally degraded unless they can aberrantly aggregate (as in poly-glutamine or poly-asparagine in-frame insertions). On the other hand, subtler variations, leading for instance to an oncogenic deregulation of structural elements, may still be exploitable from the vantage point of the drug designer. Thus, while such accidents are unlikely to alter the functionally-competent topology of the protein, they may affect its wrapping, as shown below. We may thus speculate that wrapping patterns may well be on their way to become molecular biomarkers for drug personalization in the

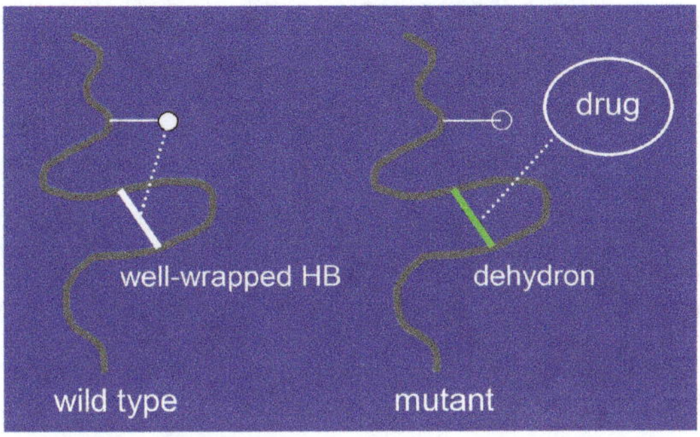

Figure 7.20. An idiosyncratic variation substituting a good hydrogen-bond wrapper (solid circle) for a bad wrapper (empty circle) can produce a new dehydron in the protein structure. This "idiosyncratic dehydron" may in turn be targeted or wrapped intermolecularly by a purposely designed drug.

particular context where a genetic accident or idiosyncrasy impacts a coding region and produces a change in the microevironment of a preformed hydrogen bond (Fig. 7.20).

In other words, a single amino acid substitution can turn a wrapping residue into a bad wrapper (that is, one of the following amino acids: G, A, N, D, S, T or P) and hence generate a dehydron in *lieu* of the well-wrapped hydrogen bond in the wild type. Thus, a mutation can produce a new dehydron, actually an "idiosyncratic dehydron", which in turn may be wrapped intermolecularly by a purposely designed drug, as shown schematically in Fig. 7.20.

Conversely, an amino acid substitution that generates a well-wrapped hydrogen bond by increasing the number of nonpolar groups in the bond microenvironment may not yield a productive opportunity from the perspective of the wrapping designer: if the bond is well wrapped, the wrapping drug would sterically clash with the intramolecular wrappers and has nothing to add in terms of hydrogen-bond stabilization (dehydration). Yet, there is a conspicuous exception arising in the case where the augmentation in the number of wrapping side-chain groups triggered by the mutation *induces* a dehydron that was absent in the wild type due to a local scarcity of wrapping residues (the $\rho < 7 \rightarrow \rho \geq 7$ transition upon drug binding).

To illustrate this case, we focus on the Asp816 → Val substitution in the activation loop that confers resistance to the C-Kit kinase against the powerful anticancer drug imatinib. This substitution renders imatinib ineffective to treat the gastrointestinal stromal tumor (GIST), which has C-Kit as the primary target. Yet, Val is a good wrapper residue while Asp is not. Hence, the Val816-Kit mutant is able to sustain the dehydron Phe811-Ala814, which is absent or unstable in the wild-type Kit kinase due to insufficient wrapping. In turn, the induced dehydron may be exploited to design a wrapping variant of imatinib with an extra methyl group, as needed to target the idiosyncratic dehydron Phe811-Ala814 by contributing to its dehydration upon association (Fig. 7.21). This wrapping modification has been named WBZ_7 and has been shown in cellular assays to be highly effective against imatinib-resistant GISTs [47].

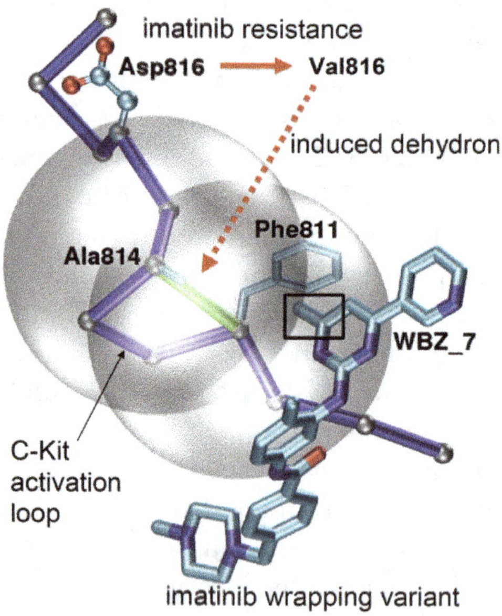

Figure 7.21. Imatinib wrapping modification engineered to overcome drug resistance in the C-Kit kinase. This resistance is promoted by the somatic mutation Asp816 → Val. The mutation induces the dehydron Phe811-Ala814, in the activation loop which in turn can be targeted or wrapped by suitably modifying imatinib at the position highlighted by the rectangle.

Thus, the subpopulation of GIST patients with the Asp816 → Val substitution in the C-Kit kinase domain may potentially be treated with a drug that targets the induced dehydron arising from the single-site mutation.

The impact on protein structure of amino acid substitutions stemming from oncogenic mutations has not been systematically studied. In the particular context of cell signaling related to mitosis or to the onset of anti-apoptotic pathways, it is likely that many such mutations will promote deregulation, yielding constitutively active kinases. Under normal conditions, these enzymes typically become activated through phosphorylation of specific residues in the activation loop. This is a reversible event that fundamentally alters the conformation of the loop, making it more soluble and less obstructive, thereby promoting ATP binding. Thus, a single aminoacid substitution within the activation loop turning a nonpolar residue into a negatively charged one can promote the deregulation of the kinase, turning it into a constitutively active signal transducer. This accident can of course promote tumor development and cancer progression, depending on whether the transduced signal recruits pathways leading to mitosis, cell immortalization, focal adhesions, etc.

On the other hand, since the oncogenic substitution solubilizes the activation loop, it should promote a loss of structure. This process is likely to yield a loop conformation far worse wrapped than that of the autoinhibited state and hence, far richer in dehydrons (Fig. 7.22). Ergo, a constitutively deregulated kinase should be more susceptible to be targeted by wrapping/crating drugs than the wild type. This operational hypothesis begs a validation in the light of the ideas described in this book.

By interfering with cell signaling pathways, single-molecule kinase inhibitors hold great promise as anticancer agents and probably hold potential for the molecular targeted treatment of other diseases. Yet, their therapeutic efficacy and clinical benefit is typically limited to a fraction of the treated patients. Genomic variations across patients and idiosyncratic patterns of drug resistance are likely to contribute significantly to such differences in clinical outcome.

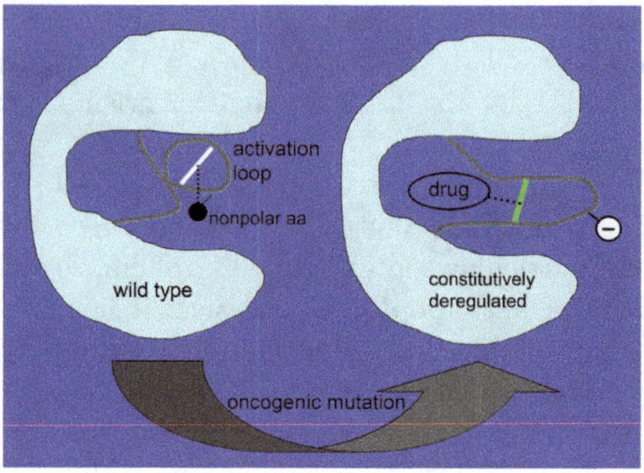

Figure 7.22. An oncogenic mutation in a kinase domain produces a constitutively active signal transducer by permanently solubilizing the activation loop. Being less structured, this deregulated kinase is richer in dehydrons than the wild type in its autoinhibited state and hence may be targeted by a wrapping drug.

The acknowledgment of these facts has triggered the need for a personalized drug design. Perhaps this challenge is not so daunting in so far as we can translate idiosyncratic or disease-related variations into molecular differences that can be systematically targeted by molecular engineers. The wrapping pattern may prove to be a transformative concept that may be brought to fruition in this key area of molecular medicine.

7.18 Epistructural drugs as blockers of targeted functions

The discovery of the chemical functionality of dehydrons (Chapter 6) forces us to contemplate a shift in paradigm for drug design, as we are not only targeting dehydrons as sticky non-conserved sites but also as catalytic enablers/stimulators. Many oncogenic mutations affect regulation of the signal transducers, often creating constitutively deregulated or constitutively active kinases. For instance, a mutation that substitutes a phosphorylation-susceptible residue (Ser, Thr, Tyr, or His) for a negatively charged one at physiological pH (Glu, Asp) often creates a constitutively active kinase whose lack

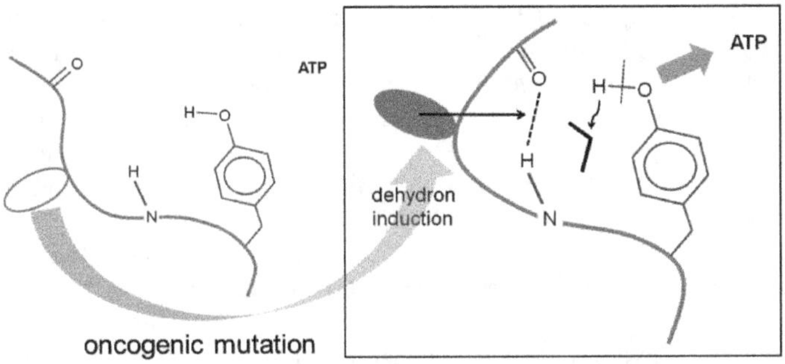

Figure 7.23. General scheme of oncogenic mutation generating a catalytically stimulating dehydron, yielding a constitutively active signal transducer. The dehydron occurs in a disordered region in the wild type as a result of a germline or somatic mutation that improves the wrapping quality of a residue (enhancing its hydrophobicity as represented by the unfilled-to-filled ellipse). The proximity of the dehydron to a phosphorylation-susceptible residue (Tyr) enables and stimulates the catalytic activity of the latter, with dramatic physiological consequences.

of regulation constitutes the molecular ethiology of the oncogenic activity. A far less studied type of mutation that, in light of the results in Chapter 6, may promote deregulated activity is the one that would lead to the creation of a dehydron in the vicinity of a phosphorylation site (Fig. 7.23). By inducing nucleophilicity in a vicinal group through proton abstraction, such mutation-induced dehydrons become enablers and stimulators of an inordinate level of catalytic activity, with dramatic physiological consequences. Thus, the therapeutic implications of targeting such a transformative mutation are immediately apparent, as a dehydron-wrapping drug is likely to prevent the functionalization of nearby groups thus blocking the aberrant activity stemming from dehydron-promoted nucleophilicity.

References

1. Fernández A (2005) Incomplete protein packing as a selectivity filter in drug design. *Structure* 13:1829–1836.
2. Fernández A, Scott R, Berry RS (2004) The nonconserved wrapping of conserved folds reveals a trend towards increasing connectivity in proteomic networks. *Proc Natl Acad Sci USA* 101:2823–2827.

3. Fernández A, Berry RS (2004) Molecular dimension explored in evolution to promote proteomic complexity. *Proc Natl Acad Sci USA* 101:13460–13465.
4. Fernández A, Berry RS (2002) Extent of hydrogen-bond protection in folded proteins: a constraint on packing architectures. *Biophys J* 83:2475–2481.
5. Fernández A, Berry RS (2003) Proteins with hydrogen-bond packing defects are highly interactive with lipid bilayers: Implications for amyloidogenesis. *Proc Natl Acad Sci USA* 100:2391–2396.
6. Fernández A, Rogale K, Scott LR, Scheraga HA (2004) Inhibitor design by wrapping packing defects in HIV-1 proteins. *Proc Natl Acad Sci USA* 101:11640–11645.
7. Deremble C, Lavery R (2005) Macromolecular Recognition. *Curr Opin Str Biol* 15:171–175.
8. Fernández A, Scheraga HA (2003) Insufficiently dehydrated hydrogen bonds as determinants of protein interactions. *Proc Natl Acad Sci USA* 100:113–118.
9. Ban Y-E, Edelsbrunner H, Rudolph J (2006) Interface surfaces for protein-protein complexes. *J Ass Comp Mach* 53:361–378.
10. Adesokan AA, Roberts VA, Lee KW, Linz RD, Briggs JM (2004) Prediction of HIV-1 Integrase/Viral DNA interactions in the catalytic domain by fast molecular docking. *J Med Chem* 47:821–828.
11. Kortemme T, Baker D (2004) Computational design of protein-protein interactions. *Curr Op Chem Bio* 8:91097.
12. Kortvelyesi T, Silberstein M, Dennis S, Vajda S (2003) Improved mapping of protein binding sites. *J Com Aid Molec Des* 17:173–186.
13. Lu L, Lu H, Skolnick J (2002) Multiprospector: An algorithm for the predction of protein-protein interactions by multimeric threading. *Proteins Str Fn Gen* 49:350–364.
14. Sen TZ, Kloczkowski A, Jernigan RL, *et al.* (2004) Predicting binding sites of hydrolase-inhibitor complexes by combining several methods. *BMC Bioinformatics* 5:205–215.
15. Huber R (1979) Conformational flexibility in protein molecules. *Nature* 280:538–539.
16. Dunker KA, Brown C, Obradovic Z (2002) Identification and function of usefully disordered proteins. *Adv Prot Chem* 62:25–49.
17. Verkhivker G, Bouzida D, Gehehaar D, Rejto P, Freer ST, Rose P (2003) Simulating disorder-order transition in molecular recognition of unstructured proteins: Where folding meets binding. *Proc Natl Acad Sci USA* 100:5148–5153.
18. Fernández A, Crespo A (2008) Protein wrapping: a molecular marker for association, aggregation and drug design. *Chem Soc Rev* 37:2372–2382.
19. Stevens RC (2004) Long live structural biology. *Nature Str Mol Biol* 11:293–295.
20. Fauman EB, Hopkins A, Groom C (2003) Structural bioinformatics in drug discovery. In: Bourne P, Weissig H (eds) Structural Bioinformatics, Wiley-Liss, New York.

21. Wlodawer A, Vondrasek J (1998) Inhibitors of HIV-1 protease: A major success of structure-assisted drug design. *Annu Rev Biophys Biomol Struc* 27:249–284.
22. Arkin MR, Wells JA (2004) Small-molecule inhibitors of protein-protein interactions: progressing towards the dream. *Nature Rev Drug Dis* 3:301–317.
23. Katz BA (2000) Structural basis for selectivity of a small molecule, S1-Binding, submicromolar inhibitor of urokinase-type plasminogen activator. *Chem Biol* 7:299–307.
24. Steinmetzer T, Hauptmann J, Sturzebecher J (2001) *Expert Opin Invest Drugs* 10:845–864.
25. Nicholls A, Sharp KA, Honig B (1991) Protein folding and association: insights from the interfacial and thermodynamic properties of hydrocarbons. *Proteins Str Fn Gen* 11:281–196.
26. Liang J, Edelsbrunner H, Woodward C (1998) Anatomy of protein pockets and cavities: measurement of binding site geometry and implications for ligand design. *Protein Sci* 7:1884–1897.
27. Lee B, Richards FM (1971) The interpretation of protein structures: estimation of static accessibility. *J Mol Biol* 55:379–400.
28. Fernández A, Scott LR (2003) Adherence of packing defects in soluble proteins. *Phys Rev Lett* 91:18102.
29. Fernández A, Scott LR (2003) Dehydron: a structure encoded signal for protein interactions. *Biophys J* 85:1914–1928.
30. NIH/NCBI website for the structural alignment program Cn3D: http://www.ncbi.nlm.nih.gov/structure/CN3D/cn3d.shtml.
31. Munshi S, Chen Z, Li Y, *et al.* (1998) Rapid X-ray diffraction analysis of HIV-1 protease-inhibitor complexes: inhibitor exchange in single crystals of the bound enzyme. *Acta Crystallogr. D* 54:1053–1060.
32. Mount DW (2001) Bioinformatics, Cold Spring Harbor Laboratory Press, New York.
33. Karaman MW, Herrgard S, Treiber DK, *et al.* (2008) A quantitative analysis of kinase inhibitor selectivity. *Nat Biotech* 26:127–132.
34. Dancey J, Sausville EA (2003) Issues and progress with protein kinase inhibitors for cancer treatment. *Nature Rev Drug Discov* 2:296–313.
35. Levitski A, Gazit A (1995) Tyrosine kinase inhibition: an approach to drug development. *Science* 267:1782–1788.
36. Tibes R, Trent J, Kurzrock R (2005) Tyrosine kinase inhibitors and the dawn of molecular cancer therapeutics. *Annu Rev Pharm Tox* 45:357–84.
37. Gibbs J, Oliff A (1994) Pharmaceutical research in molecular oncology. *Cell* 79:193–198.
38. Donato NJ, Talpaz M (2000) Clinical use of tyrosine kinase inhibitors: Therapy for chronic myelogenous leukemia and other cancers. *Clin Cancer Res* 6:2965–2966.
39. Fabian MA, Biggs WH, Treiber DK, *et al.* (2005) A small molecule kinase interaction map for clinical kinase inhibitors. *Nature Biotech* 23:329–336.

40. Gambacorti-Passerini C, le Coutre P, Mologni L, *et al.* (1997) Inhibition of the ABL kinase activity blocks the proliferation of BCR/ABL+ leukemic cells and induces apoptosis. *Blood Cells Mol Dis* 23:380–394.
41. Schindler T, Bornmann W, Pellicena P, *et al.* (2000) Structural mechanism for STI-571 inhibition of Abelson tyrosine kinase. *Science* 289:1938–1942.
42. Attoub S, Rivat C, Rodrigues S, *et al.* (2002) The c-kit tyrosine kinase inhibitor STI-571 for colorectal cancer therapy. *Cancer Res* 62:4879–4883.
43. DeMatteo RP (2002) The GIST of targeted cancer therapy: a tumor (gastrointestinal stromal tumor), a mutated gene (c-kit), and a molecular inhibitor (STI571). *Ann Surg Oncol* 9:831–839.
44. Skene RJ, Kraus ML, Scheibe DN, *et al.* (2004) Structural basis for autoinhibition and STI-571 inhibition of C-kit Tyrosine kinase. *J Biol Chem* 279:31655–31663.
45. Tuveson DA, Willis NA, Jacks T, *et al.* (2001) STI571 inactivation of the gastrointestinal stromal tumor c-Kit oncoprotein: biological and clinical implications. *Oncogene* 20:5054–5058.
46. Chen JP, Zhang X, Fernández A (2007) Molecular basis for specificity in the druggable kinome: sequence-based analysis. *Bioinformatics* 23:563–572.
47. Fernández A, Sanguino A, Peng Z, Ozturk E, Chen J, Crespo A, Wulf S, Shavrin A, Qin C, Ma J, Trent J, Lin Y, Han HD, Mangala LS, Bankson JA, Gelovani J, Samarel A, Bornmann W, Sood AK, Lopez-Berestein G (2007) An anticancer c-Kit kinase inhibitor is reengineered to make it more active and less cardiotoxic. *J Clin Invest* 117:4044–4054.
48. Kerkela R, Grazette L, Yacobi R, *et al.* (2006) Cardiotoxicity of the cancer therapeutic agent imatinib mesylate. *Nature Med* 12:908–916.
49. Druker BJ (2004) Molecularly targeted therapy: have the floodgates opened? *Oncologist* 9:357–360.
50. Vivas-Mejia P, Benito JM, Fernández A, Han HD, Mangala L, Rodriguez-Aguayo C, Chavez-Reyes A, Lin YG, Carey MS, Nick AM, Stone RL, Kim HS, Claret FX, Bornmann W, Hennessy BT, Sanguino A, Peng Z, Sood AK, Lopez-Berestein G (2010) c-Jun-NH2-kinase-1 inhibition leads to antitumor activity in ovarian cancer. *Clin Cancer Res* 16:184–194.
51. Fernández A, Scheraga HA (2003) Insufficiently dehydrated hydrogen bonds as determinants of protein interactions. *Proc Natl Acad Sci USA* 100:113–118.
52. Barker S, Kassel D, Weigl D, *et al.* (1995) Characterization of $pp^{60c\text{-}src}$ tyrosine kinase activities using a continuous assay: autoactivation of the enzyme is an intermolecular autophosphorylation process. *Biochemistry* 34:14843–14851.
53. Songyang Z, Carraway KL, Eck M, *et al.* (1995) Catalytic specificity of protein-tyrosine kinases is critical for selective signalling. *Nature* 373: 536–539.
54. Clarkson B, Strife A, Wisniewski D, Lambek CL, Liu C (2003) Chronic myelogenous leukemia as a paradigm of early cancer and possible curative strategy. *Leukemia* 17:1211–1262.

55. Prenen H, Deroose C, Vermaelen P, Sciot R, Debiec-Rychter M (2006) Establishment of a mouse gastrointestinal stromal tumour model and evaluation of response to Imatinib by small animal positron emission tomography. *Anticancer Res* 26:1247–1252.
56. Baines CP, Molkentin JD (2005) Stress signaling pathways that modulate cardiac myocyte apoptosis. *J Mol Cell Cardiol* 38:47–62.
57. Scheuermann-Freestone M, Simon Freestone N, Langenickel T, *et al.* (2001) A new model of congestive heart failure in the mouse due to chronic volume overload. *Eur J Heart Fail* 3:535–543.
58. Gazdar A (2009) Personalized medicine and inhibition of EGFR signaling in lung cancer. *New Eng J Med* 361:1018–1020.
59. Janne PA, Gray N, Settleman J (2009) Factors underlying sensitivity of cancers to small molecule kinase inhibitors. *Nat Rev Drug Disc* 8:709–723.

Chapter 8

Anticancer treatment synergizing targeted therapies with immune responses

As most clinicians would acknowledge, targeted drug-based therapies have met only moderate success in cancer treatment. This is partly because of the evolutionary substrate of the disease that typically selects for resistant phenotypes, and partly because of the drug-induced suppression of the adaptive immune response. In this chapter we shall address the second issue and develop immuno-synergistic targeted agents. The discussion focuses on epistructural tuning of extant targeted therapeutic agents to make them compatible with immunotherapy.

8.1 Epistructural tuning of targeted anticancer agents to remove drug-induced immunosuppression

We aim at developing molecular design strategies to empower drug-based anticancer therapy by aligning engineered immune responses with drug-induced antigenic activity. We first focus on re-engineering immunosuppressive anticancer drugs where the impact on the immune system is an undesirable outcome. Subsequently, we outline genetic engineering strategies to tailor an adoptive immune arm to the antigenic repertoire generated by the drug-based treatment. The first goal is to remove the immunosuppressive effects caused by drug treatment through molecular redesign, more specifically, to restore the adaptive T-cell-related immune response and natural killer (NK) cell cytotoxicity compromised by the drug treatment. The redesign strategy enables us to create synergies that may empower drug-based anticancer therapy, aligning the immune response with the molecularly targeted treatment. The second goal is to ensure therapeutic success of synergistic immunotherapies based on the genetic manipulation and infusion of autologous or allogeneic immune cells into patients subject to antigen-generating drug therapy. This success hinges on the ability to genetically tailor the modified T-cell receptor (TRC) and chimeric antigen receptor (CAR) to the antigenic repertoire of the drug-based treatment.

As described in chapter 7, kinase inhibitors (KIs) that interfere selectively with cell signaling pathways represent a therapeutic opportunity for cancer treatment [1–11]. Yet, most drug-based anticancer therapies are incomplete and do not provide a decisive cure [12]. A well-known culprit for the ultimate failure arises from the somatic evolution of patterns of drug resistance that often materialize as site mutations or constitutively deregulated chimeras. Somatic mutations compromise the affinity of the drug for its target or, alternatively, increase the affinity for the kinase natural ligand ATP, in the case of ATP-competitive inhibitors [12]. A far less acknowledged culprit for drug failure arises because these targeted therapies are typically not tailored to operate synergistically with the immune system, and often antagonize it in spite of generating antigenic activity [13–16]. KIs are often of limited applicability, since drug treatments are marred by episodes of relapse and by the development of drug resistance and intolerance [12, 17]. One reason for this incomplete success is the lack of synergy between the drug and the immune system, with the latter often incapacitated at crucial junctures during treatment due to antagonistic drug-induced effects [13, 14, 18–21]. In fact, these immune-antagonistic effects are prevalent because of the multiple roles that a protein target may play in off-target cellular contexts, as described in Chapter 7. Thus, a therapeutic imperative arises from the need to recruit cooperative immune responses concomitant with the molecular targeted treatment. The goal is to design anticancer drugs that inhibit targeted cellular functions and steer the immune system to harness the antigenic products of the drug-induced apoptosis of tumor cells. To fulfill this imperative of therapeutic integration, we propose re-designs of anticancer drugs that fulfill three constraints: a) nanomolar activity against anticancer targets; b) reversal of tumor-induced immunomodulation; and c) removal of drug-induced immunosuppressive activity.

The drug-design strategies introduced to address the therapeutic imperative of immuno-synergy have the potential to revolutionize cancer treatment and the understanding of the adaptive immune response by steering it with molecular targeted therapy. We are counting on the premise that by restoring the adaptive immune response to drug-induced antigenic activity, we shall be able to create synergies that will reciprocally empower the immune system and drug-based anticancer treatment. Novel therapeutic possibilities to harness and manipulate the immune system will probably transpire from the evaluation of immuno-synergic drugs, as described in the subsequent sections.

8.2 Drug-induced immunosuppression

The level of molecular fine tuning required to redesign an anticancer drug into an immuno-synergic drug cannot be achieved within the current drug-discovery paradigm [17, 22]. Rather, a rational design approach is needed [23], an area where novel molecular filters can be exploited to better control drug specificity [24,25]. Thus, an unprecedented control of specificity [17] is required to design therapeutic agents capable of discriminating between cancer-related targets and immunosuppressive targets. The reward in building immuno-synergic molecular therapies through rational design is potentially immense, since these targeted therapies will then engage a formidable ally-the immune response- in their anticancer activity.

Well established anticancer KIs like *imatinib* [1–3] or *dasatinib* [4–9] are also known to be directly immunosuppressive [13, 14, 18–21] through their powerful blockade of upstream signaling in the adaptive immune response, and yet, as shown in this chapter, they hold promise as chemical scaffolds that can be turned into immuno-synergic drugs. The choices are justified since these KIs are nanomolar inhibitors of the major anticancer target c-Kit kinase [2, 3, 8, 9], the kinase of the stem-cell factor (SCF) receptor, and hence the KI treatment is expected to have the additional effect of reversing tumor-induced immunosuppression, at least in certain tumor environments where tumor-secreted SCF is deployed to hijack the immune system [26]. The latter effect is promoted by the accumulation of myeloid derived suppressor cells (MDSC) and T-regulatory cells (Tregs), whose development/activation requires the SCF expressed by the tumor cells. However, both KIs are also direct immunosuppressants [13–15, 18–21], and this role is clearly antagonistic to their anticancer activity, thus requiring careful removal through a molecular remodeling of the parent compounds using stringent selectivity filters [23–25].

More precisely, these KIs are powerful (nanomolar) inhibitors of two crucial kinases implicated as upstream signal transducers controlling the immune response: the lymphocyte-associated kinase Lck and the colony-stimulating factor-1 receptor (CSF1-R) kinase [17, 22]. In fact, dasatinib is the most powerful inhibitor of Lck known to date ($K_D = 0.2nM$) [22]. Specifically, Lck is a signal transducer for the signaling cascade that originates in the CD4/8 receptors (CD = cluster of differentiation) expressed on the surface of T-cells in antigen-triggered T-cell differentiation (Fig. 8.1(a), from KEGG, the Kyoto Encyclopedia of Genes and Genomes) and in natural killer (NK) cell-mediated cytotoxicity (Fig. 8.1(b), KEGG) [27]. On the other hand, the CSF1-R kinase is implicated in the development of the monocyte/macrophage (M/M) lineage [27]. Hence, both KIs suppress antigen-specific T-cell effector functions and NK cytotoxicity and inhibit the hematopoietic development of crucial components of the immune response.

Both imatinib and dasatinib are likely to hamper the adaptive immune response triggered by the very antigenic activity they generate, and compromise the antigen presentation by precluding macrophage development. The profound inhibition of all antigen-specific T-cell effector functions at therapeutically relevant concentrations has been mechanistically tracked down to the early

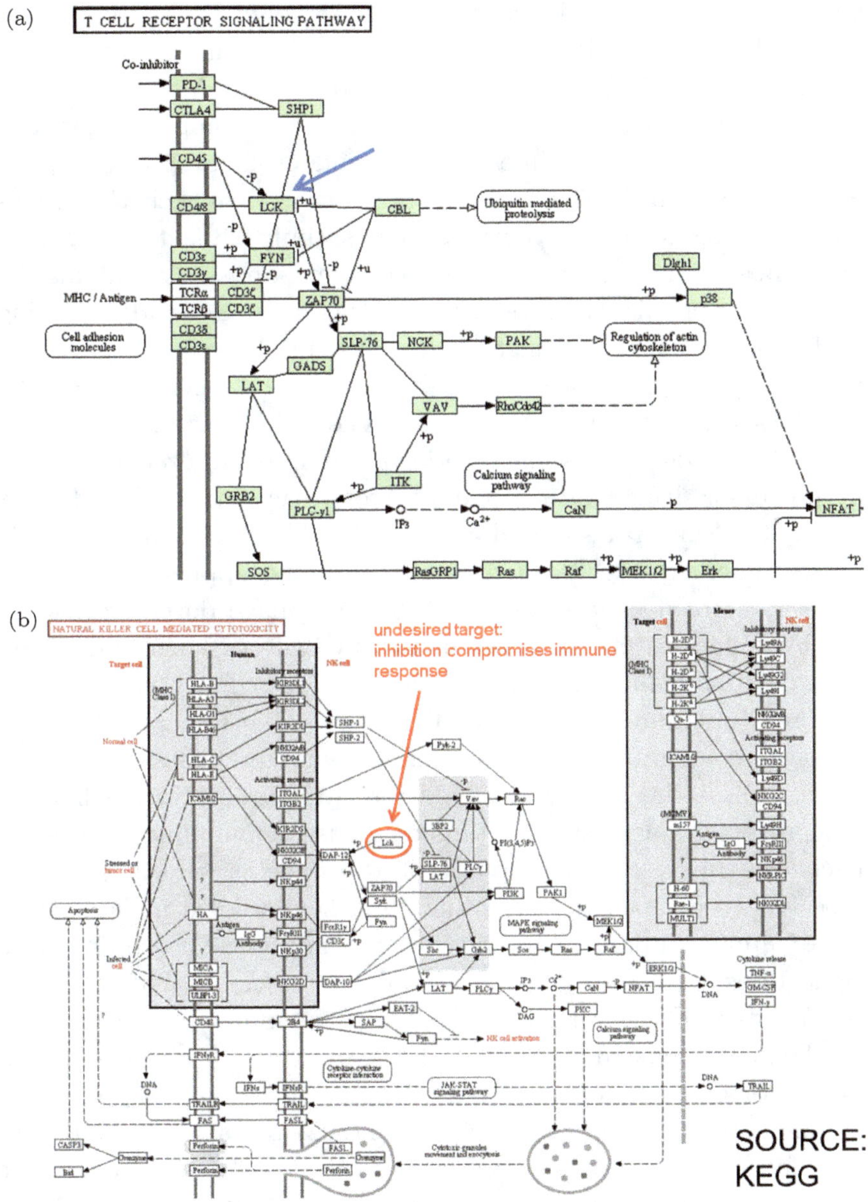

Figure 8.1. **(a)** Receptor Signaling pathways implicating Lck in the antigen-triggered T-cell response (adaptive immune response, source: KEGG, Kyoto Encyclopedia of Genes and Genomes). **(b)** The role of Lck in signaling pathways recruited in natural killer (NK) cell-mediated cytotoxicity (source: KEGG, Kyoto Encyclopedia of Genes and Genomes).

blockade of signal transduction events promoted by Lck inhibition [13, 14]. In fact, Lck is central in the transduction of T-cell receptor (TCR) signaling in response to MHC-I and MHC-II antigen presentation (MHC = major histocompatibility complex) that ultimately promotes T-cell differentiation and proliferation. Thus, the drug-induced immunosuppressive effects caused by Lck inhibition-purposely engineered in the case of dasatinib [28]-actually betray the purpose of these drugs as anticancer agents, possibly enabling the development of episodes of relapse and drug resistance and impacting the frequency of opportunistic infections. In the case of *dasatinib*, the original drug-discovery pursuits seemed to focus squarely on modulating the immune response [28]. The repositioning of *dasatinib* as an anticancer agent seemed to have arisen as an afterthought, as the precursor drug *imatinib* showed cross-reactivity against Lck as well as the cancer-associated targets Bcr-Abl, c-Kit and PDGFR kinases. Furthermore, the Lck-related immunosuppression by both KIs is reinforced by the blockade of macrophage development-and thereby of antigen presentation- caused by CSF1-R kinase inhibition (both compounds are nanomolar inhibitors of CSF1-R).

These immuno-antagonistic effects are ostensibly at odds with the need to maintain an uncompromised immune response to fight cancer, unless the kinases targeted for immunosuppression happen to be also relevant anticancer targets. Thus, the immunosuppressive effects are likely to doom much of the ongoing efforts to apply these KIs to combat cancers other than hematologic malignancies, where immunosuppression may become adjuvant. Even in those applications for which FDA approval has been obtained, i.e. the treatment of CML and Philadelphia chromosome-positive acute lymphoblastic leukemia (Ph + ALL), opportunistic infections have been reported in patients treated at therapeutic doses [19].

A kinome-wide screening of KIs [17, 22] reveals that potential side effects and immunosuppressive complications due to nanomolar inhibition of Lck (dissociation constant $K_D < 50$nM) are likely to be a concern for several compounds of therapeutic interest. Thus, a significant drug-induced impairment of adaptive immune responses, mostly affecting T-cell and NK-cell activation, is readily expected for the following KIs (K_D's from [22]): NVP-AST487 (Novartis, K_D = 11nM); *nintedanib* (BIBF-1120, Vargatef®, Boehringer-Ingelheim, K_D = 6.2nM); *crizotinib* (Xalkori®, Pfizer, K_D = 30nM); *dasatinib* (Sprycel®, Bristol-Myers Squibb, K_D = 0.2nM); *foretinib* (GSK1363089, GlaxoSmithKline (K_D = 6nM), *imatinib* (Gleevec®, Novartis, K_D = 40nM); *nilotinib* (Tasigna®, Novartis, K_D = 47nM); PD-173955 (Parke-Davis, K_D = 1.1nM); *bosutinib* (SKI-606, Bosulif®, Wyeth/Pfizer, K_D = 0.59nM); NVP-TAE684 (Novartis, K_D = 49nM); and *vandetanib* (Caprelsa®, AstraZeneca, K_D = 17nM).

While anticancer activity is a desired clinical outcome for these KIs, the reported structural similarities between Lck and validated anticancer targets like c-KIT, PDGFR and Src-family kinases, introduce extremely undesirable cross-reactivities. In fact, while these KIs are being actively evaluated as anticancer agents, their nanomolar inhibition of Lck truly compromises the immune system, depriving the patient of a key endogenous resource to fight the disease. This adverse aspect of treatment seems to have been overlooked except in the cases of *imatinib* and *dasatinib*, as indicated previously. This chapter advocates then for the need to address the imperative of building a therapeutic alliance between immune response and molecularly targeted therapy. This goal may be achieved by exploiting a selectivity filter purposely created to guide the re-design of anticancer drugs to dial out targets related to immunosuppression.

8.3 Molecular tuning of kinase inhibitors to make them immuno-synergic

To redesign an anticancer drug to make it immuno-synergic, an unprecedented level of control of drug specificity, well beyond the current drug-discovery standard, is required. This is so because anticancer activity must be retained while targets related to immunosuppression must be selectively removed from the drug affinity profile. In this regard, we may exploit the effective selectivity filter provided by the protein's unique dehydron pattern to guide the molecular re-design [12, 23–25, 29], as described in chapter 7. As we know, the dehydron pattern of proteins is not conserved even in cases of very high structural similarity, as between anticancer targets like c-Kit, PDGFR or c-Src kinases, and immunosuppression-related targets like Lck.

Thus, the problem of target discrimination tailored to our therapeutic challenge may well exploit this new selectivity filter that can transcend structural similarity (cf. Figs. 8.2, 8.3). Thus, if a dehydron is present in an anti-cancer target protein (i.e. c-Kit) while the hydrogen bond at the same location in a homologous off-target protein (i.e. Lck) is well-wrapped, we may re-design the original drug with its undesired cross-reactivity into a new drug that can tell apart the two targets, binding only to the desired target. As described in Chapter 7, the "dehydron-wrapping" drug, whereby the drug improves the dehydron packing upon association, becomes an expansion of the original chemical scaffold and is intended to locally exclude water from the specific dehydron present in the desired target and absent in the undesired target at the same location [12]. Specifically, the dehydron-wrapping capability of a drug is built by expanding the original parental compound with the addition of a nonpolar group (usually methyl) that can penetrate the desolvation domain of the preformed targetable dehydron upon drug-target association. Since the incorporation of a methyl group usually compromises bioavailability, a compensatory change increasing drug solubility is often introduced at an innocuous site removed from the protein/ligand interface [12].

To illustrate this operational strategy, let us consider the problem of redesigning *imatinib* into a new drug that retains anticancer efficacy against gastrointestinal stromal tumor (GIST) [2] and other c-Kit-dependent cancers (c-Kit dependent melanoma) [24] while becoming immune-synergic by selective removal of *imatinib*'s anti-Lck activity. The dehydron patterns for the *imatinib*-binding region of the desired target c-Kit (PDB accession code 1T46) and the undesired target Lck (PDB accession code 2PL0) are displayed in Figs. 8.2 and 8.3, respectively. Of crucial importance as guidance to *imatinib* remodeling is the dehydron (green stick) pairing

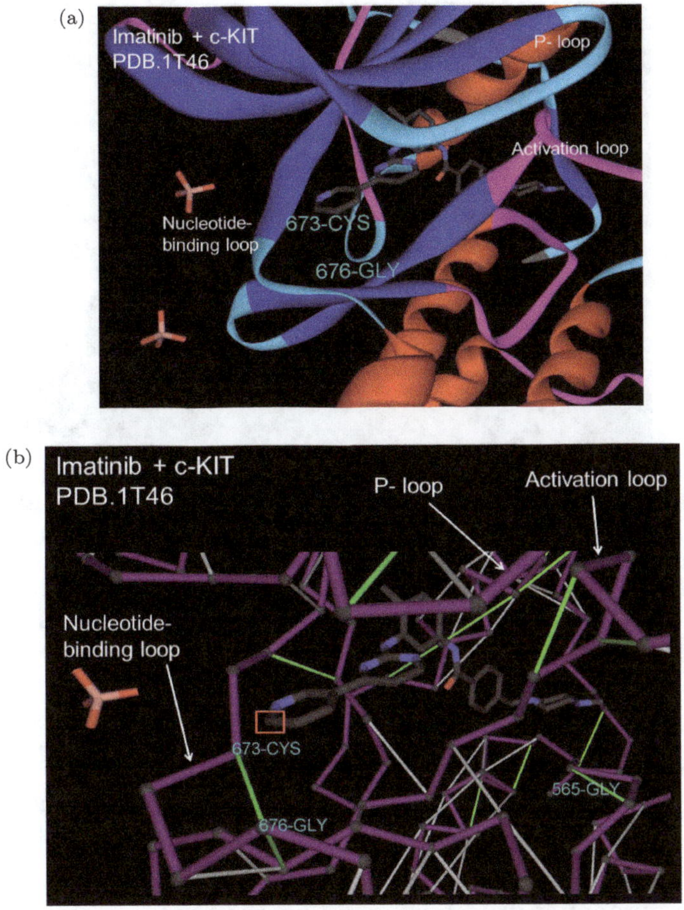

Figure 8.2. Structure and dehydron pattern of anticancer target c-Kit kinase in the complex with KI *imatinib* (PDB entry 1T46). **(a)** The protein is displayed in ribbon representation colored conventionally according to the secondary structure motif (red = α-helix, blue = β-strand, light blue = turn, pink = loop) while the drug is displayed in bond-sticks colored conventionally according to chemical element (grey = carbon or hydrogen, blue = nitrogen, red = oxygen, pink = phosphorus). **(b)** Dehydron pattern for the protein in complex with the drug. The protein backbone is displayed in magenta, with virtual bonds joining adjacent α-carbons, well wrapped (buried) hydrogen bonds are represented as grey sticks joining the α-carbons of the paired residues, while dehydrons are shown as green sticks. Of interest is the dehydron Cys673-Gly676 present in the c-Kit kinase that becomes a well-wrapped hydrogen bond pairing residues Met319 and Gly322 in Lck. This selectivity feature unique to c-Kit directs the remodeling of the *imatinib* chemical scaffold by methylation at the location highlighted by the red rectangle. Reprinted from [36], copyright 2014 with permission from Elsevier.

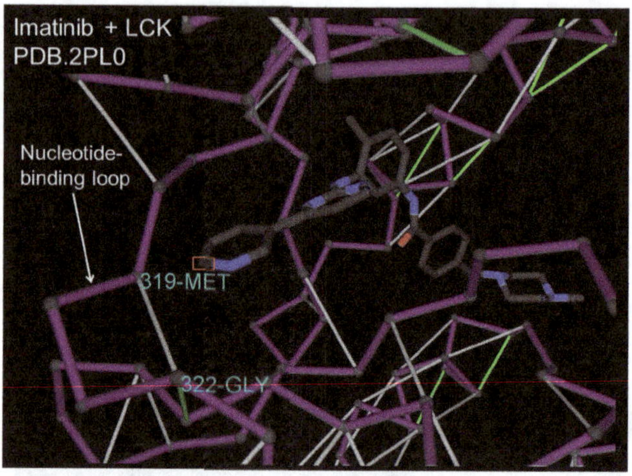

Figure 8.3. Dehydron pattern for Lck within the complex with *imatinib* with structural coordinates obtained from PDB entry 2PL0. The representation convention of Fig. 14.2(b) is followed. Upon structural alignment, the dehydron Cys673-Gly676 in the c-Kit kinase becomes the well wrapped hydrogen bond Met319-Gly322 in Lck. Reprinted from [36], copyright 2014 with permission from Elsevier.

residues Cys673 and Gly676 in the nucleotide-binding loop of c-Kit (Fig. 8.2(b)). This dehydron becomes a well-wrapped hydrogen bond (grey segment) pairing residues Met319 and Gly322 in the *imatinib* target Lck (Fig. 8.3). Thus, the uniqueness of the c-Kit Cys673-Gly676 dehydron guides us to re-design *imatinib* into a more selective dehydron-wrapping drug by expanding the chemical scaffold at the position highlighted in the terminal ring (Figs. 8.2(b) and 8.3). Thus, the resulting compound WBZ_4 [30] arises from methylation of *imatinib* at the position indicated in Figs. 8.2(b), 8.3 and its chemical structure is given in chapter 7. As shown in Chapter 7, WBZ_4 is a dehydron-wrapping drug that stabilizes the dehydron 673-676 of the c-Kit kinase upon association with the target, whereas it unfavorably promotes water removal from the surroundings of the well-wrapped 319-322 hydrogen bond in off-target Lck. Therefore, WBZ_4 retains nanomolar activity against c-Kit while showing no detectable inhibitory activity against Lck [25]. The immuno-synergic properties of WBZ_4 await validation but its higher selectivity relative to the parent compound is indicative that there will be no impairment of the adaptive immune response triggered by the antigenic activity generated during drug treatment.

Similarly, a re-design of *imatinib* discriminating between desired target SCFR (c-Kit) and CSF1-R kinases is essential to secure development of the macrophage lineage during molecular therapy and may be also carried out by exploiting the dehydron filter. We can take advantage of local differences in the dehydron patterns and align this wrapping representation for PDB entries 1T46 (c-Kit) and 3LCO (CSF-1R kinase).

8.4 Pre-clinical evaluation of immuno-synergic drugs

The immuno-synergic drugs should undergo testing at all levels, from *in silico* to clinical trials. Using the dehydron selectivity filter [12, 30], the parent drugs may be reworked into compound series with nanomolar affinity towards the original cancer targets with immuno-synergic properties arising from: A) removal of activity against Lck, B) removal of activity against the CSF1R kinase; C) simultaneous removal of both cross-reactivities.

To test class-A drugs, we may assay for T-cell receptor (TCR)-mediated T-cell proliferation and activation in a dose-dependent manner using the parent compounds in the control assays. Besides testing the redesigns in proliferation assays using cancer cell lines, we may test for selective removal of the inhibition of antigen-specific T-cell effector functions. In accord with the predictions set forth in this study, the impact on antigen-triggered $CD4^+$ T-cell proliferation and T-cell effector function [31] by the purportedly immune-synergic WBZ_4 should be preliminarily evaluated *ex-vivo* using *imatinib* as control. The results are expected to reveal a minimal level of modulation of the immune response exerted by WBZ_4 when compared with the parental drug [32].

Class-B compounds may be tested by examining the development of the monocyte/macrophage (M/M) lineage from bone marrow progenitors at concentrations of class-B or anticancer drugs of the order of 0.5–1 micromolar [26]. Based on the KEGG annotation cited above, we conjecture that anticancer drug impairment of M/M development is the result of drug inhibition of kinase CSF1-R, so the impairment should vanish as the hematopoietic stem cells (HSCs) are treated with class-B drugs. Class-C compounds should be tested following all the protocols mentioned above and are expected to restore antigen-induced T-cell response, M/M development and macrophage-mediated antigen presentation, hence they should be the optimally suited to be combined with immunotherapy, as they are likely to restore cross-talk between different immune responses.

In all cases, we may corroborate retention or enhancement of anticancer activity as the parent drugs are molecularly re-engineered exploiting the dehydron filter, following the same *in vitro, ex-vivo* and *in-vivo* assays that have led to assert the therapeutic value of the parent drugs.

The novel targeted therapies will bring about significant antigenic activity by promoting apoptosis of tumor cells without compromising the immune response. This will make them amenable to be synergistically combined with immunotherapies. The choice of the latter will depend on the changes in the components of the innate and adaptive immune system caused by the targeted therapy and relative to the parent drug treatment. The immune response triggered by targeted therapy should be determined in animal models and the immunotherapies will likely include depletion of regulatory T-cells by treatment with CD25 antibody, targeting the cytotoxic T-lymphocyte-associated antigen 4 (CTLA4) with monoclonal antibodies like *ipilimumab* (suited for c-Kit-dependent melanomas to be treated by class-A variants of *imatinib*) [33], etc.

8.5 Immune-aligned anticancer drugs to overcome HIV-1-promoted immunosuppression

Probably the need for immuno-synergic anticancer drugs is nowhere more pressing than in the context of viral cancers within AIDS, an immunosuppressive setting induced by the human immunodeficiency virus-1 (HIV-1) [34]. Drug-induced immunosuppression would be a highly undesirable effect especially in this therapeutic context where the immune system is already compromised by endogenous factors triggered by the HIV-1 infection. One of the primary cancers concurrent with HIV-1-induced immunosuppression is the Kaposi sarcoma, caused by a facilitated herpes viral infection [35]. As recently demonstrated, new lines of treatment to prevent the reactivation of Kaposi's sarcoma herpesvirus and invasiveness of infected endothelial cells involve targeting the inflammation-related kinase MAP4K4 [35]. Direct inspection of the screening data reported in [17,22] enables us to identify two very powerful nanomolar inhibitors of the MAP4K4 kinase: NVP-AST-487 (Novartis, $K_D = 15nM$) and *bosutinib* (SKI-606, Bosulif®, Wyeth/Pfizer, $K_D = 8.2nM$). Yet, none of them should be used in this specific therapeutic context because they are also extremely powerful inhibitors of Lck ($K_D = 11nM$ and 0.59nM, respectively), as already noted in this chapter. Thus, to treat Kaposi sarcoma in HIV-1-positive patients, one must first attempt a wrapping-based molecular remodeling of both inhibitors to retain nanomolar activity against MAPK4K but suppress as much as possible their anti-Lck activity. This molecular re-engineering would entail assessing the differences in the dehydron patterns for the on-target kinase MAPK4K versus the off-target kinase Lck, and redesign the parent chemical scaffolds to discriminate the two proteins according to the premises of the wrapping technology [12].

Most drug-based anticancer therapies are incomplete and do not provide a decisive cure. Molecularly targeted therapy aimed at blocking cancer-related signaling pathways seldom recruits the immune system but rather antagonizes it. This problem is magnified when the therapeutic context for cancer treatment involves HIV-1-induced immunosuppression, as in AIDS patients. Thus, we make it a therapeutic imperative to recruit cooperative immune responses triggered by molecularly targeted treatment. The main challenge posed in this chapter is to engineer drugs that inhibit targeted cellular functions and without an adverse interference, steer the immune system to harness the antigenic products that the drugs generate. To achieve this synergy we need to remove immuno-antagonistic effects generated by the drug treatment while retaining the anticancer potency of the drug. This goal demands a paradigm shift in drug design.

Through their inhibition of anticancer target c-Kit, drugs like *imatinib* or *dasatinib* are likely to elicit antigenic activity as they induce apoptosis of tumor cells, and evidence suggests that c-Kit inhibition may reverse tumor-induced immunosuppression. Thus, these inhibitors partially fulfill the therapeutic imperative. Yet, because they are also nanomolar inhibitors of Lck and CSF1-R kinase, they suppress antigen-specific T-cell effector functions and the development of the macrophage lineage, hampering antigen presentation. Ultimately, these drugs compromise the immune response, partially defeating their own purpose. Besides imatinib and dasatinib, this chapter reports on nine additional compounds of clinical oncological interest that are likely to also impair the adaptive immune response precisely at the juncture when it is most indispensable.

In consonance with the imperative of therapeutic integration, this chapter advocates for the design of immuno-synergic anticancer drugs. The synergic designs must fulfill three constraints: a) nanomolar inhibition of anticancer targets; b) reversal of tumor-induced immunosuppression; and c) removal of drug-induced immunosuppressive activity [36]. To fulfill these goals, an unprecedented level of control of drug specificity is required and is provided by the exploitation of an effective selectivity filter to guide molecular design: the dehydron pattern. The therapeutic challenge of immuno-synergy requires this new generation of selectivity filters for target discrimination. The proposed strategy has the potential to revolutionize anticancer treatment and the understanding of the adaptive immune response by steering it along with molecularly targeted treatment. We are counting on the premise that restoration of the adaptive immune response triggered by drug-induced antigenic activity will empower drug-based anticancer treatment [36]. Novel possibilities for therapeutic manipulation of the immune system are likely to arise from the evaluation of the immuno-synergic drugs along the lines presented in this chapter.

8.6 Adoptive immunotherapy aligned with targeted anticancer treatment

Innovative immunotherapies are being developed to optimize the cancer-targeted response through genetic modification. By harnessing and steering the function of immune cells, the possibility has materialized to enhance the immune response to achieve persistent cancer regression. Synergies of such immunotherapies with drug-based targeted therapies required to generate cancer-related antigens through induced apoptosis of the tumor cell will surely generate powerful combination treatments. Immunotherapies based on the manipulation and infusion of autologous or allogeneic immune cells into patients, have been satisfactorily tested in clinical trials. These include genetically modified T-cell immunotherapies [37]. Combinations of such T-cell based immunotherapies with antigen-generating anticancer drug therapies may prove fruitful if the latter has low or no inhibitory impact on the major signal transducer Lck of T-cell antigen response.

T-cells contain T-cell receptors (TCRs) on the cell surface. The TCR is a multi-subunit transmembrane complex that mediates the antigen-specific activation of T cells (cf. Fig. 8.1(a)). The TCR is composed of two different polypeptide chains, the TCR α and β chains. Both chains have an N-terminal variable region and a constant region. The chains are linked by a disulfide bond, with each receptor providing a single antigen-binding site. The TCR recognizes an antigen comprised of a short contiguous amino acid sequence of a protein presented on the target cell by the major histocompatibility complex (MHC) molecule. Other adhesion molecules expressed by T-cells, such as CD4 for MHC class II and CD8 for MHC class I, are also involved. The TCR interacts with the ligand by making contacts with both the MHC molecule and the antigen peptide. Signal transduction occurs through the associated CD3 complex (cf. Fig. 8.1(a)), which is composed of four different CD3 proteins that form two heterodimers (CD3$\delta\varepsilon$ and CD3$\gamma\varepsilon$) and one homodimer (CD3$\zeta\zeta$), as shown in Fig. 8.1(a). As previously noted in this chapter, signal transduction in the T-cell triggered by antigen recognition is transduced through Lck. Thus, for such synergistic combinations to become effective it becomes absolutely essential that the antigen-generating drug-based treatment avoids inhibiting Lck.

Following contact with the cognate peptides presented by the MHC, naive $CD8^+$cytotoxic T cells proliferate and acquire the phenotype of effector T cells. Thus, the adaptive immune response is directed by the TCR recognition and for this event to materialize it is essential that the antigen-generating arm of the therapy does not block the signaling pathway recruited by TCR-antigen recognition (cf. Fig. 8.1(a)).

The concept of transferring T-cells to patients (adoptive T-cell transfer) to treat disease has been now been established. Thus, the antigen specificity of T-cells can be manipulated by genetic modification and redirected to successfully target antigens that are generated by the complementary antitumor drug-based therapy. In particular, T-cells can be engineered to express modified TCRs (the so-called TCR therapies) or protein-fusion-derived chimeric antigen receptors (CARs) that have enhanced selective affinity for the drug-related antigenic repertoire. These "tailored" genetically modified T-cell-based approaches are predicted to be highly efficient at targeting tumors in synergistic combinations the antigen-generating drug treatment that induces tumor cell apoptosis.

Genetically modified TCR therapies are based on altering T-cell specificity through the expression of specific TCR α and β chains, which mediate the antigen-recognition process. On the other hand, chimeric antigen receptors (CARs) combine antibody-like recognition with T-cell-activating function [38]. They are composed of an antigen-binding region, typically derived from an antibody, and a transmembrane domain to anchor the CAR to the T-cell.

The therapeutic success of synergistic immunotherapies based on the genetic manipulation and infusion of autologous or allogeneic immune cells into patients combined with antigen-generating drug therapy will depend pivotally on the ability to genetically tailor the TRC and CAR to the antigenic repertoire of the drug-based treatment.

References

1. Druker BJ, Lydon NB (2000) Lessons learned from the development of an Abl tyrosine kinase inhibitor for chronic myelogenous leukemia. *J Clin Invest* 105:3–7.
2. Demetri GD, von Mehren M, Blanke CD, Van den Abbeele AD, Eisenberg B, Roberts PJ, Heinrich MC, Tuveson DA, Singer S, Janicek M, Fletcher JA, Silverman SG, Silberman SL, Capdeville R, Kiese B, Peng B, Dimitrijevic S, Druker BJ, Corless C, Fletcher CD, Joensuu H (2002) Efficacy and safety of imatinib mesylate in advanced gastrointestinal stromal tumors. *N Engl J Med* 347:472–480.
3. Hodi FS, Friedlander P, Corless CL, Heinrich MC, Mac Rae S, Kruse A, Jagannathan J, Van den Abbeele AD, Velazquez EF, Demetri GD, Fisher DE (2007) Major response to imatinib mesylate in KIT mutated melanoma. *J Clin Oncol* 26:2046–2051.
4. Gnoni A, Marech I, Silvestris N, Vacca A, Lorusso V (2011) Dasatinib: An anti-tumor agent via Src inhibition. *Current Drug Targets* 12:563–578.
5. Li J, Rix U, Fang B, Bai Y, Edwards A, Colinge J, Bennett KL, Gao J, Song L, Eschrich S, Superti-Furga G, Koomen J, Haura EB (2010) A chemical and phosphoproteomic characterization of dasatinib action in lung cancer. *Nature Chem Biol* 6:291–299.
6. Pichot CS, Hartig SM, Xia L, Arvanitis C, Monisvais D, Lee FY, Frost JA, Corey SJ (2009) Dasatinib synergizes with doxorubicin to block growth, migration, and invasion of breast cancer cells. *Brit J Cancer* 101:38–47.
7. Koreckij T, Nguyen H, Brown LG, Yu EY, Vessella RL, Corey E (2009) Dasatinib inhibits the growth of prostate cancer in bone and provides additional protection from osteolysis. *Brit J Cancer* 101:263–268.
8. Schittenhelm MM, Shiraga S, Schroeder A, Corbin AS, Griffith D, Lee FY, Bokemeyer C, Deininger MW, Druker BJ, Heinrich MC (2006) Dasatinib (BMS-354825), a dual SRC/ABL kinase inhibitor, inhibits the kinase activity of wild-type, juxtamembrane, and activation loop mutant KIT isoforms associated with human malignancies. *Cancer Res* 66:473–481.
9. Woodman SE, Trent JC, Stemke-Hale K, Lazar AJ, Pricl S, Pavan GM, Fermeglia M, Gopal YN, Yang D, Podoloff DA, Ivan D, Kim KB, Papadopoulos N, Hwu P, Mills GB, Davies MA (2009) Activity of dasatinib against L576P KIT mutant melanoma: Molecular, cellular, and clinical correlates. *Mol Cancer Ther* 8:2079–2085.
10. Martin P, Oliver S, Kennedy SJ, Partridge E, Hutchison M, Clarke D, Giles P (2012) Pharmacokinetics of vandetanib: Three Phase I studies in healthy subjects. *Clinical Therapeutics* 34:221–237.
11. Cui JJ, Tran-Dubé M, Shen H, Nambu M, Kung PP, Pairish M, Jia L, Meng J, Funk L, Botrous I, McTigue M, Grodsky N, Ryan K, Padrique E, Alton G, Timofeevski S, Yamazaki S, Li Q, Zou H, Christensen J, Mroczkowski B, Bender S, Kania RS, Edwards MP (2011) Structure based drug design of crizotinib (PF-02341066), a potent and selective dual inhibitor

of mesenchymal–epithelial transition factor (c-MET) kinase and anaplastic lymphoma kinase (ALK). *J Med Chem* 54:6342–6363.
12. Fernández A (2010) Transformative concepts for drug design: Target wrapping. Springer-Verlag, Heidelberg.
13. Seggewiss R, Loré K, Greiner E, Magnusson MK, Price DA, Douek DC, Dunbar CE, Wiestner A (2005) Imatinib inhibits T-cell receptor-mediated T-cell proliferation and activation in a dose-dependent manner. *Blood* 105:2473–2480.
14. Weichsel R1, Dix C, Wooldridge L, Clement M, Fenton-May A, Sewell AK, Zezula J, Greiner E, Gostick E, Price DA, Einsele H, Seggewiss R (2008) Profound inhibition of antigen-specific T-cell effector functions by dasatinib. *Clin Cancer Res* 14:2484–2491.
15. Wölfl M, Langhammer F, Wiegering V, Eyrich M, Schlegel PG (2013) Dasatinib medication causing profound immunosuppression in a patient after haploidentical SCT: Functional assays from whole blood as diagnostic clues. *Bone Marrow Transplantation* 48:875–877.
16. Heine A, Held SA, Bringmann A, Holderried TA, Brossart P (2011) Immunomodulatory effects of anti-angiogenic drugs. *Leukemia* 25:899–905.
17. Davis MI, Hunt JP, Herrgard S, Ciceri P, Wodicka LM, Pallares G, Hocker M, Treiber DK, Zarrinkar PP (2011) Comprehensive analysis of kinase inhibitor selectivity. *Nature Biotech* 29:1046–1051.
18. Wolf D, Tilg H, Rumpold H, Gastl G, Wolf AM (2007) The kinase inhibitor imatinib–an immunosuppressive drug? *Curr Cancer Drug Targets* 7:251–258.
19. Sillaber C, Herrmann H, Bennett K, Rix U, Baumgartner C, Böhm A, Herndlhofer S, Tschachler E, Superti-Furga G, Jäger U, Valent P (2009) Immunosuppression and atypical infections in CML patients treated with dasatinib at 140 mg daily. *Eur J Clin Invest* 39:1098–1109.
20. Kreutzman A, Juvonen V, Kairisto V, Ekblom M, Stenke L, Seggewiss R, Porkka K, Mustjoki S (2010) Mono/oligoclonal T and NK cells are common in chronic myeloid leukemia patients at diagnosis and expand during dasatinib therapy. *Blood* 116:772–782.
21. Ravandi F (2010) Dasatinib, an immunomodulator? *Blood* 116:673–674.
22. Karaman MW, Herrgard S, Treiber DK, Gallant P, Atteridge CE, Campbell BT, Chan KW, Ciceri P, Davis MI, Edeen PT, Faraoni R, Floyd M, Hunt JP, Lockhart DJ, Milanov ZV, Morrison MJ, Pallares G, Patel HK, Pritchard S, Wodicka LM, Zarrinkar PP (2008) A quantitative analysis of kinase inhibitor selectivity. *Nature Biotech* 26:127–132.
23. Crunkhorn S (2008) Anticancer drugs: Redesigning kinase inhibitors. *Nature Rev Drug Disc* 7:120–121.
24. Demetri G (2007) Structural reengineering of imatinib to decrease cardiac risk in cancer therapy. *J Clin Invest* 117:3650–3653.
25. Fernández A, Sanguino A, Peng Z, Ozturk E, Chen J, Crespo A, Wulf S, Shavrin A, Qin C, Ma J, Trent J, Lin Y, Han HD, Mangala LS, Bankson JA, Gelovani J, Samarel A, Bornmann W, Sood AK, Lopez-Berestein G (2007) An anticancer c-Kit kinase inhibitor is reengineered to make it more active and less cardiotoxic. *J Clin Invest* 117:4044–4054.

26. Kao J, Ko EC, Eisenstein S, Sikora AG, Fu S, Chen SH (2011) Targeting immune suppressing myeloid-derived suppressor cells in oncology. *Crit Rev Oncol/Hemat* 77:12–19.
27. Kanehisa M, Goto S, Sato Y, Kawashima M, Furumichi M, Tanabe M (2014) Data, information, knowledge and principle: Back to metabolism in KEGG. *Nucleic Acids Res* 42:D199–D205.
28. Das J, Brystol-Myers Squibb (2003) Cyclic protein tyrosine kinase inhibitors, U. S. patent 6,596,746
29. Crespo A, Fernández A (2007) Kinase packing defects as drug targets. *Drug Discovery Today* 12:917–923.
30. Fernández A, Bornmann W, Lopez-Berestein G, Sanguino A, Peng Z, Sood AK, The Board of Regents of the University of Texas System (2013) Methods and Composition of Matter Related to Wrapping of Dehydrons. U. S. patent 8,466,154.
31. Fei F, Yu Y, Schmitt A, Rojewski MT, Chen B, Greiner J, Götz M, Guillaume P, Döhner H, Bunjes D, Schmitt M (2008) Dasatinib exerts an immunosuppressive effect on CD8+ T cells specific for viral and leukemia antigens. *Experim Hematol* 36:1297–1308.
32. Sondel P (2012) Unpublished results (personal communication).
33. Weber J (2008) Overcoming immunologic tolerance to melanoma: Targeting CTLA-4 with ipilimumab (MDX-010). *The Oncologist* 13:16–25.
34. Gallo RC, Sarin PS, Gelmann EP, Robert-Guroff M, Richardson E, Kalyanaraman VS, Mann D, Sidhu GD, Stahl RE, Zolla-Pazner S, Leibowitch J, Popovic M (1983) Isolation of human T-cell leukemia virus in acquired immune deficiency syndrome (AIDS). *Science* 220:865–867.
35. Haas DA, Bala K, Büsche G, Weidner-Glunde M, Santag S, Kati S, Gramolelli S, Damas M, Dittrich-Breiholz O, Kracht M, Rückert J, Varga Z, Keri G, Schulz TF (2013) The inflammatory kinase MAP4K4 promotes reactivation of Kaposi's sarcoma herpesvirus and enhances the invasiveness of infected endothelial cells. *PLoS Pathogens* 9:e1003737.
36. Fernández A (2014) Synergizing immunotherapy with molecularly targeted anticancer treatment. *Drug Disc Today* 19:1427–1432.
37. Maus MV, Grupp SA, Porter DL, June CH (2014) Antibody-modified T cells: CARs take the front seat for hematologic malignancies. *Blood* 123:2625–2635.
38. Maher J (2014) Clinical immunotherapy of B-cell malignancy using CD19-targeted CAR T-cells. *Curr Gene Therapy* 14:35–43.

Chapter 9

Epistructurally engineered cancer susceptibility to checkpoint immunotherapy and the AI-empowered steering of cancer evolution towards extinction

The immune checkpoint blockers have proven most successful to treat solid tumors harboring a DNA mismatch repair (MMR) deficiency or other conditions causative of high antigenic activity related to hypermutability. Using the methods of epistructural biology aided by AI, we show that it is possible to create a drug-promoted cancer phenotype akin to the MMR deficiency in solid tumors, and thereby engineer a drug-induced susceptibility to checkpoint blockers through drug-promoted metabolic stress on DNA synthesis. Issues of compatibility between checkpoint immunotherapy and targeted therapy are first sorted out in order to enable and empower the checkpoint blocker. The potential of such drug-checkpoint-blocker combinations as universal treatments for solid tumors is shown to merit clinical evaluation.

In this context, we also describe a combined therapeutic modality to handle tumor evasion or patterns of resistance. The idea is to exploit AI to steer cancer evolution with combined immunotherapy and epistructural drug treatment. Cancer is a moving target that often evolves ahead of treatment. This is in part because genomic instability is a hallmark of cancer and enables the disease to adapt and develop resistance. These characteristics stem from an evolutionary substrate of intratumoral genetic heterogeneity where therapies select for resistance. Even immune checkpoint inhibitors

(ICIs), arguably the most promising therapeutic agents, do not generally provide lasting cure, not even for responsive patients. Combinations of ICIs and epigenetic immune-priming drugs are being evaluated to expand the pool of ICI-responsive patients. Yet, the occurrence of resistance arising from immunoediting is likely to become daunting because immune surveillance imposes selection pressure on the tumor, while genomic instability induced by the epigenetic drugs creates an evolutionary substrate. In this context, this chapter addresses the problem of overcoming resistance in a quest to develop a cure for cancer.

For targeted therapy, the challenge has been addressed by identifying collateral sensitivity of first-line drug resistant populations. However, there is no guarantee that drug cycling exploiting collateral sensitivity may not ultimately promote another evasion phenotype. Focusing on immune treatments and with the aid of AI, we develop a therapy that evolves concomitantly with the disease and steers the immune-evading tumor into a resistance pathway with dwindling survival population. To address this imperative, AI reveals how to devise an immune trap where we interfere therapeutically with clonal evolution using epistructural drugs of high specificity, perturb the fitness landscape and push the prevailing cell population down a pathway towards extinction. The epistructural therapeutic strategy is shown to be validated on a humanized murine model. Additionally, we present a computational analysis of the clonal dynamics of immune evasion under the changing selection pressure imposed by the steering immunotherapy. The results discussed in this chapter uphold the validity of the proposed paradigm and invite clinical development following evaluation of the epistructural cancer-steering drugs.

9.1 Targeted anticancer therapies that enable and empower checkpoint immunotherapy

Checkpoint immunotherapies are at the forefront of clinical cancer research. They effectively harness biomarkers for tumor-induced immunosuppression and significantly improve clinical outcome in cancers like metastatic melanoma or non-small cell lung cancer (NSCLC). Thus, humanized antibodies like pembrolizumab (Keytruda®) or nivolumab (Opdivo®) (a, b), capable of inducing a checkpoint blockade in the adaptive immune response, are revolutionizing therapy. Furthermore, spectacular results irrespective of cancer type have been recently reported for patients with a DNA mismatch repair (MMR) deficiency known as Lynch syndrome.

Despite their huge success, checkpoint blockers have met only modest success when treating malignancies where peripheral regulatory T cells hinder adaptive immune responses. In the first part of this chapter (sections 9.1-9.8) we squarely address this problem as we seek to turn checkpoint immunotherapy into a universal cancer cure. To that effect, we engineer combinations with targeted agents engineered according to epistructural blueprints with three overarching goals:

- help recruit the adaptive arm of the immune system without adverse superseding effects resulting from direct drug-induced immunosuppression,
- block tumor-induced immunosuppression,
- enhance the antigenicity of the tumor to further stimulate the adaptive response

In chapter 8 we developed molecular design strategies to empower the immune response through drug-induced antigenic activity in monotherapy. Thus, we focused on re-engineering anticancer drugs where a direct off-target impact on the immune system is an undesirable outcome. The goal was to remove drug-induced immunosuppressive effects through molecular redesign, more specifically, to restore the adaptive T-cell-related immune response through anticancer drug treatment. In this way we empowered drug-based anticancer therapy, aligning the patient immune response with the molecularly targeted treatment.

In the first part of this chapter we investigate compatibility issues affecting synergistic efficacy when combining targeted therapy based on kinase inhibitors (KIs) with checkpoint immunotherapy that blocks tumor-induced immunosuppression. Immunogenic cellular debris arising from drug-induced apoptosis needs to be harnessed by the immune system, so immune stimulation through checkpoint blockade appears *in principle* to provide a suitable complement to targeted therapy. Yet, the undesired cross-reactivity of KIs may create incompatibilities between the two therapeutic modalities, particularly if the KI shows nanomolar affinity towards LCK, a key signal transducer in T-lymphocyte activation. Molecular optimization of KIs may be essential to avert anti-LCK activity while retaining affinity towards clinically relevant targets. This chapter advocates for the implementation of epistructural selectivity filters for drug re-design capable of telling apart LCK from on-target kinases to guarantee effective synergy.

Thirdly, we focus on cancers where checkpoint immunotherapy has not proven effective. In such contexts, checkpoint blockers have not elicited a vigorous immune response, mainly because immunosuppressive regulatory T cells (T_{regs}) overwhelm effector T cells (T_{eff}) in the tumor periphery. To address this problem, we engineer combinations with immune-compatible KIs designed to lower the peripheral T_{regs}:T_{eff} ratio. The combinations enhance both the efficacy of the checkpoint blockade and the contribution of the immune system to the anti-tumor impact of targeted therapy.

Finally, in the context of MMR deficiency, Keytruda has proven effective regardless of cancer type probably because of the superior antigenic activity of such condition. Accordingly, in this chapter we propose to engineer targeted therapies geared at *inducing* the MMR deficiency and administer them in combination with Keytruda to seek universal cure for cancer, or at least for all solid tumors irrespective of their origin.

9.2 Compatible combinations of checkpoint immunotherapy with targeted drugs

With the remarkable success of immune checkpoint blockades in cancer treatment, the recruitment of immune-based anticancer activity has become a key asset in the therapeutic arsenal [1, 2]. A checkpoint blockade is achieved by removing a negative signal for the immune system. The "brake release" operates through an antibody

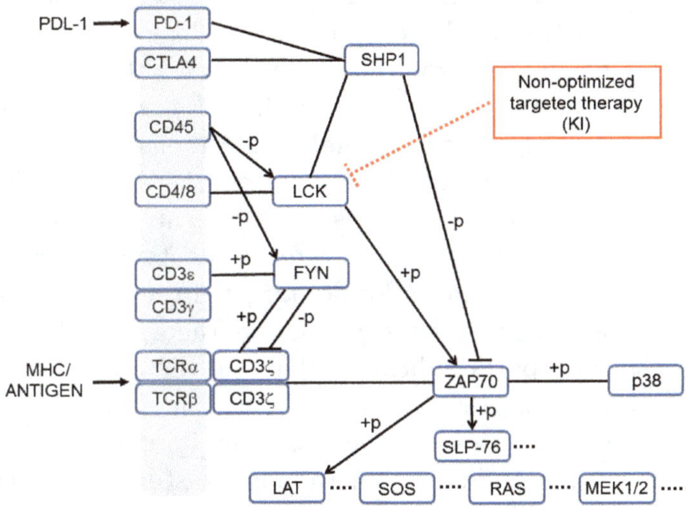

Figure 9.1. Signaling network for activation and downregulation of antigen-triggered T-cell activation. Adapted from Kyoto Encyclopedia of Genes and Genomes, T-cell receptor signaling pathway — Homo sapiens. url: http://www.genome.jp/kegg-bin/show_pathway?hsadd04660 Reprinted from [Fernández A (2017) Making Targeted Therapy Compatible with Checkpoint Immunotherapy. Trends Biotech 35:582-584], copyright 2017 with permission from Elsevier.

recognizing the programmed death-1 (PD-1) receptor (or its ligand PDL-1), which promotes downregulation of the adaptive immune response. Thus, humanized monoclonal antibodies like nivolumab (Opdivo®) (a), or pembrolizumab (Keytruda®) (b) prevent the PD-1-receptor from binding its natural ligand PDL-1 and thereby prevent the receptor from recruiting the repressive SHP1 phosphatase (Fig. 9.1) [1, 2]. When recruited, SHP1 de-phosphorylates and thereby deactivates ZAP70, a downstream signal transducer. In this way, the biologics hinder the suppression of antigen-triggered T-cell activation (Fig. 9.1). PD-1 blockade is meant to restore the adaptive immune response that is suppressed by tumors capable of expressing PD-1 ligands. Other T-cell-repressive receptors like CTLA4 may be also targeted (cf. Fig. 9.1) with similar therapeutic efficacy. This general strategy has proven successful for treating metastatic melanoma and metastatic non-small cell lung cancer, and it has succeeded as a second-line treatment for head and neck squamous cell carcinoma and renal cell carcinoma.

Recently, combinations of checkpoint immunotherapies with targeted therapies based on kinase inhibitors (KIs) are being vigorously pursued, particularly when oncogenic mutations or other genetic accidents occur at the onset of the disease [4, 5]. Although KI-based treatment often improves prognosis, most patients relapse due to the emergence of secondary mutations as drug resistance develops. This effect demonstrates the limitations of targeted therapy as monotherapy, suggesting the need for combination therapies. For example, there have been reports indicating that the therapeutic efficacy of the KI dasatinib (Sprycel®) in the c-KIT mutant P815 mastocytoma relies significantly on components of the immune response [6]. Thus, combinations of dasatinib with immuno-stimulators have been pursued. Such combinations lead to a potent therapeutic synergy with demonstrated tumor clearance in animal models [4–6]. The rationale for such combinations is that they mitigate the broad relatively short-lived effect of targeted therapy with the narrower but longer-term impact of immunotherapy. Additionally, immune stimulation harnesses the immunogenic molecular debris arising from cancer cell death promoted by targeted therapy. Some examples of combinations that are currently being clinically evaluated include:

I) imatinib/pembrolizumab in metastatic melanoma with mast/stem cell growth factor receptor (c-KIT) mutation or amplification (ClinicalTrials.gov Identifier NCT02812693),
II) crizotinib/pembrolizumab in anaplastic lymphoma kinase (ALK)-positive advanced non-small cell lung cancer (ClinicalTrials.gov Identifier NCT02511184), and
III) dabrafenib/nivolumab in BRaf-mutated metastatic melanoma (ClinicalTrials.gov Identifier NCT02910700).

However, as indicated in chapter 8, the off-target cross-reactivity of many KIs against the lymphocyte specific kinase (LCK) is likely to compromise the efficacy of such combinations because through LCK inhibition, KIs suppress precisely the antigen-triggered

T-cell response that the PD-1 inhibitors are supposed to boost. As shown in Fig. 9.1, while PD-1 blockade prevents the PD-1-recruitable phosphatase SHP1 from suppressing antigen-triggered T-cell response, drug-induced upstream LCK inhibition would exert an equivalently suppressive activity. This finding suggests that KIs with nanomolar LCK affinity are *a priori* incompatible with checkpoint immunotherapy.

Recent kinome-wide screening reveals that imatinib, crizotinib and dabrafenib are nanomolar LCK inhibitors, with dissociation constant $K_D = 40$, 20 and 180nM, respectively (c). This pharmacological-level affinity, particularly for imatinib and crizotinib, makes them intrinsically unsuitable to synergize with checkpoint blockers. Dasatinib, possibly the most powerful LCK inhibitor known ($K_D = 0.2$nM) (c), would be *a priori* the worst candidate to synergize with a PD-1 blocker, notwithstanding past efforts to combine them [4–6]. This article argues that molecular optimization of the KIs is required to synergize them with immune-based PD-1 blockers.

9.3 Epistructural optimization of KIs for combination with checkpoint immunotherapy

One of the most valuable lesson from this book is that while homologous on-target and off-target kinases are structurally similar and therefore difficult to tell apart through molecular recognition, their patterns of packing defects (dehydrons) make them distinguishable [7]. Interfacial water molecules surrounding dehydrons are constrained (Chapter 2), and hence easily removable and a payoff for such dehydration is the strengthening and stabilization of the underlying electrostatic interaction [7]. This observation has prompted the design of highly selective drugs that act as "dehydron wrappers", removing water upon drug-target association from around unique non-conserved dehydrons. This design principle has been used to rework imatinib into a more selective drug named WBZ_4 (chapters 7, 8). This compound has enhanced affinity against the primary imatinib target c-KIT while presenting a significantly reduced affinity against LCK (K_D = 800nM, compared with K_D = 40nM for imatinib) [7]. Compound WBZ_4 is a methylated version of imatinib capable of wrapping the dehydron that pairs Cys673 with Gly676 in the KIT kinase (PDB file 1T46). Since this dehydron aligns with the well wrapped backbone hydrogen bond Met319-Gly322 in LCK (chapters 7, 8), the affinity of WBZ_4 for LCK is compromised, while its affinity for on-target c-KIT is enhanced (Chapter 7). Based on this analysis, WBZ_4 is *a priori* expected to be a better KI than imatinib to synergize with pembrolizumab in the treatment of KIT-dependent melanoma, an observation that invites clinical evaluation of the novel combination.

Generally, we argue that the anti-LCK-anti-PD-1 antagonism may be removed through redesign of the KI by adopting the target's unique dehydron pattern as a selectivity filter. In this way, an optimized KI that avoids LCK while retaining on-target activity at parental-drug levels may be engineered to synergize with checkpoint blockers. The optimization strategy may be implemented by structurally aligning the dehydron pattern of the on-target protein with that of LCK. For example, due to its potency as an LCK inhibitor, crizotinib is likely to be incompatible for combination with immune-based checkpoint therapy. It would be desirable to redesign crizotinib into a compound that retains the parental nanomolar affinity for ALK, while significantly reducing LCK affinity. Structural alignment of ALK and LCK reveals that the dehydron Met1199-Gly1202 in ALK aligns with the well-wrapped Met319-Gly322 backbone hydrogen bond in LCK (Fig. 9.2). While the residues (Met, Gly) paired by the backbone hydrogen bonds are conserved, the dielectric environments around the bonds are different, with the ALK hydrogen bond significantly more exposed to water. The pre-existing wrapping difference prompts a redesign of crizotinib in order to contribute upon binding to the wrapping of dehydron Met1199-Gly1202 in ALK. This wrapping modification may be realized, for example, through methylation at the position highlighted in Fig. 9.2. The wrapping modification is expected to enhance affinity for ALK beyond parental levels since exclusion of interfacial water surrounding an electrostatic amide-carbonyl interaction enhances

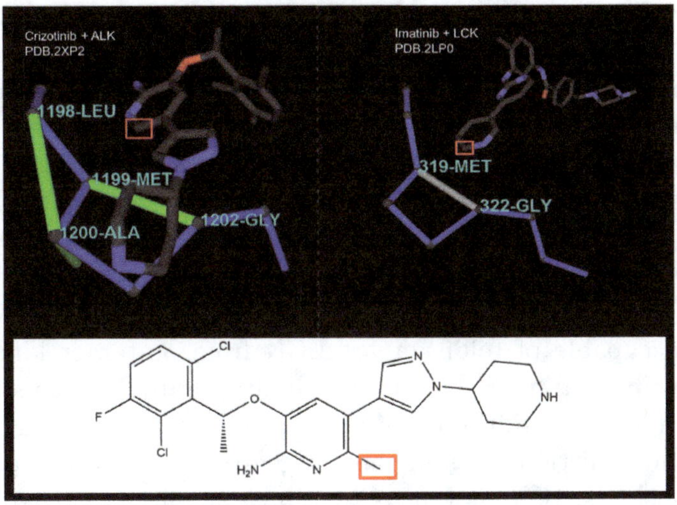

Figure 9.2. Differences in dehydron patterns apparent upon structural alignment of ALK and LCK structures enable the redesign of KI crizotinib to retain activity against on-target ALK while significantly reducing activity against LCK. The protein backbone region is represented by virtual bonds joining α-carbons of aligned residues, dehydrons are marked as green lines joining the α-carbons of the paired residues and well-wrapped (dehydrated) backbone hydrogen bonds are marked by white lines. The sites of the LCK-discriminating methylation in crizotinib and imatinib are highlighted in red. The chemical structure of the crizotinib redesign able to tell apart ALK from LCK is presented in the bottom panel.

and stabilizes the preformed hydrogen bond, and drug affinity is controlled by the free energy content of the drug-target complex. On the other hand, just like in the case of WBZ_4 versus imatinib, the proposed wrapping modification of crizotinib will decrease affinity for LCK, a desirable outcome to create a synergic combination with the anti-PD-1 antibody.

9.4 Synergies that enable immunotherapy

The adaptive arm of the immune response is a key ally of KI-based targeted therapy in the cure for cancer. Immunogenic cellular debris arising from drug-induced apoptosis needs to be harnessed by the immune system, so immune stimulation through checkpoint blockade appears *prima facie* to provide a suitable complement to targeted therapy. Yet, as discussed previously, the undesired cross-reactivity of KIs may create incompatibilities between the two therapeutic modalities, particularly if the KI shows nanomolar affinity towards LCK, a key signal transducer in T-lymphocyte activation. Molecular optimization of KIs to control their specificity has proven possible, and may be essential to avert anti-LCK activity while retaining affinity towards clinically relevant targets. This chapter advocates for the implementation of epistructural selectivity filters in drug re-design capable of telling apart LCK from on-target kinases. As discussed in Chapter 8, only compatibility-optimized KIs should be utilized in combination therapies with immune-based PD-1 blockers [8], as antagonistic effects in the antigen-triggered activation of the T-cell must first be removed to guarantee an effective synergy.

Resistance patterns are likely to emerge for the optimized combinations, impairing KI or antibody affinity, or competitively enhancing kinase or receptor affinity for their natural ligands. On targeted kinases, resistance is likely to be promoted by mutations that are not necessarily the same as those identified when the KI is used as a monotherapy. In fact, differences in resistance patterns may be informative of the synergistic mechanism of the combination therapy. Molecular wrapping re-designs of the KI may be successfully introduced to address the "moving target" problem posed by the emergence of kinase resistance mutations [9, 10], as long as the latter alter the targetable pattern of packing defects (dehydrons) of the protein.

9.5 Deficiencies of monotherapy in cancer treatment

Targeted anticancer therapy has not proven curative, since resistance involving secondary mutations eventually arises [10]. Given this reality, combinations with immunotherapy are being evaluated [5]. This modality becomes attractive since targeted agents like kinase inhibitors (KIs) behave like vaccines, generating antigenic activity as they promote tumor-cell apoptosis, while immunotherapy stimulates the antigen-triggered adaptive immune response. Thus, the broad short-lived effect of targeted therapy may be offset by the narrow long-term impact of immunotherapy.

Immunotherapies based on T cell checkpoint blockades have shown success as monotherapy against cancers like metastatic melanoma [2]. However, they have met modest success against other types of cancer like ovarian cancer [8]. In such contexts, antibody inhibitors of cytotoxic T lymphocyte-associated protein 4 (CTLA-4) or programmed death receptor 1 (PD-1) have not stimulated a vigorous immune response, mainly because immunosuppressive regulatory T cells (T_{regs}) overwhelm effector T cells (T_{eff}) in the tumor periphery. It should be noted that Tregs promote tumor-induced immune tolerance and hence hinder immunotherapy. Thus, researchers are currently evaluating combination therapies to lower the peripheral T_{regs}:T_{eff} ratio [11].

This analysis advocates combination therapy to enhance both the efficacy of the checkpoint blockade and the contribution of the immune system to the anti-tumor impact of targeted therapy. However, KIs that have succeeded as monotherapy are often *unsuitable* for such combinations, as shown subsequently. Accordingly, we propose an epistructural remodeling of KIs to promote the kind of synergistic activity that foils tumor-induced immunosuppression without adverse superseding effects.

9.6 Empowering checkpoint immunotherapy by combination with targeted therapy

We first focus on immune-synergies involving imatinib, an effective KI to treat GIST, the gastrointestinal stromal tumor [11–13]. The efficacy of the targeted agent is traced to its activity on the c-KIT (stem cell receptor) and PDGFRA (platelet growth factor receptor alpha) kinases, both susceptible to become constitutively active through mutation [12, 13]. Although imatinib improves median survival, it is not curative since secondary mutations eventually develop conferring target resistance. Combinations of imatinib with checkpoint blockers are being evaluated to improve clilnical outcome under the assumption that imatinib will reduce tumor-induced immunosuppression through inhibition of c-KIT, precisely the same target associated with its antitumor activity. Expression array analysis of GIST tumors in animal models identified how imatinib affected tumor-infiltrating $CD8^+$ T cells and T_{regs}. Differences in expression patterns caused by imatinib revealed that c-KIT promotes tumor cell expression of the immunosuppressive enzyme indoleamine 2,3-dioxygenase (Ido), which, in turn, promotes conversion, stabilization and activation of T_{regs}. Thus, *prima facie*, c-KIT inhibitory activity made imatinib suitable to synergize with immunotherapy [11].

However, as highlighted in chapter 8, it is doubtful that imatinib will succeed in combination therapies. Imatinib is almost as powerful an inhibitor of c-KIT or PDGFRA as it is of the lymphocyte-specific kinase LCK (K_D = 13, 31 and 40nM, respectively) (c). The latter off-target activity compromises the efficacy of combination therapies because LCK is a major signal transducer of the antigen-triggered adaptive response of T cells [13]. In other words, the anti-LCK activity of imatinib makes it *directly immunosuppressive*, overwriting its blockade of tumor-induced immunosuppression.

A structural remodeling of imatinib to increase c-KIT affinity while removing affinity for LCK is possible [12, 13], as discussed in chapter 8. This remodeling is guided by local epistructural differences arising in kinome-wide alignment [12, 13] combined with requirements of immuno-synergy. Specifically, the solvent-exposed backbone hydrogen bond (dehydron) C673-G676 in c-KIT becomes solvent-shielded bond M319-G322 in LCK and induced-upon-association bond M111-N114 in JNK (chapter 7) [12, 13]). Thus, a single methylation of imatinib at the position indicated in Fig. 9.3, yielding compound WBZ_4, turns the drug into a selective dehydron-stabilizer of c-KIT with superior affinity (K_D = 10.4nM). Like dasatinib, this activity would in principle make WBZ_4 eminently suitable to treat ovarian cancer [14, 15]. In turn, WBZ_4 has no significant affinity towards LCK due to the high thermodynamic cost of excluding water from the periphery of well-wrapped M319-G322 bond [12, 13], while possessing nanomolar affinity towards JNK, which is a key clinical target for ovarian cancer [16].

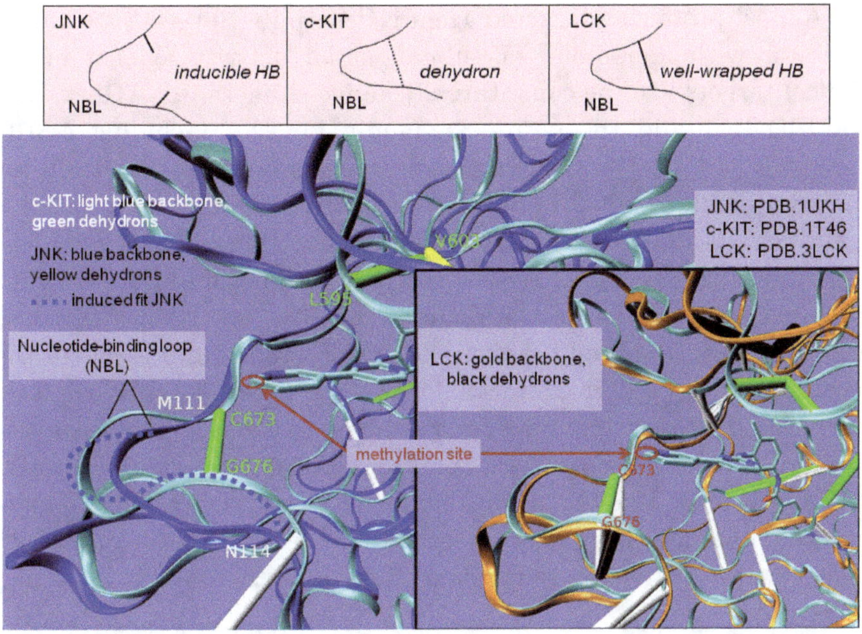

Figure 9.3. Epistructural analysis of structurally aligned c-KIT/JNK and c-KIT/LCK (inset). Epistructural differences in the nucleotide-binding loop (NBL) are indicated schematically in the upper panel and steer imatinib redesign.

Compound WBZ_4 is thus engineered to block tumor-induced immunosuppression more efficiently than imatinib through its enhanced c-KIT inhibition. Furthermore, peripheral T_{regs} modulation is free from superseding direct immunosuppressive effects associated with LCK inhibition. These advantages of WBZ_4 prompt clinical evaluation in combination with checkpoint blockers for treatment of GIST or metastatic c-KIT-dependent melanoma, in lieu of similar combinations with imatinib currently under evaluation (ClinicalTrials.gov Identifier NCT02812693). Furthermore, the anti-JNK and anti-c-KIT activity of WBZ_4 makes it suitable for synergic combinations to treat ovarian cancer. In this context, clinical efficacy makes it mandatory to reduce the T_{regs}:T_{eff} ratio at the tumor periphery, a goal achievable through c-KIT inhibition, while the concurrent antigenic activity is guaranteed through JNK inhibition [16].

A most promising targeted agent is dasatinib (Sprycel®), a kinase inhibitor with nanomolar or subnanomolar activity against major clinical targets like the constitutively active chimera bcr-ABL, c-KIT and PDGFR and the entire Src-family kinases, including c-SRC and LCK [14, 15, 17]. Ongoing clinical trials evaluate dasatinib for the treatment of solid tumors, including GIST (ClinicalTrials.gov Identifier NCT02776878) and ovarian cancer (ClinicalTrials.gov Identifier NCT02059265). However, a combination of dasatinib with immunotherapy to achieve a definite cure has not been attempted and may be forbiddingly challenging because dasatinib is one of the most powerful LCK inhibitors known (K_D = 0.2nM)(c). Therefore, the level of direct immunosuppression is extreme [17], making it dangerous even as monotherapy. Yet, dasatinib is a more powerful c-KIT inhibitor than imatinib, hence its potential to block tumor-induced immunosuppression is probably greater. These properties make it imperative to re-engineer dasatinib to make it immune-synergic.

To address the challenge, we aligned all dasatinib targets and examined epistructural differences. Like with WBZ_4 target JNK, the major dasatinib target c-SRC presents an inducible backbone hydrogen bond at position M341-G344 (Fig. 9.4) that aligns with dehydron C673-C676 in c-KIT and with solvent-secluded M319-G322 bond in LCK (Fig. 9.3). Methylation at the position indicated in Fig. 9.4 induces the M341-G344 c-SRC hydrogen bond, enhancing the anti-c-SRC inhibitory power of dasatinib by further stabilizing the drug/target complex [13]. This chaperone role through wrapping of a preformed hydrogen bond inspired the term "*wrapperone*". The drug alteration also selectively removes LCK affinity following the same rationale that holds for WBZ_4 (cf. Fig. 9.3). Furthermore, the wrapperone augments the wrapping of dehydron C673-G676 upon binding to c-KIT, hence stabilizing the drug/target complex. Thus, the wrapperone is expected to curb tumor-induced immunosuppression more strongly than dasatinib. The fact that this crucial effect is not overwritten by direct LCK-related immunosuppression makes the wrapperone an ideal agent to synergize with immune-stimulating checkpoint blockades. Reciprocally, the checkpoint immunotherapies,

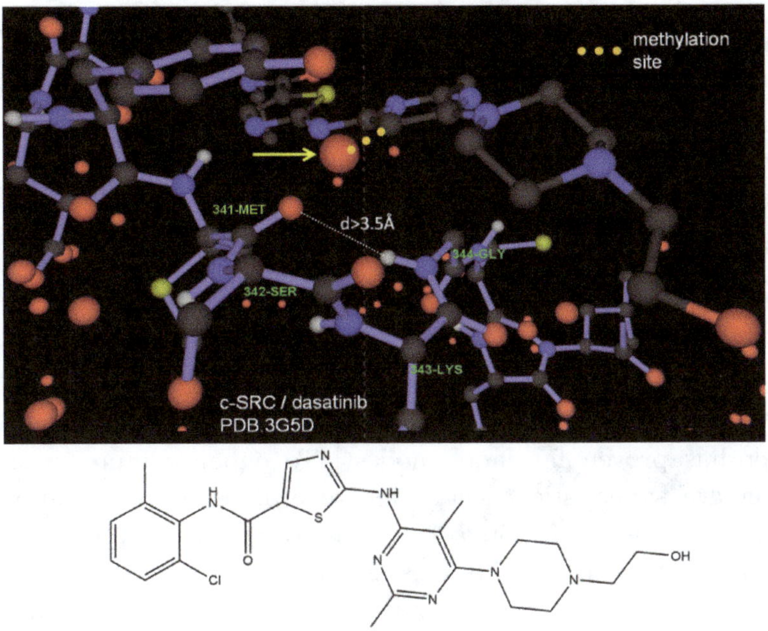

Figure 9.4. Region in dasatinib/c-SRC complex containing inducible M341-G344 backbone hydrogen bond that structurally aligns with dehydron C673-G676 in c-KIT. To induce the M341-G344 bond, the exogenous wrapping must be augmented through methylation of dasatinib at the position indicated, yielding the wrapperone compound. The resulting compound excludes the water molecule (oxygen as red ball, arrow) that disrupts M341-G344 bond formation. The chemical structure of the *wrapperone* is shown in the lower panel.

that have proven only moderately successful to treat ovarian cancer [8], will be rescued through the wrapperone combination, since the potent and now unfettered anti-c-KIT activity significantly reduces the peripheral T_{regs}:T_{eff} ratio.

9.7 Checkpoint immunotherapy made operative in ovarian cancer and other malignancies impervious to treatment

In many malignancies like ovarian cancer, targeted therapy is not curative while checkpoint immunotherapy is not fully operative. Combinations of both treatments may succeed if tumor-induced immunosuppression is reduced without introducing adverse overwriting effects. Available KI cannot achieve such goals and some structural remodeling is needed. There are limitations to the approach arising from structural correlations among KI targets. We offer a selectivity filter that may be exploited to engineer combination therapies that fulfill the therapeutic imperatives. This strategy should prompt evaluation in clinical contexts exhibiting dominant T_{regs} population in the tumor periphery (d).

Checkpoint blockade has proven extremely successful in the treatment of cancers with high immunogenicity, such as metastatic melanoma, NSCLC, RCC, etc. By contrast, with response rates of 10-15%, the clinical efficacy of checkpoint immunotherapy in ovarian cancer has proven far more modest. To enhance immunogenicity and create synergistic effects, we are evaluating combinations of checkpoint PD-1 inhibitors and targeted therapy based on KIs. The rationale for such combinations is that they mitigate the broad relatively short-lived effect of targeted therapy with the narrower but longer-term impact of immunotherapy. Additionally, immune stimulation harnesses the immunogenic molecular debris arising from cancer cell death promoted by targeted therapy.

To test the improvement in outcome for the treatment of ovarian cancer beyond the levels achieved by checkpoint blockers, we evaluated a combination therapy in animal models, synergizing the immune-compatible inhibitor WBZ_4 with an anti-mouse PD-1 checkpoint blocker (a-PD-1). Cohorts of 10 syngenic mice were first inoculated i. p. with five million cells from mouse ovarian epithelial papillary serous adenocarcinoma line ID8. One week after inoculation, a survival therapy began with daily dose of 50mg/mouse of WBZ_4 (in other cohorts, imatinib or IgG(1) were used as controls at the same dose). Beginning 30 days after tumor cell inoculation, mice were injected i. p. on alternate days for 1 week with 200mg/mouse of a-PD-1 antibody (in a control cohort, the a-PD-1 antibody was administered as monotherapy at the same dose after 30 days after tumor cell i. p. inoculation). Tumor maturation point is reached 52 ± 2 days after inoculation, and at that point, specimens in one cohort were subject to debulking surgery to extract the tumor

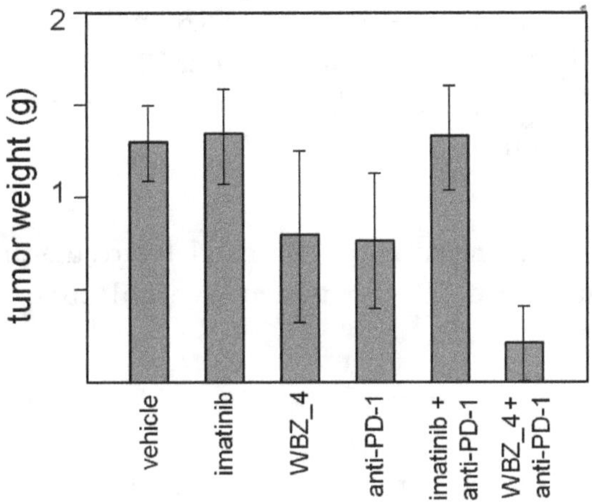

Figure 9.5. Tumor weight in murine model of ovarian cancer on the 52nd day after inoculation. Specimens in a 10-mice cohort were subject to debulking surgery to extract the tumor from the peritoneal cavity.

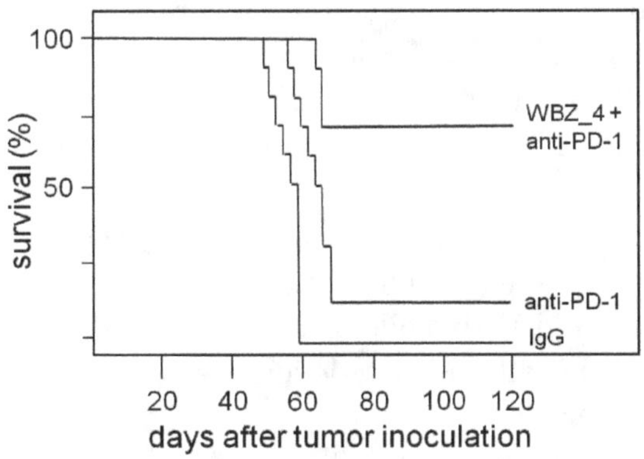

Figure 9.6. Survival experiments in single cohorts for murine model for ovarian cancer.

from the peritoneal cavity and determine its weight (Figure 9.5). Survival experiments on a single cohort of 10 mice are reported in Figure 9.6.

The results explicitly reveal synergistic effects and significant therapeutic efficacy for the WBZ_4-checkpoint blocker combination therapy, highlighting the value of epistructural analysis that dictated the design of the immune-compatible JNK inhibitor. The encouraging results in Figures 9.5, 9.6 make it imperative to clinically evaluate WBZ_4 in combination with checkpoint blockers to seek a definite cure for ovarian cancer.

9.8 Cancer immunotherapy primed by drug-induced hypermutation: Towards a universal cure for solid tumors

As described in the previous sections, Merck's drug Keytruda (pembrolizumab) unleashes antitumor immunity by suppressing a negative signal: the checkpoint of the adaptive immune response. On the other hand, Vogelstein, Diaz and colleagues showed that cancer gene mutations can be presented in surface protein fragments by the major histocompatibility complex recognized by T cells, and conjectured that hypermutated tumors would stand out, especially those harboring the DNA mismatch repair (MMR) deficiency [18]. This condition is known as Lynch syndrome and its ultra-antigenic activity is well documented ([18, 19] and references therein). Such tumors stimulate the adaptive immune response by accruing 100 to 1000 times more mutations than typical tumors, thus displaying a vastly higher antigenic activity. By releasing the brakes of T cells that become activated through recognition of the mutant proteins, Vogelstein, Diaz and their colleagues realized that Keytruda would make most tumors with MMR deficiency highly susceptible to an immune attack [18].

In a recent clinical trial [19], researchers identified a cohort of 86 advanced cancer patients with 12 tumor types including colorectal, breast, prostate, and pancreatic cancer, all with MMR deficiency. These cases were all unyielding to standard tumor-specific treatment. After bimonthly dose of Keytruda, cancer remission was observed in the majority of the patients. In 18 patients, including two with advanced pancreatic cancer - that yield a dismal prognosis -, complete responses were achieved, whereas objective radiographic responses were observed in 53% of patients. Responses were durable with median progression-free and overall survival limit not reached three years after the study was initiated. The data supports the hypothesis that the significantly large antigenic activity in MMR-deficient cancers makes them hypersensitive to immune checkpoint blockade, regardless of the originating tumor.

The data in support of such striking conclusions were provided to FDA months prior to publication and won Keytruda approval through priority review, enabling the monoclonal antibody to be used in any solid tumor on patients harboring the MMR deficiency (e). Spectacular as these findings are, the MMR deficiency phenotype is somewhat rare (although probably underdiagnosed) in cancer, with a 3–5% occurrence [18–20]. Thus, the striking results reported in [19] prompt the following question:

> *Is it possible to induce the MMR deficiency in any solid tumor, for example through targeted drug-based therapy, and thereby enhance the cancer antigenic activity and diversity to turn the Keytruda-drug combination into a universal cure?*

The likely answer to this question is yes. The key to the problem resides in identifying a major signaling pathway recruited to promote MMR and finding a therapeutically relevant KI that would block that pathway. It turns out that the alpha-isoform of phosphoinositide 3-kinase (PI3Kα) is a key signal transducer for the MMR-associated signaling pathway [20]. In this capacity, PI3Kα plays a metabolic role as it mediates carbohydrate uptake so that the anti-metabolic role of PI3K inhibition is the depletion of nucleotides. This depletion is a consequence of reduced flux through glycolysis that results in a decrease in R5P required for base ribosylation. Ultimately, the nucleotide depletion induces the DNA damage phenotype [20]. Thus, treatment with a PI3K inhibitor, specifically with a PI3Kα inhibitor, leads to nucleotide depletion in rapidly proliferating cancer cells that could result in replication stress within hours. This metabolic effect appears to be specific to tumor cells since they rely more heavily on de novo nucleotide biosynthesis than normal cells. This specificity explains the therapeutic benefit of PI3K inhibitors.

The interference with DNA synthesis in tumor cells through nucleotide depletion induced by PI3Kα inhibitors results in replication stress, as tumor cells enter the S phase but DNA synthesis is compromised. Thus, nucleotide shortage leads to error-prone DNA replication, which in turn overloads the cell reliance on MMR mechanisms.

In this way, treatment with PI3Kα inhibitors [20] may realize the Vogelstein-Diaz scenario for enhanced antigenic activity and checkpoint hypersensitivity, mimicking the MMR condition and thereby making the tumor susceptible to an adaptive immune attack promoted by Keytruda.

In light of this argument, the clinical evaluation of a combined Keytruda+PI3Kα inhibitor treatment is likely to become an imperative in the quest for a definite universal cure for solid tumors.

9.9 The evolutionary substrate of cancers susceptible to checkpoint immunotherapy

Endowed with the evolutionary substrate of genomic instability, cancer evolves, adapts and ultimately develops resistance to therapy, hence constituting a moving target. In this evolutionary context, current therapies select for resistance and therefore do not effectively deal with the problem. This chapter squarely and boldly addresses the problem of overcoming cancer resistance to immunotherapy. To that effect, we introduce a dynamic immunotherapy that evolves concomitantly with the disease, steering the tumor into a resistance pathway of dwindling cell population. As in the two previous chapters, we exploit immune checkpoint inhibitors (ICIs), at present some of the most promising therapeutic agents. We are aware that ICIs do not provide lasting cure, not even for the subpopulation of responsive patients. Immune surveillance imposes selection pressure on the tumor and the genomic instability induced by immune-priming agents creates the substrate for cancer evolution and adaptation articulated through immunoediting. This scenario leads to patterns of immune resistance that ultimately cause relapse. Thus, it becomes imperative that the immunotherapy avoids maintaining a fixed selection pressure and rather evolves to steer the immune evasion pattern towards extinction. This chapter addresses this imperative and implements a solution to the moving target problem. We thus introduce Lethal Immune Complementarity (LIC). LIC is somewhat akin to synthetic lethality but differs since the complementary subtherapies are not administered simultaneously but rather in an alternating fashion due to their opposing effects. Parallels with collateral sensitivity also exist but the therapeutic context is entirely different and the complementarity of immune-evasion phenotypes ensures that the tumor would be steered into an immunogenic trap. To assess efficacy, we first present a computational analysis of the clonal dynamics of immune evasion under the changing selection pressure imposed by the steering immunotherapy. The results are subsequently validated using a preclinical experimental model and shown to uphold the proposed paradigm.

As said, genomic instability is a hallmark of cancer, enabling the disease to evolve and develop resistance to treatment [21, 22]. To overcome resistance, we implement a choreographed immunotherapy guided by an analysis of the clonal dynamics of cancer cells under a variable selection pressure arising from switching targeting of evasion phenotypes. As in the previous chapter and in the previous sections, we exploit immune checkpoint inhibitors (ICIs)[23, 24], and this time we combine them with immune-priming drugs to promote responsiveness [25–27] and, furthermore, we incorporate a switching targeted therapy to steer the immune-evading phenotype into an immunogenic trap. As emphasized, resistance needs to be circumvented since immune surveillance imposes selection pressure, while genomic instability induced by priming drugs [28–30] creates an evolutionary substrate for relapse of the disease. The therapy implemented interferes with clonal evolution, perturbs the fitness landscape and pushes the cell population down an immune-evasion pathway towards extinction. Therapeutic efficacy is established on a humanized murine model, validating the mathematical analysis of clonal dynamics and inviting clinical development.

With the ability to block tumor-induced immunosuppression, ICIs hold promise as anticancer agents [23, 24]. However, responsiveness to ICI remains low, mostly restricted to patients with highly immunogenic conditions [23]. Even when impressive results are achieved, restoration of T cell function is transient, usually followed by relapse as a consequence of resistance to treatment [24]. The crux of the problem is that the genomic instability that promotes immunogenicity also provides the evolutionary substrate for evasion. In this therapeutic context, we address the challenge of achieving lasting cure, overcoming resistance through a timed immunotherapy that evolves concomitantly with the disease, steering the immune-evasion phenotype towards extinction. The therapy is choreographed based on a mathematical analysis of clonal dynamics under a variable (steering) selection pressure.

To enhance ICI-responsiveness, combinations with epigenetic drugs (epidrugs) are implemented [25–27]. Such epidrugs are usually chromatin-unraveling promoters like inhibitors of DNA methyltransferases (DNMTi) or inhibitors of histone deacetylases (HDACi) that impact significantly the regulation of chromatin restructuring, with multiple immune-priming effects [28–30]. Thus, epidrugs upregulate expression of checkpoint ligands PD-L1/PD-L2 (programmed death ligands 1 and 2) in cancer cells, embryonic antigens like the cancer testis antigen (CTA) not expressed in adults, and genes involved in antigen processing and presentation along the MHC (major hystocompatibility complex) pathway. In particular, the DNMTi reactivates endogenous retroviral (ERV) repetitive elements that restore interferon (IFN) pathways that in turn lead to expression of checkpoint ligands, antigen-presentation complexes, and pro-apoptotic and anti-proliferative genes [31]. In spite of such immune-priming effects conducive to the enhancement of ICI efficacy, tumors subject to ICI + epidrug combination therapy are likely to develop resistance, especially since epidrugs like DNMTi's promote genomic instability [28–30], creating an evolutionary substrate for immune evasion.

9.10 Overcoming the immune evasion of the immune-susceptible tumor

To overcome the selection of an immune evading phenotype, we outline an evolving therapy that avoids maintaining a fixed selection pressure by cycling the tumor through two alternatives for immune evasion: a) recruitment of immunosuppressive T regs (regulatory T cells) [32] and TAMSCs (tumor-associated myeloid suppressive cells) within the tumor microenvironment (TME) [33]; and b) impairment of antigen presentation through beta2-microglobulin (B2M) [34] mutation or mutational deactivation of the JAK1/2 kinase, transducer in the IFN pathway that induces expression of MHC-I [31, 34]. There is evidence that under a suitable evolutionary substrate enabling selection and adaptation, i.e. genetic instability provided by the Lynch syndrome, the (T reg, TAMSC)-recruiting phenotype a and the antigen-presentation deficient phenotype b compete with each other [34]. Thus, expression levels of mutated B2M in cancer cells are anticorrelated with expression levels of the transcription factor FOXP3 in tumor-adjacent T regs that controls gene expression programs for T reg function. In principle, nonadaptive immune evasion may take other alternative pathways, such as the JAK1-impairing mutation. However, this impairment of the IFN pathway does not to occur in our preclinical setting or in quintessential models of ICI responsiveness [34], as shown below. Should it become operational in other systems under investigation, it can be incorporated into the mathematical modeling through an additional variable for an alternative evasion phenotype.

The immune-evading phenotype can be steered into pattern b by complementing the ICI + epidrug combination with a PI3K inhibitor specific for γ,δ-isoforms, such as *duvelisib*. This targeted agent enables the immune system to eliminate cancer cells that adopted evasion pattern a [35], while the residual population that survived by adopting pattern b may be partly eliminated by switching to a β-isoform-specific PI3K inhibitor [35], like GSK2636771 or AZD8186, that promotes elimination of phenotype b [36]. Thus, the evolving therapy cycles the tumor back and forth between the two immune-evading phenotypes by alternating between the PI3K(γ,δ)-inhibitor and the PI3Kβ-inhibitor, so that the selected phenotype becomes susceptible in the next iteration (Figure 9.7). In this way, we outline a timed immunotherapy choreographed to steer cancer evolution into a lethal immunogenic trap furnished by alternating the selection of immune-evasion phenotypes.

(a)

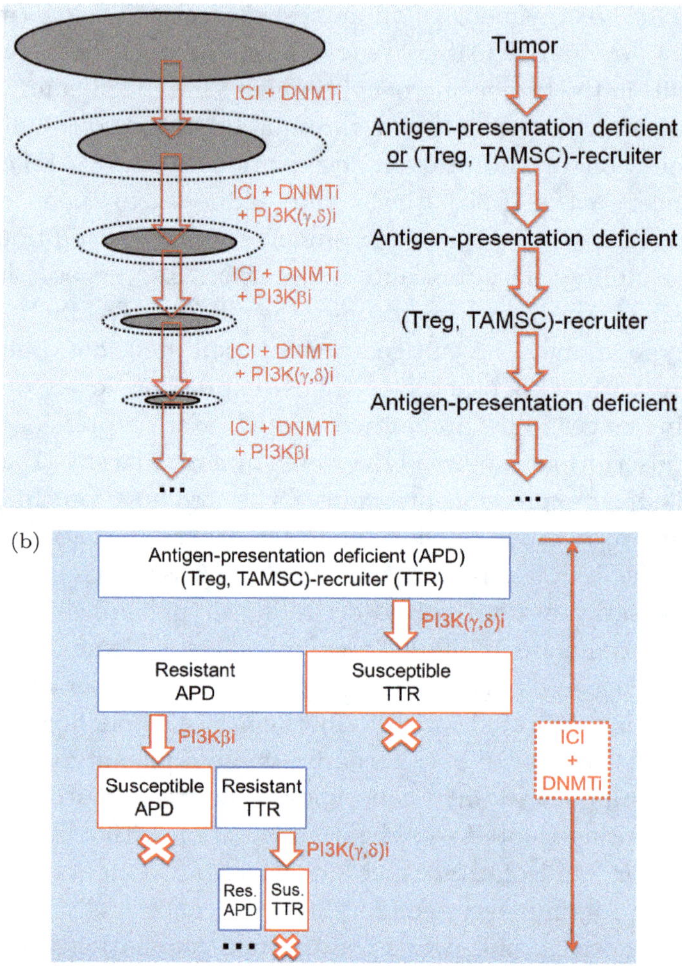

(b)

Figure 9.7. *Lethal Immune Complementarity, choreographed therapy to steer immune evasion.* (a) Evolving therapy promoting immune attack and steering the tumor back and forth between two immune-evading phenotypes with dwindling surviving population. The therapy involves three components: 1) ICI-induced blockade of tumor-induced immunosuppression; 2) immune priming by an epidrug, here represented by DNA methyltransferase inhibitor (DNMTi), or other targeted agent; 3) alternation between two isoform-selective PI3K inhibitors (PI3K(γ,δ)i, PI3Kβi) needed to respectively suppress two competing resistant phenotypes arising from immunoediting. Immune surveillance creates a selection pressure that promotes adaptive change in the tumor. Adaptive change

Figure 9.7. (*Continued*) is realized by two immune-evading competing phenotypes: a) The recruiter of immunosuppressive T cells (Tregs) and tumor-associated myeloid suppressive cells (TAMSCs); b) the antigen-presentation deficient cell. After the initial immune attack fostered by the ICI+DNMTi combination, the tumor is cycled between the two immune-evasion phenotypes, so that phenotype b prevails in the (ICI+DNMTi)-resistant population when the PI3K(γ,δ)i is administered placing selective pressure on phenotype a, while prevailing phenotype b in the smaller (ICI+DNMTi+PI3K(γ,δ)i)-resistant population is under selection pressure when PI3K(γ,δ)i is switched to PI3Kβi. The alternation between PI3K(γ,δ)i and PI3Kβi funnels the cancer cell population towards extinction. The prevailing phenotype at each stage is indicated. (b) Alternating targeted therapies (PI3K(γ,δ)i, PI3Kβi) within an immune-priming background (ICI+DNMTi) setting an immunogenic trap, so that the cell subpopulation selected by one targeted therapy becomes susceptible to the other. The initial batch contains the evasion phenotypes selected by immune surveillance. During subsequent alternating treatment, immune resistance provides a selective advantage with one therapy but the selective advantage turns into a handicap as the therapy is switched. In this way, the selected cancer phenotype becomes susceptible to drug treatment in the next iteration, and therefore subject to selection pressure. For each iteration that follows after immune priming, the susceptible and resistant subpopulations and their respective fate are indicated.

The choice of evasion-steering agents is justified. Pharmacological inactivation of PI3Kγ reduces integrin-mediated adhesion of myeloid-derived cells and T regs, hampering their infiltration into the TME, while PI3Kδ-inhibition in T regs is known to impair their maintenance and function within the TME [35]. On the other hand, PI3Kβ-inhibition in tumor cell impairs MHC-I mediated antigen presentation while stimulating the innate immune response of natural killers (NK), themselves responsive to cells lacking MHC-I antigen presentation [36].

The centrality of the PI3K-AKT-mTOR pathway in maintaining homeostasis in normal cells makes pan-PI3K inhibitors toxic and therapeutically inefficient, since the tolerable dose is insufficient to fulfill their inhibitory role [37]. Furthermore, nonspecific PI3K inhibition would create counterproductive effects, as PI3Kβ-inhibition suppress the adaptive immune response promoted by PI3K(γ,δ)-inhibition [35]. These opposing effects justify the need to use isoform-specific PI3K inhibitors in the proposed alternating manner.

9.11 AI defines mathematical and preclinical experimental models of cancer evolution to assess the efficacy of the evolutionary immunotherapy

To assess *a-priori* the efficacy of the proposed evolutionary immunotherapy, we need to verify that a route to extinction indeed materializes. Thus, fed by experimental time series data, AI delineates the clonal dynamics of the complementary immune-evasion phenotypes a, b under the selection pressure imposed by the steering immunotherapy. Thus, a deep learning (DL) system gets trained with the time series of P_a = [FOXP3] and P_b = [B2Mmut], respectively the density of immunomodulatory gene FOXP3 expression in tumor peripheral T lymphocytes and density of mutated B2M in tumor cells. Other routes for nonadaptive immune evasion, such as JAK1 impairing mutation discussed previously, should be considered *a priori* but have been shown not to be viable for the system adopted or for the system archetypical of ICI responsiveness [34].

The DL CNN trained with time series reporting the clonal dynamics of immune-evading phenotypes a, b yields the proper mathematical model for steered tumor evolution. The CNN parameter optimization reveals that the clonal dynamics is essentially enslaved or entrained by what is known as a center manifold dynamics [41–43]. Thus, the model stems from a symbolic regression enabled by the scaling symmetry subsumed in the center manifold. The latter is governed by the autocatalytic rate constants for clonal expansion k_a, k_b, the rate constant f_{ab} for the $a \to b$ transition, the time periods $t_{m-1} < t < t_m (m = 1, 2, \ldots)$ for administration of the PI3K(γ,δ)-inhibitor labeled n = n(m) = 1 or the PI3Kβ-inhibitor (n = n(m) = 2), and the phenotype-suppression coefficients $g_{i,n}$ quantifying the impact of the n = 1, 2 targeted sub therapies on phenotypes a, b. Subsuming the center manifold $P_a - P_b$-dynamics, there is an extended dynamical system that includes the proportion of unselected tumor cells, whose fate is adaptation or death induced by the adaptive immune response. As selection becomes operative, the extended dynamics becomes entrained by the $P_a - P_b$-dynamics over long ($\sim k_a^{-1}, k_b^{-1}$) timescales. Thus, the steered clonal evolution, a projection of the extended dynamics, is described by a matrix system of ordinary differential equations:

$$\dot{\boldsymbol{P}} = \begin{pmatrix} \dot{P}_a \\ \dot{P}_b \end{pmatrix} = \underline{\boldsymbol{A}} \begin{pmatrix} P_a \\ P_b \end{pmatrix}$$

$$\underline{\boldsymbol{A}} = \begin{pmatrix} k_a - f_{ab} - \left\{ \sum\limits_{m=1}^{\infty} g_{a,n(m)} G_m(t) \right\} & 0 \\ f_{ab} & k_b - \left\{ \sum\limits_{m=1}^{\infty} g_{b,n(m)} G_m(t) \right\} \end{pmatrix}$$

Where $G_m(t) = H(t - t_{m-1}) - H(t - t_m)$, with $H(t') = 0$ *if* $t' \leq 0$, $H(t') = 1$ *if* $t' > 0$; $n(m) = 1$ *when m is odd m*; $n(m) = 2$ *when m is even*; $g_{a,1} > 0$; $g_{a,2} = g_{b,1} = 0$; $g_{b,2} > 0$; $f_{ab} > 0$ while $f_{ba} = 0$ ($a \to b$ transition is irreversible). The switching between the two targeted subtherapies $n = n(m) = 1, 2$ with no cross-reactivity ($g_{a,2} = g_{b,1} = 0$) is captured by the terms $\sum_{m=1}^{\infty} g_{a,n(m)} G_m(t)$, $\sum_{m=1}^{\infty} g_{b,n(m)} G_m(t)$ defined by the plateau functions $G_m(t) = 1$ if $t \in (t_{m-1}, t_m)$, $G_m(t) = 0$ otherwise. The constraints on the parameters to warrant tumor extinction follow from the eigenvalue analysis of matrix $\underline{\boldsymbol{A}}$:

$$\lambda_a = k_a - f_{ab} - g_{a,1} < 0 \quad for\, t_{m-1} < t < t_m, m\ odd$$

$$\lambda_b = k_b - g_{b,2} < 0 \quad for\, t_{m-1} < t < t_m, m\ even$$

yielding inequalities $g_{a,1} > (k_a - f_{ab})$, $g_{b,2} > k_b$.

To ensure net depletion of both phenotypes, we need the more stringent conditions:

$$-(k_a - f_{ab} - g_{a,1}) > k_a - f_{ab} \text{ or } g_{a,1} > 2(k_a - f_{ab}) \quad \text{and}$$

$$-(k_b - g_{b,2}) > k_b \text{ or } g_{b,2} > 2k_b$$

A humanized mouse model with patient-derived tumor engraftment [38–40] was also developed to enable testing of the therapeutic steering of immune evasion described by the clonal dynamics. The compatibility between tumor and stroma and the preservation of essential human components of adaptive and innate immune response provide an ideal setting to validate the proposed evolutionary immunotherapy. In this preclinical context, a set of parameters fulfilling the relations derived has been numerically and experimentally verified to drive the tumor to extinction.

The system of ODEs defined by matrix $\underline{\boldsymbol{A}}$ entrains or subordinates the clonal dynamics after the selection pressure imposed by therapy-induced immune surveillance sets in, causing depletion of unselected (nonadapted) cancer cells. The $P_a - P_b$-dynamics are actually subsumed into an extended dynamical system including the additional variable P_q that measures the proportion of unselected cancer cells. The extended dynamics are given by

$$\dot{\boldsymbol{P}} = \begin{pmatrix} \dot{P}_q \\ \dot{P}_a \\ \dot{P}_b \end{pmatrix} = \underline{\boldsymbol{E}} \begin{pmatrix} P_q \\ P_a \\ P_b \end{pmatrix}$$

$$\underline{\boldsymbol{E}} = \begin{pmatrix} k_q - f_{qa} - f_{qb} - g_q & 0 & 0 \\ f_{qa} & k_a - f_{ab} - \left\{ \sum_{m=1}^{\infty} g_{a,n(m)} G_m(t) \right\} & 0 \\ f_{qb} & f_{ab} & k_b - \left\{ \sum_{m=1}^{\infty} g_{b,n(m)} G_m(t) \right\} \end{pmatrix}$$

Where $\sigma(\underline{\boldsymbol{A}}) \subset \sigma(\underline{\boldsymbol{E}})$ ($\sigma \equiv$ *spectrum*), and the parameters k_q, f_{qa}, f_{qb}, g_q represent respectively growth rate constant, rate coefficient for conversion into adapted phenotype a, conversion into adapted phenotype b, and rate constant for destruction due to adaptive immune attack. Thus, as selection pressure due to immunotherapy (ICI + epidrug treatment) becomes operative, the clonal dynamics are enslaved by the center manifold dynamics [41–43], i. e., the $P_a - P_b$-dynamics that entrains the whole dynamical system on larger ($\sim k_a^{-1}, k_b^{-1}$) timescales.

This center manifold reduction discovered by the CNN works because the evolutionary adaptation that arises as therapy selects for resistance implies a significant separation of timescales between nonadapted and adapted cell net depletion resulting from marked differences in susceptibility to immune attack. This timescale separation is reflected in the eigenvalue relations:

$$|\lambda_q|^{-1} = |k_q - f_{qa} - f_{qb} - g_q|^{-1} \ll |\lambda_a|^{-1}, |\lambda_b|^{-1}$$

Thus, in the generic time interval $t_{m-1} < t < t_m$, with $t_{m-1} \gg |\lambda_q|^{-1}$ the center-manifold reduced dynamics representing clonal evolution is described by the solution to the differential equation system

$$\begin{pmatrix} \dot{P}_a \\ \dot{P}_b \end{pmatrix} = \underline{\boldsymbol{A}} \begin{pmatrix} P_a \\ P_b \end{pmatrix}$$

given by

$$\begin{pmatrix} P_a \\ P_b \end{pmatrix} = c_{am} e^{\lambda_{am} t} \begin{pmatrix} \frac{(\lambda_{am} - \lambda_{bm})}{f_{ab}} P_b(t_{m-1}) \\ P_b(t_{m-1}) \end{pmatrix} + c_{bm} e^{\lambda_{bm} t} \begin{pmatrix} 0 \\ P_b(t_{m-1}) \end{pmatrix}$$

Where $\lambda_{am}, \lambda_{bm}$ are the eigenvalues of matrix $\underline{\boldsymbol{A}}$ for the time interval $t_{m-1} < t < t_m$, and $c_{am}\, c_{bm}$ are m-dependent coefficients defined by initial conditions.

The adopted humanized murine model (Fig. 9.8) supports the therapeutically steered clonal dynamics (Fig. 9.9). As discussed, the efficacy of checkpoint blockade (α-PD-1 antibody) requires a level of immune stimulation furnished by high mutational load. The epidrug treatment on the murine model is plagued with uncertainty and thus we induced immune stimulation through a PI3Kα inhibitor known to cause a DNA mismatch repair (MMR) deficiency resulting in a level of hypermutability akin to the Lynch syndrome [40]. The evolution substrate created by PI3Kα inhibition and the therapeutically steered evolutionary trajectory emerging thereof are illustrated in Figs. 9.8, 9.9 where a competition becomes apparent between impairment of HLA class-I-mediated antigen presentation and expression of immunomodulatory gene FOXP3, a hallmark of the effector-to-regulatory T cell transformation. Other routes of evasion based on JAK1-impairment are not viable. Thus, upon PI3Kα-inhibition, there is enough mutational diversity to get significant impairment of

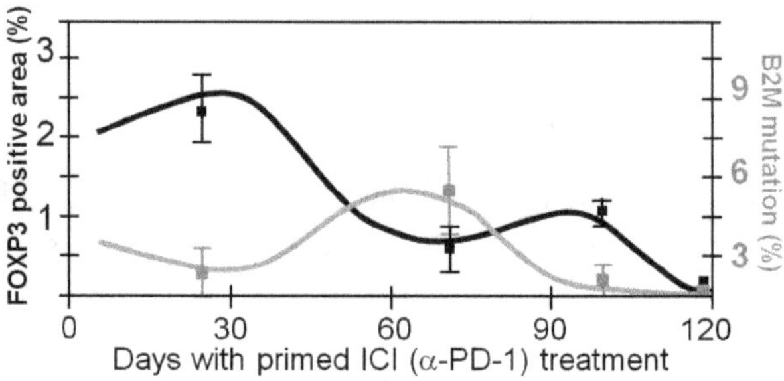

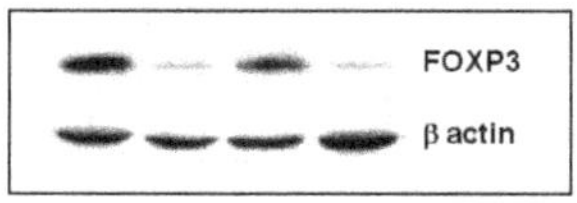

Figure 9.8. Agreement of mathematical and experimental models of clonal dynamics for steering immunotherapy. Parametrization: $t_m - t_{m-1} = 30\,days$ for all m; $k_a = 1.0 \times 10^{-3}h^{-1}$; $f_{ab} = 3 \times 10^{-4}h^{-1}$; $g_{a,1} = 1.7 \times 10^{-3}h^{-1}$; $k_b = 2.5 \times 10^{-3}h^{-1}$; $g_{b,2} = 5.5 \times 10^{-3}h^{-1}$ The parametrization was obtained using a CNN that performed a least-squares (Euclidean distance) curve fitting of the experimental datapoints to the center-manifold solution [41–44]. The parametrization for the center-manifold dynamics is indicated above, while the fast relaxation mode parameters obtained from the least-squares curve fitting are $k_q = 1.4 \times 10^{-2}h^{-1}$, $f_{qa} = 2.0 \times 10^{-3}h^{-1}$, $f_{qb} = 3.6 \times 10^{-3}h^{-1}$, $g_q = 1.2 \times 10^{-2}h^{-1}$. The steering into a lethal immunogenic trap is evident by examining the clonal evolution of the immune-evading phenotypes. The results are validated experimentally (R^2 =0.83) on four cohorts of Hu-CD34 NSG humanized immunocompetent mice engrafted with a patient-derived xenograft (PDX, JAX) TM00091 of breast invasive ductal carcinome. Error bars represent dispersion over five specimens collected at the four selected points during treatment. Western Blots for FOXP3 expression in TILs, the biomarker of adaptive immune evasion, are shown for four specimens (black square datapoints) harvested at the selected points during treatment. The assessment of B2M mutation and JAK1-impairing mutation (negative) were performed. Experimental data were obtained from a humanized preclinical model. Four cohorts of five Hu-CD34 NSG (JAX) immunocompetent mice, humanized through myeloablation followed by inoculation of human CD34+ hematopoietic stem cells, are engrafted at week 12 with patient-derived xenograft (PDX, JAX) TM00091 (breast invasive ductal carcinome). Tumor and stromal cells are compatible, enabling evaluation of immunomodulatory anti-cancer agents. Three weeks after engraftment, survival therapy began with daily dose of 50mg/mouse of PI3K(α) inhibitor *alpelisib*. Through nucleoside depletion, this targeted kinase inhibitor induces DNA mistmatched repair deficiency [45, 46] mimicking Lynch-syndrome immunogenic conditions, thereby promoting susceptibility to ICI[40]. Beginning five weeks after engraftment, mice were also injected on alternate days with 200 mg/mouse of α-PD-1 antibody. Thirty days after initiation of treatment with the combination

HLA class-I-mediated antigen presentation but the impairment does not correlate with suppression of FOXP3 expression, an expected result since there is no selection pressure introduced as yet. After combining the PI3Kα-inhibitor with the α-PD-1 antibody, selection pressure due to immune surveillance is imposed and tumor cells capable of antigen presentation are forced to promote expression of FOXP3 in T cells in order to avoid immune surveillance. The MMR deficiency that stimulates the adaptive immune system also enables the onset of the immune-evading phenotype arising from natural selection. Once the tumor host is treated with the combined PI3Kα and PI3K(γ, δ)-inhibitors, the possibility of recruiting immunomodulatory adaptive components gets suppressed and the alternative to evade immunosurveillance becomes impairment of antigen presentation. This immune-evading phenotype becomes susceptible to destruction by NK-mediated cytolysis upon switching to the PI3Kβ-inhibitor [35, 36]. Fig. 9.8 reports the effect on cancer evolution of the alternation every 30 days between PI3K(γ, δ) and PI3Kβ inhibitors upon the immune-primed surveillance generated by the combination α-PD-1 antibody + PI3Kα-inhibitor. Thus, the

---

Figure 9.8. (*Continued*) α-PD-1 antibody + PI3Kα-inhibitor, alpelisib is supplemented with PI3K(γ, δ) inhibitor *duvelisib* at identical dose and 30 days later duvelisib is replaced with PI3Kβ-inhibitor AZD8186 at identical dose. An inhibitor switch is repeated every thirty days as specified in the dynamic model outlined previously. On days 25, 70, 100 and 120 after initiation of treatment with the α-PD-1 antibody + PI3Kα-inhibitor combination, tumor specimens in each cohort were subject to debulking surgery. Sets of 5 specimens were obtained from each of the four cohorts. Resection of a region of 1mm^2 of tumor-adjacent tissue was performed on each specimen and subject to immunohistochemical staining and quantification of T cell infiltration, utilizing the anti-beta-2 microglobulin antibody [4H5L5], ABfinity^{TM} Rabbit Monoclonal (Invitrogen, Cat.: 701250) and anti-FOXP3 antibody [5H10L18], ABfinity^{TM} Rabbit Monoclonal (Invitrogen, Cat.: 700914). The nuclear FOXP3-positive areas were counted when correlated with CD3-positive TIL surfaces, as marked by mouse anti-CD3 monoclonal antibody AM12005PU-N (Acris-ORIGENE). In this setting, no adaptive immune evasion via JAK1-impairing mutation has been detected using anti-JAK1 monoclonal antibody [413104] CBMAB 0200-WJ (Creation Biolabs).

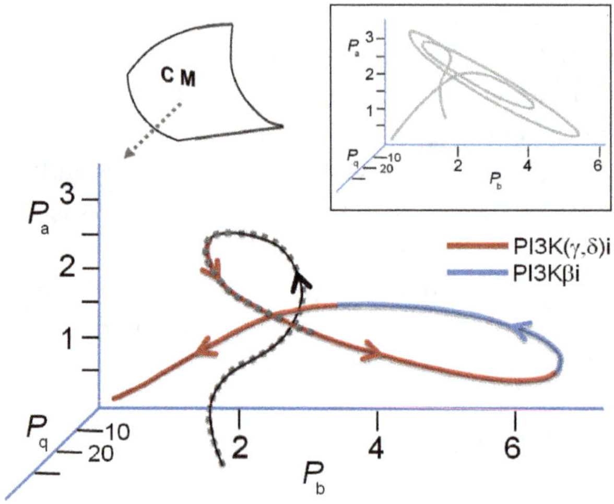

Figure 9.9. *Extended dynamics of clonal evolution under the steering immunotherapy.* The dashed line represents the portion of the trajectory prior to entrainment by the therapeutically induced selection process that steers the dynamics into the center manifold (CM). The projection onto the CM region is the trajectory shown in Fig. 9.8. This projection constitutes a good representation of the dynamics at long timescales, as described. For comparison, the inset illustrates the clonal dynamics under a suboptimal parametrization (R^2 =0.55) that does not fulfill $g_{a,1} > 2(k_a - f_{ab})$ and $g_{b,2} > 2k_b$.

preclinical experimental results (Figs. 9.8, 9.10–9.13) validate the clonal evolutionary model shown in Fig. 9.9.

9.12 AI delineates the principle of lethal immune complementarity as a paradigm to achieve lasting cancer cure

The emergence of resistance represents a major setback in the development of cancer therapies. Most cancers have an evolutionary substrate and the adapted phenotypes arising clearly suggest that evolution selects for resistance. Proposing and developing a strategy to overcome resistance is precisely the overarching goal of this chapter. The implemented hybrid immunotherapy exploits ICIs in a priming context, the most promising treatment to-date, and deals effectively with resistant phenotypes arising from immunoediting by

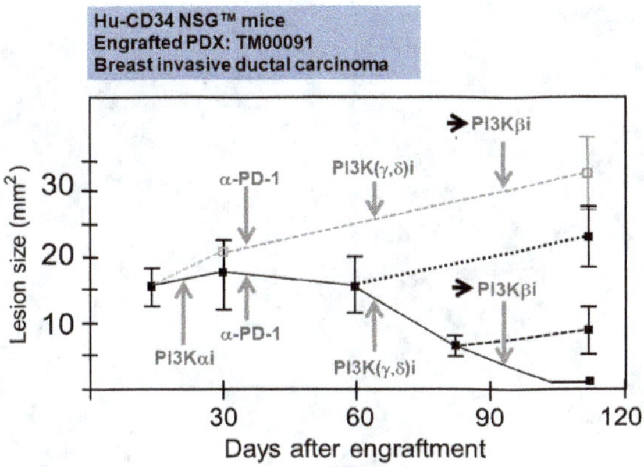

Figure 9.10. Lesion size at different stages of therapeutic treatment contrasted against different control runs. The points of inoculation of isoform-specific PI3K inhibitors and anti-PD-1 antibody are marked by grey arrows (missing arrow indicates no inoculation). The lack of mutational load translated into insufficient immunogenicity, rendering the α-PD-1 antibody ineffective (control in grey hyphen). Horizontal dark arrows indicate inhibitor switching, as per text. No inhibitor switching results in relapse (control in dark dashed line).

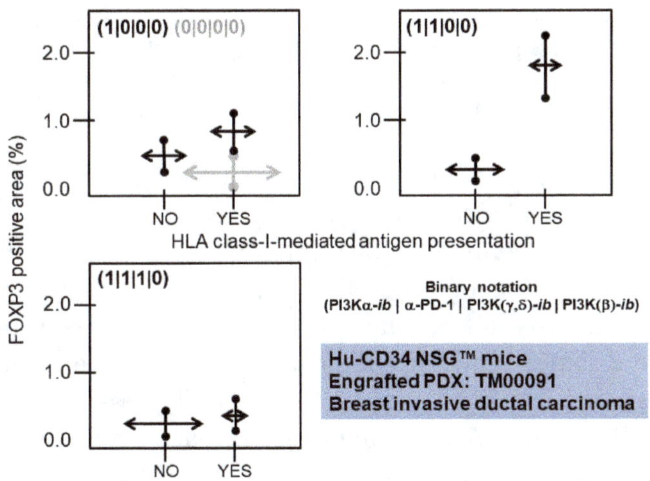

Figure 9.11. Expression levels for immunomodulatory gene FOXP3 in T lymphocytes plotted against impairment or enablement of HLA class-I-mediated antigen presentation at different stages of therapy. The dumbbell error bars represent dispersion in FOXP3 expression level, while the double-arrow error bars indicate % impairment or enablement of antigen presentation. A binary vector notation is adopted as indicated in the figure to represent different stages of treatment.

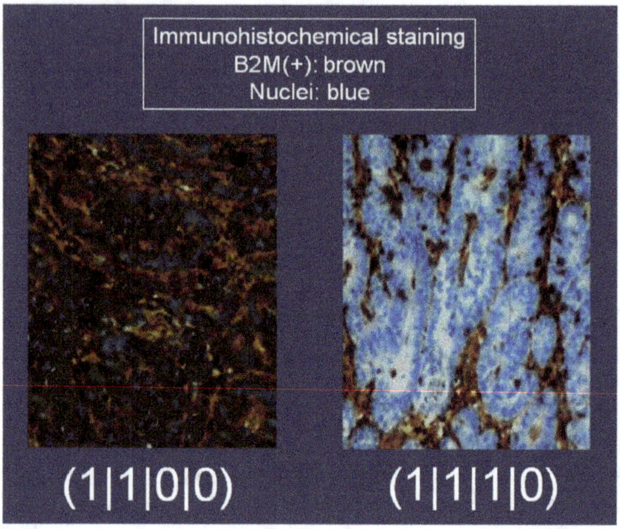

Figure 9.12. B2M expression levels on cancer cells, TILs and stroma before and after treatment with PI3K(γ,δ) inhibitor *duvelisib,* 25 and 70 days after initiation of primed ICI treatment. At stage (1|1|0|0), B2M expression is ubiquitous in cancer cells, TILs and stroma, while at stage (1|1|1|0), B2M has been substantially wiped out from cancer cells, remaining only in TILs and stroma. Cell nuclei have been counterstained with NucBlue^{TM}, Live Ready Probe Reagent (ThermoFisher, Cat. 37605).

avoiding to maintain a single pattern of selection pressure imposed by immune surveillance. Instead, it steers the tumor back and forth through two complementary immune-evasion phenotypes with progressive shrinking of the selected population, so that the cell subpopulation resistant to one therapy becomes susceptible to the other. The resistance phenotype provides a selective advantage with one therapy but becomes subject to selection pressure as therapies are switched (Figure 9.7(b)). We name this paradigm Lethal Immune Complementarity (LIC).

Clinical experience shows that the evading phenotype resulting from treatment cannot be fully anticipated or eliminated when a single source of selection pressure is maintained. To avoid resistance, therapy must be choreographed to steer cancer evolution and LIC may well be the underlying paradigm.

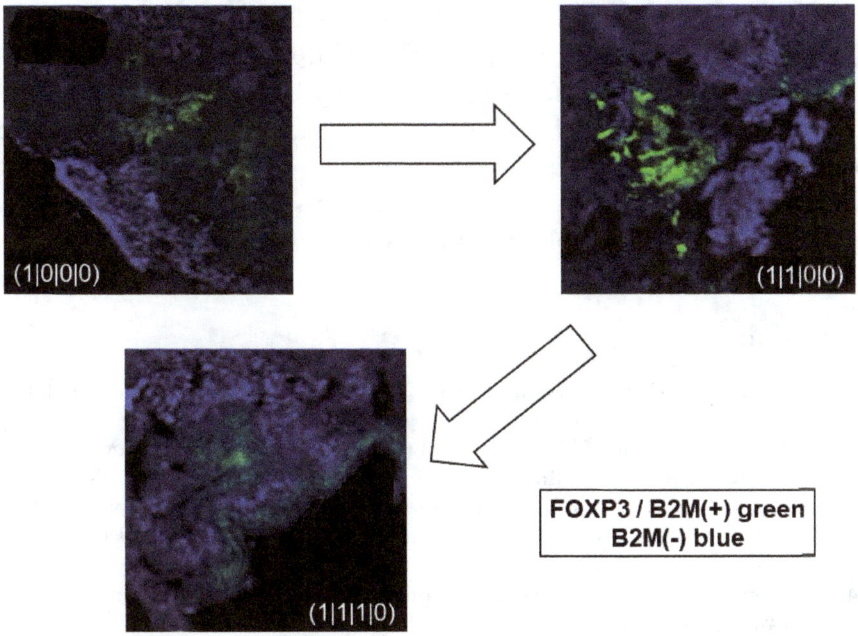

Figure 9.13. Immunohistochemical staining at different stages of treatment (*ut supra*). Specimens were obtained as specified in text.

The key contention in this chapter that it is possible to overcome resistance to ICI-based immunotherapy by a second-stage drug-based steering of tumor evolution into an immunogenic trap. The hybrid therapy developed unleashes the adaptive immune response and subsequently chases the evading phenotype into an immunogenic trap wherein the tumor is driven to extinction. This trap involves steering the tumor into an alternation between the adaptive and nonadaptive routes of immune evasion through the periodic switching of two isoform-specific PI3K inhibitors. The competing/complementary routes of evasion have been identified by examining through AI the evolutionary substrate of a representative cancer for ICI responsiveness.

Clinical development reliant on properly identified endpoints and proper scheduling of drug inoculation upon the immune-priming substrate will then become an essential future direction.

New areas of research will likely emerge, focusing on the immunologic counterpart of synthetic lethality and collateral sensitivity. In this chapter we have demonstrated that, with the aid of AI, it is possible to steer cancer evolution in the context of immunoediting. Our results presented will surely invite innovative ways of implementing lethal complementarities in a manner akin to collateral sensitivity with the ultimate goal of achieving lasting cancer cure.

References

1. Johnson DB, Peng C, Sosman JA (2015) Nivolumab in melanoma: latest evidence and clinical potential. *Ther Adv Med Oncol* 7:97–106.
2. Redman JM, Gibney GT, Atkins MB (2016) Advances in immunotherapy for melanoma. *BMC Med* 14:20.
3. Druker BJ, Lydon NB (2000) Lessons learned from the development of an Abl tyrosine kinase inhibitor for chronic myelogenous leukemia. *J Clin Invest* 105:3–7.
4. Vanneman M, Dranoff G (2012) Combining immunotherapy and targeted therapies in cancer treatment. *Nature Rev Cancer* 12:237–251.
5. Hughes PE, Caenepeel S, Wu LC (2016) Targeted Therapy and Checkpoint Immunotherapy Combinations for the Treatment of Cancer. *Trends Immunol* 37:462–476.
6. Marabelle A, Caux C (2012) Combined targeted and immunotherapy: the future of personalized medicine. *Blood* 120:4454–4455.
7. Fernández A, Scott LR (2017) Advanced Modeling Reconciles Counterintuitive Decisions in Lead Optimization. *Trends Biotech* 35:490–497.
8. Gaillard SL, Secord AA, Monk B (2016) The role of immune checkpoint inhibition in the treatment of ovarian cancer. *Gyn Oncol Res Pract* 3:11.
9. Fernández A, Sanguino A, Peng Z, Crespo A, Ozturk E, Zhang X, Wang S, Bornmann W, Lopez-Berestein G (2007) Priority Report: Rational Drug Redesign to overcome drug resistance in cancer therapy: Imatinib moving target. *Cancer Research* 67:4028–4033.
10. Ferrarelli LK (2016) Tackling kinase inhibitor resistance. *Science Signal* 9:ec97.
11. Balachandran VP, Cavnar MJ, Zeng S, Bamboat ZM, Ocuin LM, Obaid H, Sorenson EC, Popow R, Ariyan C, Rossi F, Besmer P, Guo T, Antonescu CR, Taguchi T, Yuan J, Wolchok JD, Allison JP, DeMatteo RP (2011) Imatinib potentiates antitumor T cell responses in gastrointestinal stromal tumor through the inhibition of Ido. *Nature Med* 17:1094–1100.
12. Fernández Stigliano A (2015) Biomolecular Interfaces, Springer, Berlin.
13. Fernández A (2016) Physics at the Biomolecular Interface, Springer, Berlin.
14. Haltia UM, Andersson N, Yadav B, Färkkilä A, Kulesskiy E, Kankainen M, Tang J, Bützow R, Riska A, Leminen A, Heikinheimo M, Kallioniemi O,

Unkila-Kallio L, Wennerberg K, Aittokallio T, Anttonen M (2017) Systematic drug sensitivity testing reveals synergistic growth inhibition by dasatinib or mTOR inhibitors with paclitaxel in ovarian granulosa cell tumor cells. *Gynecol Oncol* 144:621–630.

15. Schittenhelm MM, Shiraga S, Schroeder A, Corbin AS, Griffith D, Lee FY, Bokemeyer C, Deininger MW, Druker BJ, Heinrich MC (2006) Dasatinib (BMS-354825), a dual SRC/ABL kinase inhibitor, inhibits the kinase activity of wild-type, juxtamembrane, and activation loop mutant KIT isoforms associated with human malignancies. *Cancer Res* 66:473–481.
16. Vivas-Mejia P, Benito JM, Fernandez A, Han HD, Mangala L, Rodriguez-Aguayo C, Chavez-Reyes A, Lin YG, Carey MS, Nick AM, Stone RL, Kim HS, Claret FX, Bornmann W, Hennessy BT, Sanguino A, Peng Z, Sood AK, Lopez-Berestein G (2010) c-Jun-NH2-kinase-1 inhibition leads to antitumor activity in ovarian cancer. *Clin Cancer Res* 16:184–194.
17. Obut F, Randall N, Young JA, Valent P, Ustun C (2015) Dasatinib-induced immunosuppression and recurrent respiratory tract infections. *Leuk Lymphoma* 56:2484–2485.
18. Le DT, Uram JN, Wang H, Bartlett BR, Kemberling H, Eyring AD, Skora AD, Luber BS, Azad NS, Laheru D, Biedrzycki B, Donehower RC, Zaheer A, Fisher GA, Crocenzi TS, Lee JJ, Duffy SM, Goldberg RM, de la Chapelle A, Koshiji M, Bhaijee F, Huebner T, Hruban RH, Wood LD, Cuka N, Pardoll DM, Papadopoulos N, Kinzler KW, Zhou S, Cornish TC, Taube JM, Anders RA, Eshleman JR, Vogelstein B, Diaz LA (2015) PD-1 Blockade in Tumors with Mismatch-Repair Deficiency. *N Engl J Med* 372:2509–20.
19. Le DT, Durham JN, Smith KN, Wang H, Bartlett BR, Aulakh LK, Lu S, Kemberling H, Wilt C, Luber BS, Wong F, Azad NS, Rucki AA, Laheru D, Donehower R, Zaheer A, Fisher GA, Crocenzi TS, Lee JJ, Greten TF, Duffy AG, Ciombor KK, Eyring AD, Lam BH, Joe A, Kang SP, Holdhoff M, Danilova L, Cope L, Meyer C, Zhou S, Goldberg RM, Armstrong DK, Bever KM, Fader AN, Taube J, Housseau F, Spetzler D, Xiao N, Pardoll DM, Papadopoulos N, Kinzler KW, Eshleman JR, Vogelstein B, Anders RA, Diaz LA (2017) Mismatch-repair deficiency predicts response of solid tumors to PD-1 blockade. *Science* 357:409–413.
20. Juvekar A, Hu H, Yadegarynia S, Lyssiotis CA, Ullas S, Lien EC, Bellinger G, Son J, Hok RC, Seth P, Daly MB, Kim B, Scully R, Asara JM, Cantley LC, Wulf GM (2016) Phosphoinositide 3-kinase inhibitors induce DNA damage through nucleoside depletion. *Proc Natl Acad Sci U S A* 113:4338–4447.
21. Andor N, Maley CC, Ji HP (2017) Genomic Instability in Cancer: Teetering on the Limit of Tolerance. *Cancer Res* 77:2179–2185.
22. Dhawan A, Nichol D, Kinose F, Abazeed ME, Marusyk A, Haura EB, Scott JG (2017) Collateral sensitivity networks reveal evolutionary instability and novel treatment strategies in ALK mutated non-small cell lung cancer. *Scientific Reports* 7:1232.

23. Le DT, Uram JN, Wang H, Bartlett BR, Kemberling H, *et al.* (2015) PD-1 Blockade in Tumors with Mismatch-Repair Deficiency. *N Engl J Med* 372:2509–20.
24. Zaretsky JM, Garcia-Diaz A, Shin DS *et al.* (2016) Mutations associated with acquired resistance to PD-1 blockade in melanoma. *N Engl J Med* 375:819–829.
25. Chiappinelli KB, Zahnow CA, Ahuja N, Baylin SB (2016) Combining Epigenetic and Immune Therapy to Combat Cancer. *Cancer Res* 76:1683–1689.
26. Hellmann M (2017) Pembrolizumab (Immunotherapy Drug) in Combination With Guadecitabine and Mocetinostat (Epigenetic Drugs) for Patients With Advanced Lung Cancer. MDClinicalTrials.gov Identifier: NCT03220477.
27. Woods DM, Sodré AL, Villagra A *et al.* (2015) HDAC Inhibition Upregulates PD-1 Ligands in Melanoma and Augments Immunotherapy with PD-1 Blockade. *Cancer Immunol Res* 3:1375–1385.
28. Sheaffer KL, Elliott EN, Kaestner KH (2016) DNA Hypomethylation Contributes to Genomic Instability and Intestinal Cancer Initiation. *Cancer Prev Res (Phila)* 9:534–546.
29. Lee JH, Choy ML, Ngo L, Foster SS, Marksa PA (2010) Histone deacetylase inhibitor induces DNA damage, which normal but not transformed cells can repair. *Proc Natl Acad Sci USA* 107:14639–14644.
30. Jin B, Robertson KD (2013) DNA Methyltransferases (DNMTs), DNA Damage Repair, and Cancer. *Adv Exp Med Biol* 754:3–29.
31. Chiappinelli KB, Strissel PL, Desrichard A *et al.* (2015) Inhibiting DNA Methylation Causes an Interferon Response in Cancer via dsRNA Including Endogenous Retroviruses. *Cell* 162:974–986.
32. Chaudhary B, Elkord E (2016) Regulatory T Cells in the Tumor Microenvironment and Cancer Progression: Role and Therapeutic Targeting. *Vaccines (Basel)* 4:28.
33. Katoh H, Watanabe M (2015) Myeloid-Derived Suppressor Cells and Therapeutic Strategies in Cancer. *Mediators Inflamm* 2015:159269.
34. Echterdiek F, Janikovits J, Staffa L *et al.* (2016) Low density of FOXP3-positive T cells in normal colonic mucosa is related to the presence of beta2-microglobulin mutations in Lynch syndrome-associated colorectal cancer. *Oncoimmunol* 5:e1075692.
35. Pons-Tostivint E, Thibault B, Guillermet-Guibert J (2017) Targeting PI3K Signaling in Combination Cancer Therapy. *Trends Cancer* 3:454–469.
36. Bommarito D, Martin A, Forcade E *et al.* (2016) Enhancement of tumor cell susceptibility to natural killer cell activity through inhibition of the PI3K signaling pathway. *Cancer Immunol Immunother* 65:355–366.
37. O' Donnell JS, Massi D, Teng MW, Mandala M (2018) PI3K-AKT-mTOR inhibition in cancer immunotherapy, redux. *Sem Cancer Biol* 48:91–103.
38. Wang M, Yao LC, Cheng M *et al.* (2018) Humanized mice in studying efficacy and mechanisms of PD-1-targeted cancer immunotherapy. *FASEB J* 32:1537–1549.

39. Rongvaux A, Willinger T, Martinek J *et al.* (2014) Development and function of human innate immune cells in a humanized mouse model. *Nature Biotech* 32:364–372.
40. Fernández A (2017) Engineering tumor hypersusceptibility to immunotherapy. *Trends Cancer* 3:675–677.
41. Fernández A (1985) Center Manifold Extension of the Adiabatic Elimination Method. *Physical Review A* 32:3070–3075.
42. Fernández A (1986) The Steady State Approximation as a Center Manifold Elimination in Chemical Kinetics. *J Chem Soc Faraday Transactions II* 82:849–855.
43. Fernández A (1987) Letter: Intrinsic Fluctuations associated with the Onset of a Center Manifold. *Journal of Physics A* 20:L579–L583.
44. Björck A (1996) Numerical methods for least squares problems. SIAM, Philadelphia.
45. Juvekar A, Hu H, Yadegarynia S, *et al.* (2016) Phosphoinositide 3-kinase inhibitors induce DNA damage through nucleoside depletion. *Proc Natl Acad Sci USA* 113:E4338–4347.
46. Michel S, Benner A, Tariverdian M, *et al.* (2008) High density of FOXP3-positive T cells infiltrating colorectal cancers with microsatellite instability. *Br J Cancer* 99:1867–1873.

Resources

(a) FDA Report: nivolumab/Opdivo® Highlights of prescribing information (revised 11/2015) url: http://www.accessdata.fda.gov/drugsatfda_docs/label/2015/125554s012lbl.pdf

(b) FDA Report: pembrolizumab/Keytruda® Highlights of prescribing information (revised 10/2016) url: http://www.accessdata.fda.gov/drugsatfda_docs/label/2016/125514s012lbl.pdf

(c) Harvard Medical School - Library of Integrated Network-based Cellular Signatures (HMS-LINCS) Kinome Scan Data/Last Update: September 15, 2016. url: http://lincs.hms.harvard.edu/kinomescan/

(d) Signaling network for activation and downregulation of antigen-triggered T-cell activation. Kyoto Encyclopedia of Genes and Genomes, T-cell receptor signaling pathway - Homo sapiens. url: http://www.genome.jp/kegg-bin/show_pathway?hsadd04660

Chapter 10

AI-empowered molecular dynamics

Molecular dynamics (MD) remains the most valuable tool for the predictive understanding of the behavior of biological mater at the atomistic level. However, its true potential remains largely untested because relevant timescales are often beyond reach, limited portions of conformation space can get sampled, and infrequent events of direct relevance to biophysical processes are missed. A culprit for these shortcomings is the huge informational burden that is required to iterate the integration steps in order to generate an MD trajectory. To address the problem, we apply deep learning to a) encode the dynamics into a simplified embodiment that retains only essential topological features of the vector field that steers MD integration, and b) to propagate the simplified trajectory beyond the timescales accessible to atomistic MD. We simplify the flow via an equivalence relation that identifies conformations within basins of attraction in potential energy and encodes the dynamics onto a modulo-basin "quotient space" where fast motions are averaged out. Encoding MD-generated information in quotient space enables coverage of physically meaningful timescales while unraveling the underlying dynamic hierarchy. Deep learning is exploited to propagate the coarse grained state and to reconstruct it back at the atomistic level at a later time. As shown, the quotient-encoding-propagating-decoding scheme generates within few GPU hours protein folding pathways with experimentally verified outcomes. By contrast, MD computations covering comparable timespans would take hundreds of days on today's fastest special-purpose supercomputers. Thus, quotient space constitutes a generative model that provides hierarchical understanding of MD simulation while enabling access to realistic timescales and the capture of physically meaningful rare events.

10.1 A deep learning platform to hierarchical extract dynamic features in the protein folding processes

This chapter places additional demands on behalf of the reader, as it requires a certain level of familiarity with abstract mathematical thinking. The goal here is to empower molecular dynamics (MD) by placing it within an AI platform to enable the investigation of physically relevant phenomena. This empowerment requires that we introduce a simplified version of conformation space, an adiabatic version of the space, where fast motions are hierarchically averaged out within a mathematical construct named *quotient space*. The mathematical process needed to simplify the informational universe is akin to an adiabatic approximation that casts the vector field that steers MD integration as a topological simplification. Thus, the quotient space retains only the topological determinants of the flow that become operative at relevant (long) timescales. The canonical projection of the MD trajectory in quotient space may be digitally represented in a spatial tensor-like array, hence it can be subsumed into TensorFlow, the underlying operational scheme for deep learning platforms (cf. Chapter 1). This adiabatic version of the trajectory living in quotient space may be readily propagated with enough training of the underlying neural network. In this way, the mathematical procedure of transference to quotient space places within reach the physically relevant timescales that would be otherwise inaccessible to MD computations.

Molecular dynamics (MD) computation has been widely adopted as a primary method to obtain an atomistic understanding of observable kinetics, thermodynamic properties and for inferring singular events in biological matter [1–3]. Yet, its full potential has not been realized and its efficacy remains essentially untested. Several factors contribute to this state of affairs, especially the huge informational burden that needs to be carried over from one move to the next as the equations of motion are stepwise integrated, a process requiring full atomistic description of the starting state at each stage [4–7]. Thus, only a limited sampling of conformation space is feasible, physically relevant timescales are usually beyond reach [4–9] and rare events remain largely undiscovered [4–9]. In addition to these shortcomings, the accurate physical picture of key biomolecular processes such as protein folding or ligand-induced folding gets further befuddled by a morass of seemingly elusive systematic and conceptual errors that get amplified as the MD trajectories are propagated in time.

To overcome such problems, various procedures have been introduced, all geared at promoting the escape from basins of attraction in the potential energy surface, thereby inducing interbasin transitions that presumably improve the efficiency of conformational sampling [4–7, 9–11]. Here we describe a different construct that stems from the inherent topological architecture of the MD-steering vector field, hence expediting exploration of conformation space without resorting to *ad-hoc* assumptions or heuristic topological models whereupon coarse-graining encoders need to be variationally optimized [12]. The simplification introduced requires an equivalence relation "$\sim$", whereby two microstates/conformations are regarded as equivalent if and only if the respective local conformations of the constitutive subunits lie in the same basins of attraction in the local potential energy surface. This "modulo basin" representation constitutes a quotient space made up of equivalence classes [13]. In generic terms, if x_i indicates a microstate of a system of N subunits, the modulo-basin class (state) to which x_i belongs is denoted $\bar{x}_i$ and may be expressed as a Cartesian product of N basins designating the basin occupancies for the individual subunits: $\bar{x}_i = \prod_{n=1}^{N} B(i,n)$ where $B(i,n)$ is the basin of attraction occupied by subunit n when the system is in microstate x_i. Thus, for any two microstates x, y : $x \sim y \Leftrightarrow \bar{x} = \bar{y}$. Since the products of basins $B = \prod_{n=1}^{N} B(n)$ constitute a denumerable set, the classes/states in quotient space may be conveniently designated by encoding vectors or even represented as points on a real line interval, as shown below.

Because the quotient space averages out fast motions (intrabasin equilibrations) respecting the inherent topology of the dynamical system, it represents a generative model providing a hierarchical predictive understanding of MD simulations. Evidence in support of this key point is provided in this work, as protein folding pathways with experimentally verified outcomes are generated using the quotient space construct.

To enhance the focus, from now on we consider protein folding trajectories defined by the evolution of backbone torsional coordinates $\{\phi_n, \psi_n\}_{n=1,\dots N}$ [4–7]. Conformation space Ω thus becomes a 2N-dimensional torus, i.e. the product of 2N unit circles, one of each dihedral coordinate of the protein backbone. In this context, the modulo-basin quotient space, denoted $\Omega/\sim$, is made up of Cartesian products of the so-called Ramachandran basins [13, 14], that is, the allowed low-energy regions in the potential energy surface of each residue along the protein chain of length N (Fig. 10.1). The topology of $\Omega/\sim$ is inherited from that of Ω, in the sense that a subset $Q \subset \Omega/\sim$ is open if and only if $\pi^{-1}Q \equiv \bigcup_{\bar{y}\in Q} \pi^{-1}\bar{y}$ is open in Ω, where $\pi : \Omega \to \Omega/\sim$ is the canonical projection that associates each microstate with its modulo-basin class: $\pi y = \bar{y}$. A state in $\Omega/\sim$ may be labeled with a 4N-vector $(\mathbf{b}_1|\mathbf{b}_2|\cdots|\mathbf{b}_n\cdots)$ consisting of N binary 4-tuples $\mathbf{b}_n$ ($\mathrm{n} = 1, 2, \dots, \mathrm{N}$) indicating the Ramachandran basin occupancy for each residue, so the value 1 at entry m in $\mathbf{b}_\mathrm{n}$ ($\mathrm{b}_\mathrm{nm} = 1$) indicates that residue n occupies basin m ($\mathrm{m} = 1, 2, 3, 4$) (Fig. 10.1). For example, (1000|0001) indicates the state of a dipeptide with first residue in basin 1 and second residue in basin 4. The classes/states in $\Omega/\sim$ constitute a denumerable set ordered by associating the 4N-vector with the rational number $0.\mathrm{b}_{11}\mathrm{b}_{12}\mathrm{b}_{13}\mathrm{b}_{14}\mathrm{b}_{21}\mathrm{b}_{22}\mathrm{b}_{23}\mathrm{b}_{24}\cdots$ in decimal representation, where b_nm is the binary m-th entry for the n-th 4-tuple. By adopting this representation, the states in $\Omega/\sim$ may be plotted on a one-dimensional axis as an ordered set of rational numbers contained in the real line interval $[0.00010001\dots, 0.10001000\dots]$.

Within this mathematical construct, we may project the MD trajectory on the quotient space and then adopt deep learning to propagate the encoded "shorthand" dynamics to simplify computations and make them more agile. The shorthand dynamics carry far

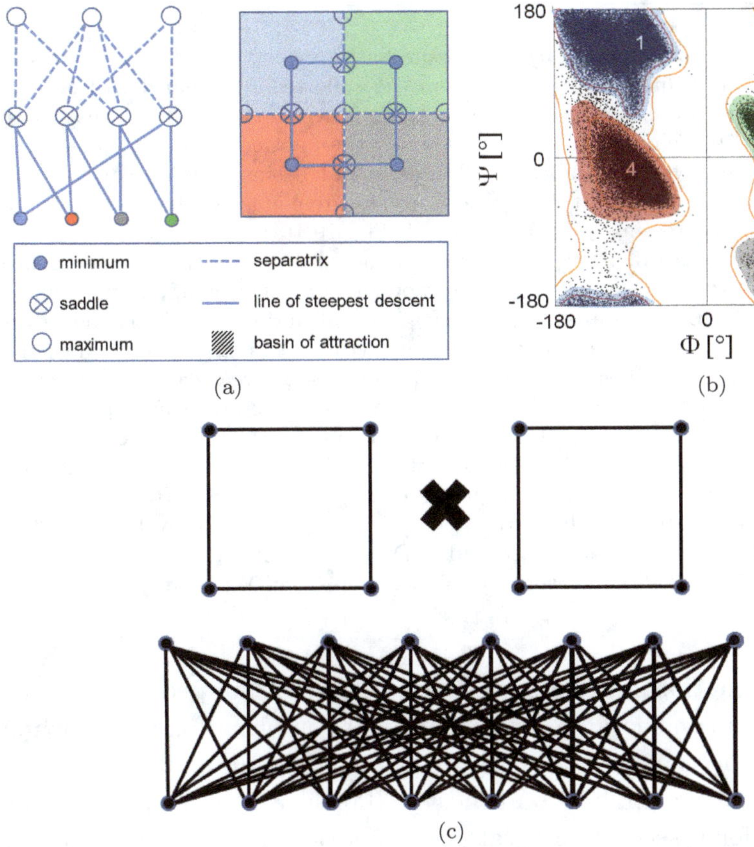

Figure 10.1. Quotient space simplification of the vector field integrated in MD computations. **(a)** Topological representation of the vector field steering the backbone torsional dynamics of a generic residue in the protein chain. Opposite sides of the square are identified as per the $\pm 180^{\circ}$ identification of ϕ, ψ dihedrals determining the local torsional state of the backbone. Thus, the residue conformation space constitutes a 2-torus, i.e. the Cartesian product of two circles. The four colored sectors morph topologically into the allowed valleys in the Ramachandran potential energy plot. Except for glycine (G), the grey sector is energetically inaccessible to other residues due to steric clash with the side chain. Other accessibility restrictions apply to geometrically constrained proline (P) and adjacent residues. The basin topology with its distribution of critical points (minima, saddles, maxima) is compatible with the underlying 2-torus. The graph on the left describes the topological organization of the basins of attraction of the critical points (minima and saddles). The basins of attraction of saddles are 1-dimensional separatrices of the 2-dimensional basins of minima.

Figure 10.1. (*Continued*) **(b)** The actual basin regions 1,2,3,4 and equipotential lines in the Ramachandran plot from the collected torsional data from the MD simulations described in this work. **(c)** Quotient space for two consecutive residues on a protein chain. For each residue, the quotient space is represented by a graph with vertices indicating 2-dimensional basins, and an edge linking two vertices indicates that the respective basins are connected through a line of steepest descent crossing a saddle point (cf. Fig. 10.1(a)) and orthogonal to the separatrix at the saddle. For two residues, denoted 1 and 2, the quotient space graph is a tensor product where vertices now denote basin pairs (B_1, B_2) where basin pair (B_1, B_2) is connected with (B'_1, B'_2) if and only if B_1 is connected with B'_1 or $B_1 = B'_1$, and B_2 is connected with B'_2 or $B_2 = B'_2$. Thus, the quotient space for two residues consists of 16 vertices, where each vertex connects via one edge with 8 other vertices and connects via two adjacent edges to the 7 remaining vertices. The quotient space for two consecutive residues is shown at the bottom. An MD trajectory projected onto the quotient space becomes a walk on the graph, that is, a sequence of adjacent vertices. Reprinted from [Fernández A (2020) Rapid Research Letter: Deep Learning Unravels a Dynamic Hierarchy While Empowering Molecular Dynamics Simulations. Annalen der Physik (Berlin) 532:1900526] with permission from John Wiley and Sons.

lower information burden as conformations are lumped into classes that entail a considerable simplification of conformation space, while the transition timescale for each iteration is the minimal Ramachandran intrabasin equilibration time $\tau = 100$ps [13], considerably larger than the femtosecond integration timescales used in MD. Hence, since intra-basin events are lumped together within the equivalence classes and the iteration timescale is five orders of magnitude longer, the propagated modulo-basin dynamics has a far better chance of capturing the infrequent or rare interbasin transitions, a highly sought after goal and a significant shortcoming in MD.

10.2 AI framework to learn and propagate MD data

Since modulo-basin states are denumerable and the time step for the dynamics in quotient step is τ, the propagation actually indicates iterations of a transition matrix operator Γ_τ that satisfies the commutative diagram:

$$\begin{array}{ccc} x(t) & \xrightarrow{\pi} & \overline{x(t)} \\ \downarrow MD & & \downarrow \Gamma_\tau \\ x(t+\tau) & \xrightarrow{\pi} & \overline{x(t+\tau)} \end{array}$$

The diagram commutativity informs us that at any time t, running MD for a time period τ takes microstate $x(t)$ to $x(t+\tau)$, and the modulo-basin class for this destiny microstate, $\overline{x(t+\tau)}$, is identical to $\Gamma_\tau \overline{x(t)}$.

To determine the transition operator Γ_τ that satisfies the diagram commutativity we exploit a deep learning platform trained on MD data. To that effect, we break up the MD trajectory spanning a time period $[0, \mathrm{t_f}]$ into two regions, a training portion with simulated timespan in the interval $[0, \mathrm{t_0}]$ and an optimization portion covering the time interval $(\mathrm{t_0}, \mathrm{t_f}]$. With the trajectory statistics drawn for the region $[0, \mathrm{t_0}]$ we can obtain a first approximation to Γ_τ as a maximum likelihood estimation [15]. Thus, the probability for the transition $\bar{x}_i \to \bar{x}_j$ is estimated at $[\Gamma_\tau]_{ij} = \frac{M_{ij}(\tau)}{M_i}$, where $M_{ij}(\tau)$ is the number of transitions $\bar{x}_i \to \bar{x}_j$ that occurred for the projected trajectory between t and $t+\tau$ within the time period $0 \leq t \leq t_0 - \tau$, and M_i is the number of times state $\bar{x}_i$ is visited within the same training time frame. Once this first estimation is at hand, the optimization of the transition operator requires deep learning as the projection of each MD-generated microstate $x(t_0 + n\tau)$ for $n = 1, \ldots, W$ and W satisfying $(t_0 + W\tau) \leq t_f < [t_0 + (W+1)\tau]$ must be approximated as $[\Gamma_\tau]^n \pi x(t_0)$. In other words, the parametrization of the transition operator in quotient space is optimized to minimize the loss function $\mathcal{L}(\Gamma_\tau)$ [16] given by

$$\mathcal{L}(\Gamma_\tau) = W^{-1} \sum_{n=1}^{W} \|\pi x(t_0 + n\tau) - [\Gamma_\tau]^n \pi x(t_0)\|^2$$

We know this loss function is the correct one since $\mathcal{L}(\Gamma_\tau) = 0$ if and only if the transition operator makes the previous diagram commutative. Once the optimal $\Gamma_\tau^* = argmin\, \mathcal{L}(\Gamma_\tau)$ has been obtained from stochastic steepest descent [16], the modulo-basin projected trajectory can be propagated beyond MD-accessible timescales. At this stage, the coarse-grained modulo basin trajectory needs to be decoded back to the MD-level atomistic description. This reconstruction process also requires deep learning as we need to optimize a 1-to-1 application $\lambda : \Omega/\!\sim\, \to \Omega$ that makes the following diagram commutative in the time range $t_0 \leq t \leq t_f - \tau$:

$$\begin{array}{ccc} x(t) & \xrightarrow{\pi} & \overline{x(t)} \\ \downarrow MD & & \downarrow \Gamma_\tau^* \\ x(t+\tau) & \underset{\lambda}{\longleftarrow} & \overline{x(t+\tau)} \end{array}$$

This implies that the decoder λ must be optimized to minimize the loss function:

$$\mathcal{L}(\lambda) = W^{-1} \sum_{n=1}^{W} \|x(t_0 + n\tau) - \lambda[\Gamma_\tau^*]^n \pi x(t_0)\|^2$$

Again, the choice of loss function is correct since $\mathcal{L}(\lambda) = 0$ if and only if the decoder makes the diagram commute. Once the decoder have been obtained as $argmin\, L(\lambda)$, we can expand the MD computation as $\lambda[\Gamma_\tau^*]^n \pi x(t_0)$ for any $n \geq W$. Thus, the quotient space becomes a canonical simplification of the dynamics, and the proposed AI application is naturally tailored to access physically relevant timescales.

We have thus described a learned quotient-encoding (π) — propagating (Γ_τ^*) — decoding (λ) (QEPD) scheme that greatly simplifies and extends the MD computation, reducing significantly the informational burden at each step by learning to propagate the simplified shorthand dynamics encoded in quotient space and to decode the shorthand trajectory back to the atomistic level. In rigorous terms, the QEPD process enables to compute the MD mapping $x(0) \to x(t = n\tau), \forall n \geq 1$ as $x(n\tau) = \lambda[\Gamma_\tau^*]^n \pi x(0)$.

10.3 AI-generated protein folding pathways

The efficacy of this QEPD is illustrated by folding a protein chain. We selected an N = 57 chain known to be capable of folding autonomously: the thermophilic variant of the B1 domain of protein G from *Streptococcus* (PDB.1GB4). The thermophile was chosen over the wild type due to higher stability of the folded structure. Using the charmm package (free version of CHARMM) [3], we first generated a 220 μs-folding trajectory within the NPT (isothermal/isobaric, T = 298 K) ensemble.

To expand MD computations reaching subsecond timespans and create a generative model of the dynamic hierarchy enshrined in the multiscale simulation, we introduce a shorthand version of the dynamics obtained by projection onto a modulo-basin quotient space. The optimization of the propagation and atomistic reconstruction of the metadynamics in quotient space requires a deep learning (DL) platform which is scripted in Python [17] with TensorFlow [18]. The DL process yields the transition matrix operator Γ_τ that propagates over time the metadynamics resulting from projection of the MD trajectory onto the quotient space $\Omega/\sim$. To incorporate the training information, a multi-layer network for DL is built and exploited whereby network training involves a progressive enrichment (as defined below) of the maximum likelihood (ML) transition probability matrix $[\Gamma_{ML}]_{ij} = \frac{M_{ij}(\tau)}{M_i}$ for generic transition $\bar{x}_i \to \bar{x}_j$ within the time range $0 \leq \mathrm{t} \leq \mathrm{t}_0$. The ML transition probability matrix is generated for different MD runs I, II, $\cdots$ (I denotes the distinguished run extended through AI), where the respective coarse grained initial condition is obtained in decimal representation using random number generation of rational numbers with binary decimals in the interval $[0.00010001\ldots, 0.10001000\ldots]$ representing classes in $\Omega/\sim$. The metadynamics in quotient space is Markovian as evidenced by the fact that, if state $\bar{x}_i$ is visited, the quotients $[\Gamma_{ML}]_{ij} = \frac{M_{ij}(\tau)}{M_i}$ are identical irrespective of the MD trajectory generated. The number of layers is contingent on the extent of transition probability coverage required to construct the matrix Γ_{ML} through progressive incorporation of entries obtained from the different MD runs (Fig. 10.2(a, b)). The training limits are empirically delineated

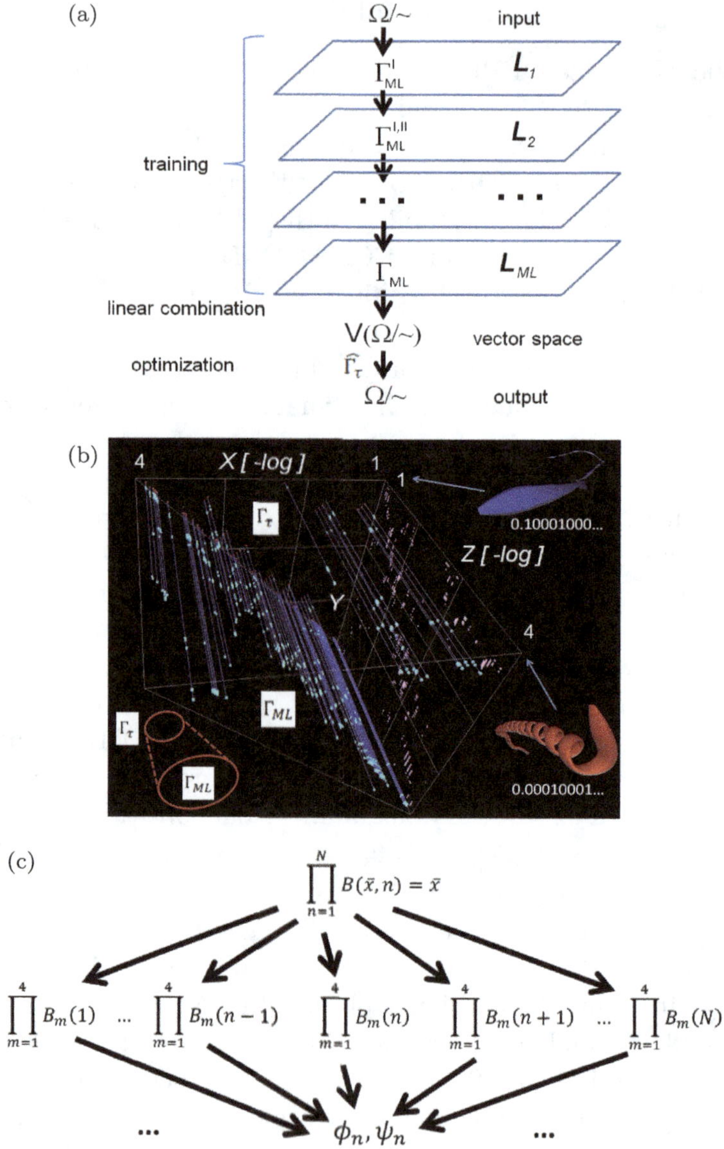

Figure 10.2. *(Continued)*

by the expediency of the propagator optimization steered by the loss function. In other words, the adequacy of the training is defined vis-à-vis the efficacy of the learning process. Clearly, multiple training runs are required for efficient learning (Fig. 10.3). The protein folding case illustrated in this chapter required 38 layers and this value corresponds to minimal but sufficient training beyond which accuracy does not improve (Fig. 10.3).

Starting at state $\overline{x(t)} = \bar{x}_i$, the destiny state of a single iteration of the modulo-basin dynamics is approximated by the fully trained network as $\overline{x(t+\tau)} \approx [\overline{x(t+\tau)}]_{ML} = \sum_j [\Gamma_{ML}]_{ij}\bar{x}_j$ where the linear combination belongs to the vector space $\mathrm{V}(\Omega/\sim)$ spanned by the set $\Omega/\sim$ of linearly independent vectors that constitutes the base. The linear combination state $[\overline{x(t+\tau)}]_{ML}$ serves as starting point for the parameter optimization, via minimization of $\mathcal{L}(\Gamma_\tau)$, of the retracting operator $\widehat{\Gamma}_\tau$, that satisfies $\Gamma_\tau = \widehat{\Gamma}_\tau \circ \Gamma_{ML}$. Thus, since the maximum likelihood matrix is fixed as obtained during the training stage, the parameter optimization of Γ_τ during the period $\mathrm{t_0} \leq \mathrm{t} \leq \mathrm{t_f}$ boils

←

Figure 10.2. Artificial Intelligence platform to propagate MD trajectories simplified through projection onto quotient space. **(a)** Scheme of multi-layer deep learning network required to generate the propagation operator $\Gamma^*_\tau = \widehat{\Gamma}^*_\tau \circ \Gamma_{ML}$ in quotient space $\Omega/\sim$. **(b)** Tensor array of transitions between modulo-basin states in $\Omega/\sim$ for the protein folding case studied. The states/classes are denoted by residue basin occupancies in decimal representation and they are plotted on axis X, Y, Z in –log scale. The transitions dictated by optimized operator Γ^*_τ are plotted as red entries on the X–Y plane, with X and Y coordinates representing originating states and destiny states, respectively. The full set of destiny states arising from maximum likelihood transitions with probabilities ≥ 0.1 learned from 38 MD runs are plotted as light blue entries along the Z-axis. **(c)** Learning flow for decoding map λ used for atomistic reconstruction. For a given state $\bar{x}$ in $\Omega/\sim$ and a generic residue n along the chain, the decoded torsional coordinate region is significantly reduced beyond the constraints imposed by basin occupancy for residue n. This is so because the basin occupancy of all other residues also impose significant constraints arising from the formation of 3D-structures compatible with $\bar{x}$.

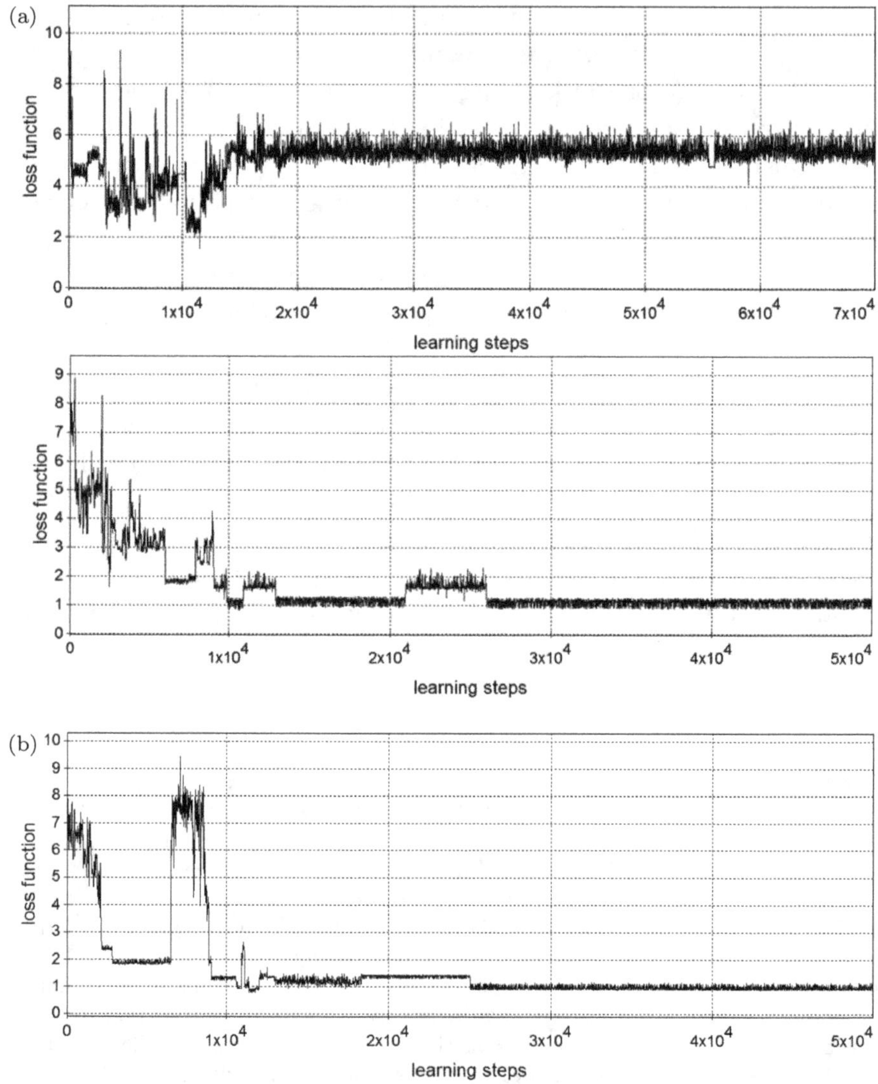

Figure 10.3. Loss function $\mathcal{L}(\Gamma_\tau)$ for the protein folding problem. **(a)** The upper plot is associated with training on a single MD run, i.e., the one whose extension is sought, while the plot in the lower panel displays an efficient optimization requiring 38 MD runs with randomly generated initial conditions. The steady state value in the optimization process plateaus as the number of layers is increased beyond 38. **(b)** Testing accuracy computed by plotting the loss function over a testing run outside the training set of 38 MD runs. This run with randomly generated initial conditions was generated to assert the convergence to the optimization steady state.

down to identifying the optimal $\hat{\Gamma_\tau}$ that minimizes the loss function

$$\mathcal{L}(\Gamma_\tau) = \mathcal{L}(\hat{\Gamma_\tau}) = W^{-1}\sum_{n=1}^{W} \|\pi x(t_0 + n\tau) - [\hat{\Gamma_\tau} \circ \Gamma_{ML}]^n \pi x(t_0)\|^2$$

Thus, the learning process is encoded in the connective weight optimization $\widehat{\Gamma}_\tau = \widehat{\Gamma}^*_\tau = argmin\, \mathcal{L}(\widehat{\Gamma}_\tau)$. The minimization of $\mathcal{L}(\widehat{\Gamma}_\tau)$ becomes a least-squares problem numerically solved with stochastic gradient descent. The set $\wp(t_0, t_f)$ of MD-generated states during the period $t_0 \leq t \leq t_f$ is sampled randomly at each iteration to compute the gradient with minibatches given by trajectory fragments spanned by randomly chosen time intervals of size $10^{-2}|t_f - t_0|$. To optimize the network connectivity given by $\widehat{\Gamma}_\tau$, the ADADELTA optimization protocol with learning rate 0.3 is adopted [19]. The operator $\widehat{\Gamma}_\tau$ acting on the maximum likelihood (ML) transition vector $[x(t+\tau)]_{ML}$ has the net effect to retract the linear combination into a single destiny vector in the base $\Omega/\sim$. Figure 10.2(b) displays the optimized retraction of the ML transition matrix Γ_{ML} onto the operator $\Gamma_\tau = \widehat{\Gamma}_\tau \circ \Gamma_{ML}$ for the protein folding problem described below. For clarity, only transitions with ML probability $\geq$0.1 are displayed. To generate the tensor description of the $\Gamma_{ML} \to \Gamma_\tau$ retraction, the decimal representation of residue basin occupancies was adopted enabling plotting the states in quotient space $\Omega/\sim$ on a 1-dimensional axis.

The full MD trajectory encoded as the shorthand version in quotient space is shown in Fig. 10.4, with selected $t_0 = 120\mu s$ as training parameter and $120\mu s < t \leq 220\mu s$ as learning period to optimize the matrix propagator in quotient space. Using the QEPD procedure, this trajectory is further extended up to $t = 7500\mu s$ (Fig. 10.5).

We note that the final state is significantly stable, prevailing since the time of its inception at $t = 3108\mu s$ detectable on Fig. 10.5(c). Furthermore, the decoded final stable state at $t = 7500\mu s$, corresponding to the eigenvector associated with eigenvalue 1 of the matrix Γ^*_τ, is topologically equivalent to the native crystallographic state, as evidenced by the high similarity in the contact maps,

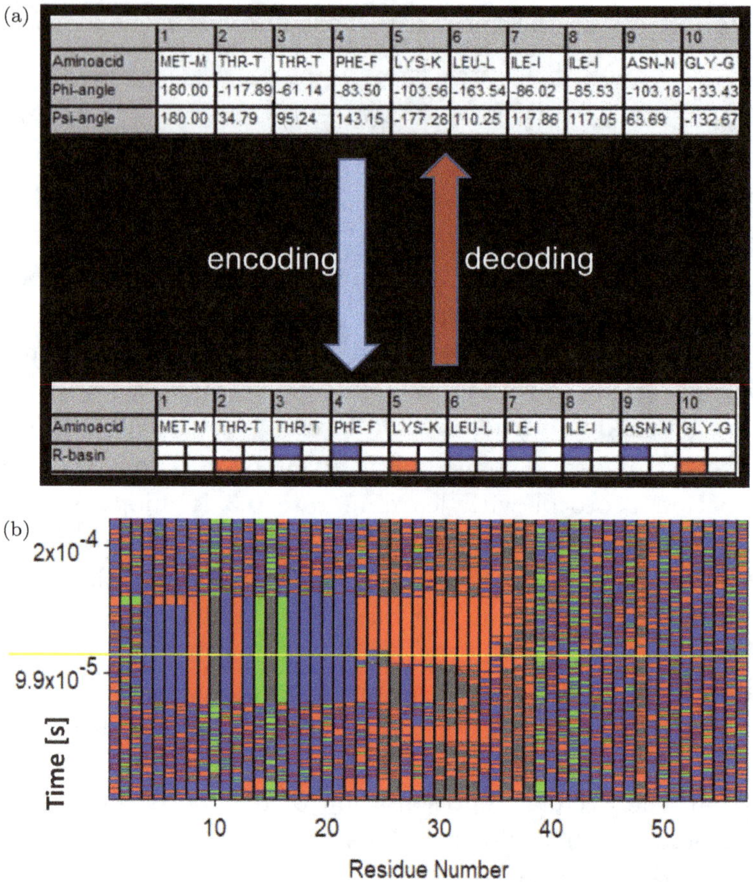

Figure 10.4. Encoding an MD trajectory in quotient space. **(a)** Encoding backbone torsional information in the modulo-basin quotient space for the first 10 residues in the thermophilic variant of the B1 domain of protein G from *Streptococcus* (chain length N = 57). The decoding process is the inverse operation and requires additional information on the whole trajectory encoded in quotient space (main text). **(b)** Quotient-space encoded MD trajectory at 1μs-resolution for the protein chain. At each time, the modulo-basin state of the chain is represented as a color sequence, where the basin for each residue is specified following the color convention established in Fig. 10.1(a). A 220 μs-folding trajectory was generated within the NPT (isothermal/isobaric, T = 298 K) ensemble, selecting the timespan interval $[0, t_0 = 120\mu s]$ as training region and the interval $[120\mu s, 220\mu s]$ as the learning period to optimize the parametrization of the matrix propagator in quotient space. Reprinted from [Fernández A (2020) Rapid Research Letter: Deep Learning Unravels a Dynamic Hierarchy While Empowering Molecular Dynamics Simulations. Annalen der Physik (Berlin) 532:1900526] with permission from John Wiley and Sons.

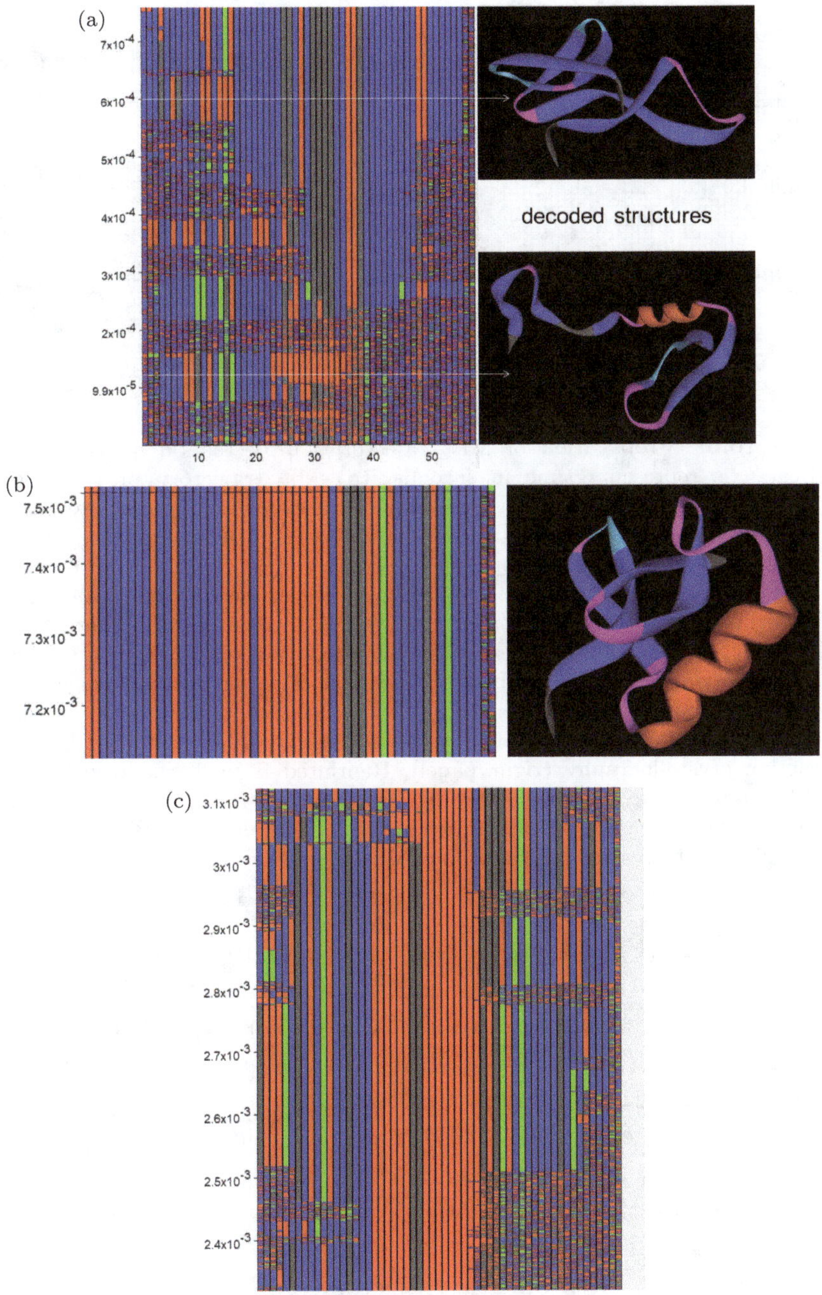

Figure 10.5. (*Continued*)

(d) 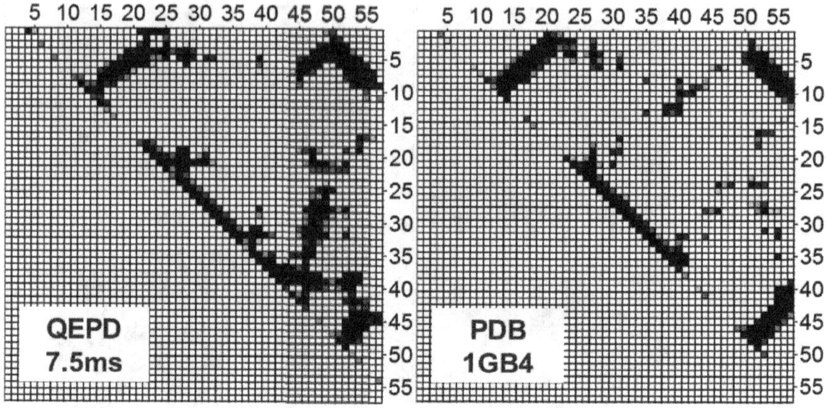

Figure 10.5. Propagation of MD trajectories projected on quotient space. Vertical axis represents time in seconds. **(a)** MD trajectory projected onto quotient space at 1μs-resolution for timespan $[0, 220\mu s]$ and propagated for an additional 7280μs, covering the time range $[0, 7500\mu s]$. **(b)** Steady state observed in the final portion of the propagation of the projected MD trajectory (full coverage: 7500μs). **(c)** Critical portion of generated trajectory in quotient space within which the native-like steady state begins to develop at around 3100μs. **(d)** Contact map for microstate obtained by decoding the steady state at final point t = 7500μs of QEPD computation (left panel), equated to the eigenvector associated with eigenvalue 1 of matrix Γ^*_τ. The decoded microstate is contrasted against the topologically equivalent native state PDB.1GB4 obtained by X-ray diffraction crystallography (right panel). Reprinted from [Fernández A (2020) Rapid Research Letter: Deep Learning Unravels a Dynamic Hierarchy While Empowering Molecular Dynamics Simulations. Annalen der Physik (Berlin) 532:1900526] with permission from John Wiley and Sons.

contact motifs (Fig. 10.5(d)), and backbone-atom RMSD at 1.9 Å. These assertions follow as the contact matrix associated with the equilibrated destiny conformation (Fig. 10.5(b)) has been compared with the native fold in PDB.1GB4. An (i, j) entry in the matrix is filled in black if the minimum Euclidean distance $d_{min}(i, j)$ between all the atoms (backbone and side chain) in residues i and j is ≤ 4 Å, grey if 4 Å $< d_{min}(i, j) \leq 6$ Å and white if $d_{min}(i, j) > 6$ Å. The two matrices reveal the same topological pattern of antiparallel and parallel β-sheets and α-helix.

We note that the atomistic trajectory obtained from the QEPD computation would take about 150 days on one of today's fastest special-purpose supercomputers covering an estimated 50μs per day [20]. By contrast, full network training and parameter optimization took approximately 12 hours on a cluster of 12 Titan RTX GPUs, while the QEPD computation required an additional 8 hours on the same resource.

10.4 Towards an AI platform for molecular dynamics

MD has been deemed essential to gain insight into the molecular basis of thermodynamic properties and detectable events in condensed phase materials and constitutes an invaluable aid in a variety of applications [1–3]. However, exhaustive or even statistically significant sampling of conformation space becomes often prohibitively costly and, consequently, crucial infrequent events are seldom captured in an MD computation. In the face of such limitations, we addressed the need to extend MD timespans by encoding the MD trajectory as a "shorthand" version in the quotient space and then learning to propagate the encoded trajectory through the use of artificial intelligence. Quotient space is a mathematical construct that enables a simplification of the dynamics by defining an equivalence relation between microstates that are related via fast intrabasin equilibration. Thus, the class partitioning constituting quotient space is dictated by the topology of the vector field that steers the MD trajectory. Equivalence classes define how the space is dynamically related, hence, significantly mitigating the information burden that needs to be carried over from one MD-integration step to the next. In this way, we introduced a scheme that makes MD computation significantly more agile, enabling coverage of physically relevant timescales while bringing meaningful insights into the dynamic hierarchy that underlies the MD computation.

In regards to extending MD timescales, coarse graining methods represent an alternative to the quotient space projection approach. Yet, their learning efficiency requires a difficult joint variational optimization of both encoding and propagation, with an *ad-hoc* delineation of the topology that constrains the variational search [12]. By contrast, the quotient space inherits the topology defined by class partitioning from the dynamic determinants of the system, while its inherent equivalence relation circumvents the need to optimize the encoder. Thus, the quotient space projection represents a considerably simplification and a rigorous generative model providing a hierarchical dynamics framework for the MD computation.

References

1. Lindorff-Larsen K, Piana S, Dror RO, Shaw DE (2011) How fast-folding proteins fold. *Science* 334:517–520.
2. Plattner N, Doerr S, De Fabritiis G, Noé F (2017) Protein-protein association and binding mechanism resolved in atomic detail. *Nature Chem* 9:1005–1011.
3. Brooks BR, Brooks III CL, Mackerell AD, Nilsson L, Petrella RJ, *et al.* (2009) CHARMM: The Biomolecular simulation Program. *J Comp Chem* 30:1545–1615.
4. Fernández A (1999) Coarse graining the soft-mode dynamics of a folding protein. *Phys Chem Chem Phys* 1:861–869.
5. Fernández A (1999) Folding a protein by discretizing its backbone torsional dynamics. *Phys Rev E* 59:5928–5934.
6. Fernández A, Colubri A, Berry RS (2000) Topology to geometry in protein folding: Beta-lactoglobulin. *Proc Natl Acad Sci USA* 97:14062–14066.
7. Fernández A, Colubri A, Berry RS (2001) Topologies to geometries in protein folding: Hierarchical and nonhierarchical scenarios. *J Chem Phys* 114:5871–5888.
8. Singhal N, Pande VS (2005) Error analysis and efficient sampling in Markovian state models for molecular dynamics. *J Chem Phys* 123:204909.
9. Zimmerman MI, Bowman GR (2015) Fast conformational searches by balancing exploration/exploitation trade-offs. *J Chem Theory Comput* 11:5747–5757.
10. Buchete NV, Hummer G (2008) Coarse master equations for peptide folding dynamics. *J Phys Chem B* 112:6057–6069.
11. Laio A, Parrinello M (2002) Escaping free energy minima. *Proc Natl Acad Sci USA* 99:12562–12566.
12. Wang W, Gómez-Bombarelli R (2019) Coarse-graining auto-encoders for molecular dynamics. *npj Comp Mat* 5:125.
13. Fernández A (2016) Physics at the Biomolecular Interface: Fundamentals for Molecular Targeted Therapy. Chapter 3. Springer International Publishing, Switzerland.
14. Altis A, Nguyen PH, Hegger R, Stock G (2007) Dihedral angle principal component analysis of molecular dynamics simulations. *J Chem Phys* 126:244111.
15. Rossi RJ (2018) Mathematical Statistics: An Introduction to Likelihood Based Inference. John Wiley & Sons, New York.
16. Stanley KO, Clune J, Lehman J, Miikkulainen R (2019) Designing neural networks through neuroevolution. *Nature Mach Intel* 1:24–35.

17. Ketkar N (2017) *Deep Learning with Python.* Apress, Berkeley, CA.
18. Rampasek L, Goldenberg A (2016) TensorFlow: Biology's gateway to deep learning. *Cell Sys* 2:12–14.
19. Zeiler MD (2012) ADADELTA, an adaptive learning rate method. arXiv:1212.5701 https://arxiv.org/abs/1212.5701.
20. Shaw DE, Grossman JP, Bank JA, Batson B, Adam Butts J, *et al.* (2014) Anton 2: Raising the bar for performance and programmability in a special-purpose molecular dynamics supercomputer. SC '14: Proceedings of the International Conference for High Performance Computing, Networking, Storage and Analysis. *IEEE ACM* 2014:41–53. DOI: 10.1109/SC.2014.9

Chapter 11

Artificial intelligence guides drug design in the absence of information on target structure and regulation and unravels the origin of cooperativity

"The future ain't what it used to be."

Yogi Berra

The absence of reported structure for a therapeutic target and the lack of information on its regulation pose major hurdles for rational drug design. This chapter delineates the exploitation of AI to steer the engineering of molecular targeted therapy in such challenging situations. The chapter focuses specifically on protein associations, where drug-based disruption of dysfunctional complexes poses a major challenge to targeted therapy. The problem becomes daunting when the structure and regulated modulation of the complex are unknown. To address the challenge, we leverage an artificial intelligence platform that learns from epistructural information and infers regulation-susceptible regions that also generate interfacial tension between protein and water, thereby promoting contextually tuned protein associations. The input consists of sequence-derived 1D-features. The network is configured with evolutionarily coupled residues and taught to search for phosphorylation-modulated binding epitopes. The discovery platform is benchmarked against a PDB-derived testing set and validated against experimental data on a therapeutic disruptor designed according to the inferred epitope for a large deregulated complex known to be recruited in heart failure.

Thus, dysfunctional "molecular brakes" of cardiac contractility get released through a therapeutic intervention guided by artificial intelligence.

11.1 Disrupting dysfunctional protein complexes with no known structure and no information on their regulation: An almost intractable problem

Protein-protein interfaces (PPIs) determine supramolecular complexes that get recruited in core biological processes in the cell, including signaling cascades, regulation of enzyme activity and control of molecular motors [1]. A deregulated or dysfunctional complex may be disrupted through a molecular targeted intervention, offering a therapeutic opportunity [1,2]. For example, the association of the negative regulator MDM2 (murine double-minute 2 homolog) to the tumor suppressor p53 constitutes an important target in cancer therapies aimed at disrupting the modulation of p53 [2]. Another important illustration from cancer immunotherapy consists of disrupting PD-1 receptor recognition of its natural ligand PD-L1, a checkpoint blockade that enables the T-cell adaptive response by curbing tumor-induced immunosuppression [2].

Despite such successes, therapeutic disruption of PPIs remains challenging, mostly because the structure and regulated modulation of the complex are usually unknown or unreported. We address this problem by developing a deep learning (DL) platform [3] trained on structural [4] and inferred epistructural [5] data to identify regions on the protein surface capable of promoting functionally regulated protein associations. Such regions are not merely binding hot spots [5] but are also endowed with enzymatic activity to enable PPI modulation via the acquisition of signals in a regulatory setting. Thus, the underlying convolutional network exploits sequence-derived 1D-features [6] as input data, learns to infer structural and epistructural information, and uses the latter to generate an output that identifies the region fulfilling the dual role of binding epitope and regulation-susceptible element. We justify subsequently the need to go beyond a structural representation of the 1D-input for the purpose of discovery to disrupt deregulated PPIs. As in DL platforms for structural inference [7–9], the input is first processed into a 2D-matrix of evolutionarily coupled residue pairs [10]. However, our approach differs fundamentally from other predictors [7–9] that are not concerned with identifying regulatory elements governing PPI modulation.

In this work, the coevolved-pair representation determines structural constraints that enable further training based on structure-derived features representing regulatory elements. The discovery platform is ultimately validated against experimental data on a therapeutic complex disruptor designed by mimicking the inferred epitope for a large dysfunctional complex [11–13] with unreported structure and poorly understood biochemical modulation.

If a binding partner in a protein complex becomes dysfunctional, complex formation may lead to disease and hence PPI disruption represents a therapeutic imperative [1, 2, 14, 15]. An illustration this work focuses on is provided by the association of the myosin motor with the myosin-binding protein C (MyBP-C), a central regulator of cardiac contractility [12, 13]. When deregulated, the association promotes heart failure, while in healthy cardiomyocytes, the PPI is modulated by phosphorylation at the MyBP-C binding epitope [12]. Thus, MyBP-C may be regarded as a "molecular brake" of the myosin motor. In the context of heart failure, a targeted intervention to release the brake constitutes an unmet therapeutic imperative [13] (Fig. 11.1. The intervention is tantamount to the drug-based disruption of a PPI, itself a major challenge [1,2]. The design problem becomes daunting because the 3D structure of the multidomain MyBP-C and the detailed regulatory context for the complex-modulation mechanism are unknown, hence key issues like interdomain binding cooperativity and induced folding [1] have remained essentially intractable.

Our goal is to steer molecular targeting by leveraging artificial intelligence (AI) technology [16,17] trained on structural data to infer leads for therapeutic disruption of large dysfunctional complexes with unreported structure and regulation. In the specific context of heart failure, the goal is to identify a fragment of MyBP-C representing a peptide-based lead[15] that mimics a regulation-susceptible binding epitope. The peptide should be suitable for emergency

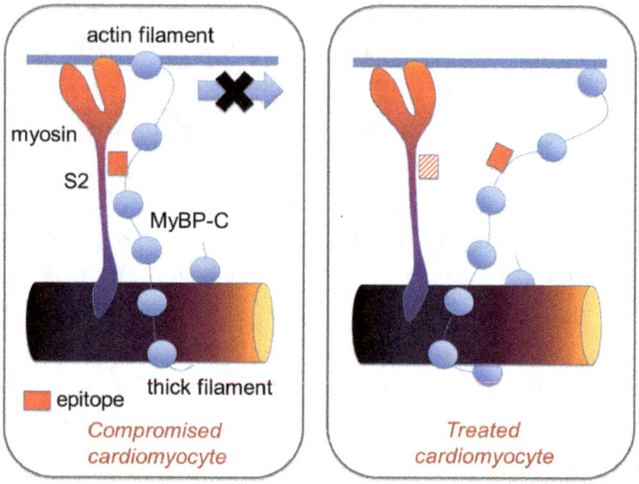

Figure 11.1. *Schematics of therapeutic intervention to treat heart failure through targeted disruption of the PDB-unreported MyBP-C/myosin complex.* The drug lead consists of a peptide reproducing the epitope region (red box) in MyBP-C. As the peptide binds to myosin competitively, it displaces the tethering/anchoring modulation inducing a 'brake release' that accelerates the cross-bridge kinetics of cardiomyocyte contractility. Reprinted from [Fernández A (2020) Artificial Intelligence Steering Molecular Therapy in the Absence of Information on Target Structure and Regulation. Journal of Chemical Information and Modeling (ACS) 60:460–466] with permission from the American Chemical Society.

interventions, administered *in situ* to displace MyBP-C from its association with myosin ([13], Fig. 11.1).

To identify phosphorylation-susceptible binding epitopes from sequence-derived 1D-input it is necessary to search beyond a structural description of the type that DL methods can achieve [7, 8], and represent the structure-solvent interface, i.e. the epistructure. To perform this task, we take advantage of the fact that the epistructural features are encoded in the structure itself [18–21], more specifically in the packing of the structure, that is, in the way backbone hydrogen bonds are shielded from structure-disruptive hydration [11]. The need to explore the epistructure is immediately apparent if we search for a binding hot spot since a binding region promotes the exclusion of interfacial water, hence it generates interfacial tension [5], as shown in Chapter 2. On the other hand, identifying a phosphorylation-susceptible region also requires an epistructural representation, since the region must be endowed with functionalized side-chain hydroxyl groups, capable of launching a nucleophilic attack on the beta-gamma phosphodiester linkage in ATP [21], as discussed in Chapter 6. So, the operative questions addressed in this work is: *what epistructural feature may be a hot spot of interfacial tension while also promoting a nucleophilic attack on ATP, hence becoming a phosphorylation-based regulatory element? And how can we infer this epistructural feature in the absence of structure or information on regulation?*

As we have learned from Chapters 2 and 6, a solvent-exposed backbone hydrogen bond (BHB), known as *dehydron*, fulfills both requirements [20, 21]. Water interfacing with a dehydron is deprived of full hydrogen-bond coordination in a manner that makes it also a proton acceptor, with hydronium becoming a good leaving group [18, 21]. Thus, due to suppressed hydrogen bonding of interfacial water, a dehydron creates interfacial tension, while it also functionalizes nearby side-chain hydroxyls (for example, from serine, threonine and tyrosine) by enhancing the basicity of coordination-deprived interfacial water to the point of accepting the hydroxyl proton [21]. As discussed subsequently, this dual role of dehydrons motivates the construction of a neural network sustaining a DL platform that provides an epistructural, rather than structural, output.

11.2 Deep learning to disrupt a dysfunctional complex

The discovery platform exploits a neural network trained on evolutionary and PDB-derived structural data [4] to represent the sequence-based 1D-input [6,7] across a hierarchy of network layers up to an epistructural [5, 18] resolution that enables the identification of regulation-susceptible binding epitopes. Drug leads may be inferred from target sequence provided DL is instructed on the epistructural characterization of the binding epitope. To that effect, we note that the MyBP-C-myosin complex is naturally disrupted upon phosphorylation of the so-called m-motif of MyBP-C, probably at loci Ser273, Ser282, Ser302 [12]. Thus, we focus on mimicking epitopes that promote water exclusion, driving protein associations, while also functionalizing spatially adjacent nucleophilic side chains of phosphorylation-susceptible residues as the epitope is exposed to water [21]. As described in Chapters 2 and 6, dehydrons are precisely the type of epistructural features endowed with the sought after dual role [18, 20].

To summarize, the overarching aim of this work is the development of DL method to expand the pharmaceutical discovery platform to cases where there is no detailed information on target structure and regulation of target activity. We focus on the most challenging cases involving rational design of molecular disruptors of deregulated protein complexes whose recruitment leads to disease. The neural network uses sequence-based 1D-input, gets trained on evolutionary and structural PDB-derived data and informed on how to generate epistructural features from structural inferences, and is capable of inferring binding regions that are also susceptible of phosphorylation-based regulation of their binding activity. This is possible because epistructural information or, equivalently, the structure-solvent dynamic relationship, which is key to infer regulated binding epitopes, is encoded in structural information, as discussed in Chapter 2 and briefly recapitulated in the next section. In turn, because of structural training, the network is able to represent the required epistructural information. Preliminarily, the deep learning discovery platform is benchmarked by establishing the accuracy of epistructural inference on a PDB-derived testing set as network connection parameters are optimized to minimize the appropriate loss function. Then, the DL platform is validated by showing it enables the identification of the clinically competent molecular disruptor of the deregulated MyBP-C-myosin complex recruited in the heart failure condition [13]. This peptide-based pharmaceutical has been tested *ex-vivo* and *in vitro* but the discovery process that led to its identification was not revealed in the patent that covered the invention.

11.3 Protein binding sites that may be susceptible to regulation

For the sake of clarity in the exposition, this section essentially recapitulates material from Chapters 2 and 6. Since BHBs are structural determinants, protein integrity is contingent on the ability of the structure, by itself or within a complex, to prevent disruptive BHB hydration. Thus, dehydrons compromise structural integrity and promote protein associations to exclude surrounding water. Dehydrons become determinants for protein association because, by decreasing charge screening, exogenous removal of water from the dehydron microenvironment strengthens and stabilizes the electrostatic interaction that underlies the BHB. Ample bioinformatics evidence on the distribution of dehydrons at interfaces of protein complexes supports this picture, pointing to dehydrons as key factors driving complex formation. Dehydrons and epistructures are computed from structural coordinates of proteins. To that end, we introduce the extent of hydrogen-bond wrapping, w, indicating the number of sidechain nonpolar groups contained within a "desolvation domain" that defines the BHB microenvironment. Being marginally wrapped, dehydrons are located in the tail of the distribution of wrapping values across BHBs in the structural database.

In their alternative role, dehydrons play an enzymatic role by promoting phosphorylation of adjacent residues, as described in Chapter 6. This chemistry is enabled since dehydrons turn interfacial water molecules into proton acceptors, thereby activating the nucleophilic hydroxyls in the side chains of phosphorylation-susceptible residues (Fig. 11.2). As the hydroxyl gets deprotonated, it is enabled to nucleophilically attack the $\beta-\gamma$ phosphoester linkage of ATP, the key step in side-chain phosphorylation.

To explain how dehydrons enhance basicity of nearby water requires a conceptual departure from the standard Debye picture where water polarization is assumed to align with electrostatic field determined by fixed charges [21]. The "Debye ansatz" breaks down under confinement of water molecules in regions of nanoscale dimensions, such as partially hydrated backbone regions at dehydron sites. The breakdown takes place since the bulk-like floppy lattice of water hydrogen bonds gets distorted to the point where water is effectively deprived of hydrogen-bond partnerships. Thus, dehydron-interfacing water molecules generate a polarization component $\overline{P\#}$ orthogonal to the electrostatic field $\vec{E}$ and arising from partially hindered BHB

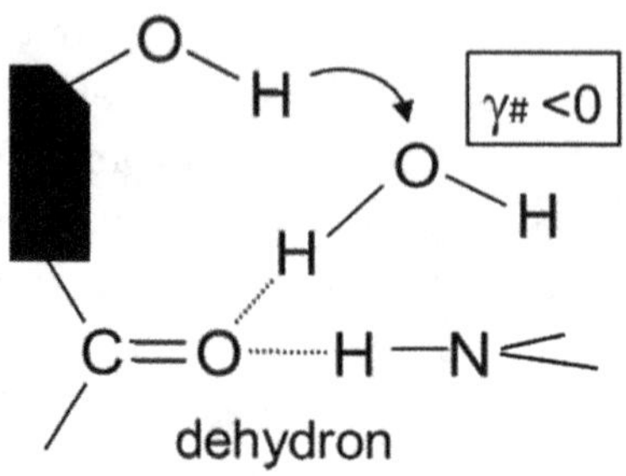

Figure 11.2. An epitope dehydron functionalizes a nearby side-chain hydroxyl by frustrating interfacial water, turning it into acceptor of the side-chain hydroxyl proton. Thus, dehydrons at epitopes can functionalize phosphorylation sites nearby, as required to modulate the MyBP-C/myosin interface.

hydration. This polarization induces an $\vec{E}$-independent net charge $\gamma^{\#} = -\vec{\nabla}.\ \overrightarrow{P^{\#}}$ not accountable by the protein chemical composition. The local dehydron-induced functionality of interfacial water is in accord with the sign of $\gamma^{\#}$, i. e. proton donor if $\gamma^{\#} > 0$ and proton acceptor if $\gamma^{\#} < 0$. It has been shown that the latter possibility $\gamma^{\#} < 0$, implying that at least one water oxygen atom remains on average unpaired to a hydroxyl proton (its orbital-localized lone electron pair is unutilized), is the one that holds at dehydron sites (Fig. 11.2). Thus, dehydron-interfacing water yields a non-Debye polarization-induced charge $\gamma^{\#} < 0$ that begets a proton-acceptor role compatible with unfulfilled hydrogen-bond coordination of water oxygen (where partial negative charge is located), turning dehydron-interfacing water into a chemical base. This result identifies dehydrons as promoters phosphorylation (Fig. 11.2).

11.4 Deep learning platform to infer phosphorylation-modulated binding epitopes in the absence of structure

Leveraging a DL platform to identify dehydron-rich regions poses constraints on the represented data that may be processed by the network. The structural/epistructural data must lend itself to a tensor representation wherein information is describable and processed on a multidimensional array (tensor) of digital entries within a layered hierarchical architecture.

As argued subsequently, the DL algorithm queries the PDB-derived repository on predetermined evolutionarily coupled residues in order to represent BHBs involving the residue pairs. The training data has structural and epistructural components arranged in a tensor. The structural components are BHBs arranged in matrix form, while the epistructural components describe the extent of BHB wrapping. Epistructural components are thus drawn upon the structural data in tensor arrangement. The implemented learning algorithm pivots on two facts: a) dehydrons constitute hot spots for phosphorylation-modulated protein association, and b) dehydron patterns lend themselves to a tensor representation whereby a 2D array (matrix) $\boldsymbol{Y}$ is constructed to indicate pairs of residues interacting through BHBs, while their respective wrapping r, is represented along $\boldsymbol{Y}$-orthogonal vectors, $\boldsymbol{z}_{ij}$ for entry $\boldsymbol{Y}_{ij}$. Thus, the data processing realizes a tensor flow, with the tensor identified by the product $\boldsymbol{Y} \otimes \boldsymbol{Z} = [\boldsymbol{Y}_{ij} \otimes \boldsymbol{z}_{ij})]_{ij}$.

The DL flowchart is [Sequence-derived 1D input features] $\rightarrow$ [$\mathbf{E}$ = Evolutionary coupling matrix compounded with 1D-features for paired residues] $\rightarrow$ [structure/epistructure tensor $\boldsymbol{Y} \otimes \boldsymbol{Z}$] $\rightarrow$ [scalar output identifying dehydron-rich region]. The DL network is trained to learn the relationship between evolutionarily coupled residues and dehydron-paired residues, with the goal of inferring dehydron-rich regions. The output gets further translated into a peptide-based drug lead that can be exploited for therapeutic disruption of specific protein associations, as illustrated in this study by the molecular targeted treatment of heart failure through disruption of the molecular brakes of cardiac contractility (Fig. 11.1). Thus, the peptide-based drug lead embodies the inferred dehydron-rich epitope and enables therapeutic disruption of the dysfunctional complex [13].

The DL discovery platform is trained by the PDB-derived ASTRAL dataset [4] filtered for sequences with less than 40% identity and parsed according to a 9:1 training:testing ratio, with no superfamilies intersecting both subsets. Network input nodes $\ldots, \boldsymbol{x}_i, \ldots, \boldsymbol{x}_j, \ldots$ contain residue amino acid identity compounded with sequence-derived 1D-features including predicted solvent accessibility and predicted secondary structure[6]. Thus, the 1D-feature nodes are constructed by incorporating two dominant input features of the contact predictor MetaPSICOV, in turn obtained from predictors SOLVPRED (solvent exposure) and PSIPRED (secondary structure probability) [6]. For weak alignments, the contact predictor tends to overwrite the coevolution contribution in favor of the two 1D-features named above. Thus, for weak alignment, MetaPSICOV operates like a standard machine learning-based contact inference, whereas for strong alignments, coevolution signals outweight the two standard 1D-features.

In the first layer (L_1), the information is transformed into a 2D-array $\boldsymbol{E}$ representing the evolutionary coupling matrix (ECM) [7]. The rationale for using the evolutionary filter is that columns coupled in a multiple sequence alignment (MSA) will likely be close in the 3D-structure. Pixel (entry) $\boldsymbol{y}_{ij}$ in the ECM informs on the extent of evolutionary correlation between residues in $\boldsymbol{x}_i$, $\boldsymbol{x}_j$, and this information is concatenated with the 1D-features in $\boldsymbol{x}_i$, $\boldsymbol{x}_j$. Once layer L_1 is constructed, the network is trained with the structural database. For each sequence/structure from the training dataset, the $\boldsymbol{E}$-matrix is computed along with the structure/epistructure information encoded in $\boldsymbol{Y} \otimes \boldsymbol{Z}$. With this training, the network learns to draw the relationship between evolutionary couplings $\boldsymbol{y}_{ij}$ and structural/epistructural features $(\boldsymbol{Y}_{ij} \otimes \boldsymbol{z}_{ij})$ (Fig. 11.3). Thus, nodes in L_2 are elements in the symmetric tensor $\boldsymbol{Y} \otimes \boldsymbol{Z} = [\boldsymbol{Y}_{ij} \otimes \boldsymbol{z}_{ij}]_{ij}$, with "wrapping vector" $\boldsymbol{z}_{ij} = [A_w(i,j)]_{w=1,2,\ldots}$, where $A_w(i,j)$ denotes the number of learned representations of BHBs pairing residues in $\boldsymbol{x}_i$, $\boldsymbol{x}_j$ with wrapping w (Fig. 11.4(a)).

The output is a descriptor of the epistructure generated by the input sequence. It is defined as the set of scalars $< w >_i$, enabling inference of the regulation-susceptible binding epitope as the region richest in dehydrons with hydroxyl-containing side chains. The value $< w >_i$ indicates the expected extent of wrapping of BHBs involving the residue in $\boldsymbol{x}_i$. The $< w >_{i-}$ values are computed by compounding inputs drawn from layer L_2 resolved in the epistructural tensor (Fig. 11.4(a)):

$$< w >_i = \left(\frac{1}{N-1}\right) \sum_{j \neq i,\, j=1}^{N} \sum_{w=1}^{M} w \frac{A_w(i,j)}{M(i,j)}$$

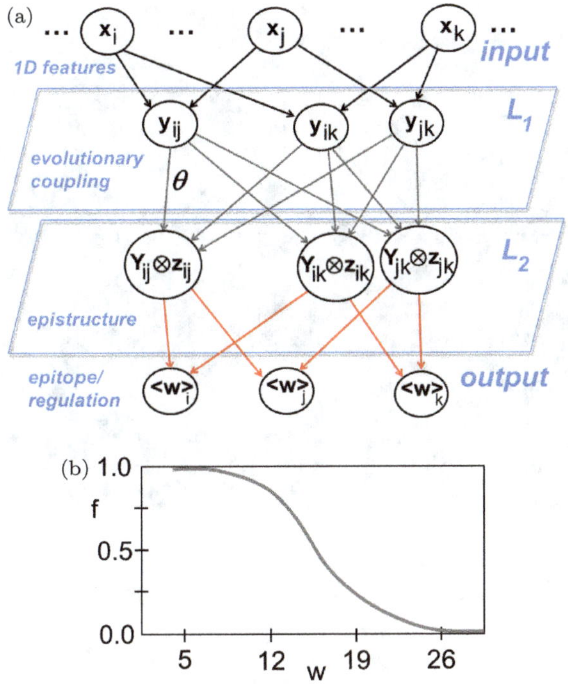

Figure 11.3. *Two-layer network for deep leaning (DL) exploited in a drug discovery platform in the absence of structure for the target protein.* **(a)** DL network enabling the processing of input sequence information on the target protein and sustaining a tensor flow. In the first layer (L_1), the information is organized on the evolutionary correlation matrix $\boldsymbol{E}= [y_{ij}]_{ij}$. The network is trained with structural and structure-derived epistructural information, yielding tensor $\boldsymbol{Y} \otimes \boldsymbol{Z}$ in layer L_2. By establishing correspondences between $\boldsymbol{E}$ and $\boldsymbol{Y} \otimes \boldsymbol{Z}$, the network learns the relationship between evolutionary coupling $\boldsymbol{y}_{ij}$ and backbone hydrogen-bond epistructure ($\boldsymbol{y}_{ij} \otimes \boldsymbol{z}_{ij}$). The output is the set of scalars $< w >_i$, indicating the expected extent of wrapping of BHBs involving the residue in $\boldsymbol{x}_i$. **(b)** Sigmoidal activation function (f) to represent the DL output. Reprinted from [Fernández A (2020) Artificial Intelligence Steering Molecular Therapy in the Absence of Information on Target Structure and Regulation. Journal of Chemical Information and Modeling (ACS) 60:460–466] with permission from the American Chemical Society.

where N is sequence length and $M(i,j) = \sum_{w=1}^{M} A_w(ij)$, with M = 32 being the maximum wrapping found in PDB. Thus, residue i is inferred to be paired by a dehydron if it belongs to the "wrapping-twilight region" $11.6 \leq < w >_i \leq 19.1$ (Fig. 11.4(b))[22].

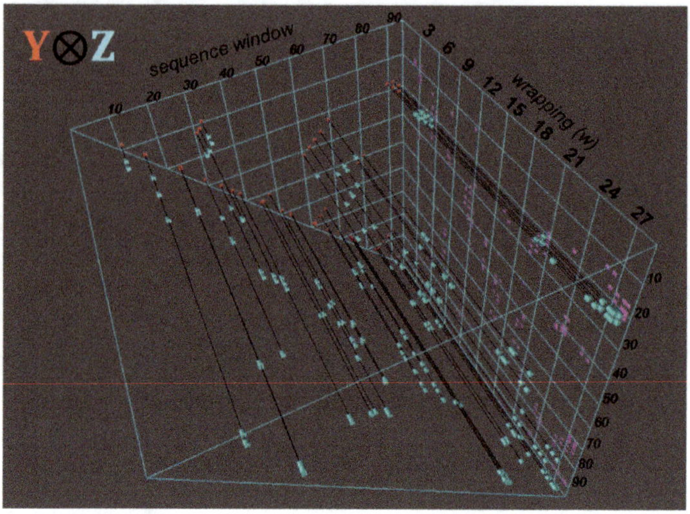

(a)

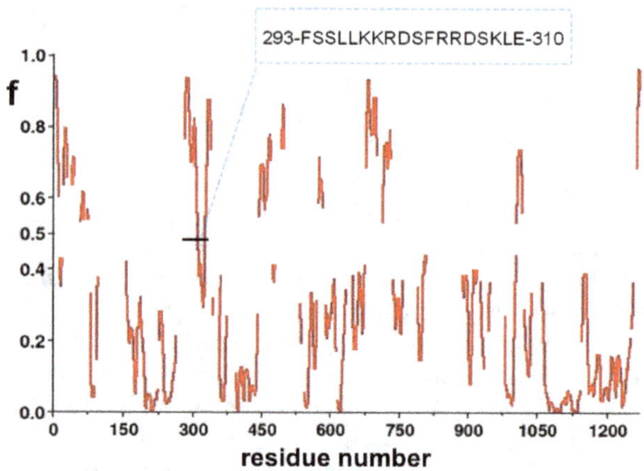

(b)

Figure 11.4. *Tensor representation of learned features and DL output for target MyBP-C sequence.* **(a)** Learned structural/epistructural $\boldsymbol{Y} \otimes \boldsymbol{Z}$ tensor for the testing 96-amino acid sequence in the initial Ig-domain (C0) of MyBP-C. The background matrix ($\boldsymbol{Y}$) features the BHB-paired windows ($\boldsymbol{Y}_{ij}$, red entries), while the learned wrapping vector $\boldsymbol{z}_{ij}$ (light blue entries) for each $\boldsymbol{Y}_{ij}$ is shown along the $\mathbf{Y}$-orthogonal axis. The domain sequence processed is: MPEPGKKPVS AFNKKPRSAE VTAGSAAVFE AETERS-GVKV RWQRDGSDIT ANDKYGLAAE GKRHTLTVRD ASPDDQGSYA VIAGSSKVKF DLKVTE. **(b)** Deep learning output $\langle w \rangle_i$ for $\boldsymbol{x}_i$ sliding along

11.5 Implementing the deep learning system for therapeutic disruption of dysfunctional deregulated protein complexes

The DL algorithm is fully scripted in Python [23] with Tensor Flow [24]. The Python script is run from a PyMol 2.3 platform (Schrödinger, LLC, https://pymol.org/2/) as previously described (https://pymolwiki.org/index.php/Python_Integration), while PyMol exploits the dehydron calculator "Wrappy" as a plugin (Appendix 1). A two-layer network for DL is built and exploited in a drug discovery platform in the absence of structure for large multi-domain target proteins. The DL network architecture enables the processing of input sequence information on the target protein and sustains the tensor flow [sequence-based 1D-input $\rightarrow \boldsymbol{E} \rightarrow \boldsymbol{Y} \otimes \boldsymbol{Z} \rightarrow$ output]. In the first layer (L_1), the information is represented in an evolutionary coupling matrix $\boldsymbol{E} = [\boldsymbol{y}_{ij}]_{ij}$ using the tool CCMPred with default parameters [10]. Sequence alignments were generated with the tool HHBlits [25] using the UNIPROT (February, 2019) sequence library [26], adopting e-value threshold at 0.001, pairwise identity cutoff at 0.99 and minimum coverage of the target sequence at 60%. The network is then trained using ASTRAL structure database [4] filtered for sequences with less than 40% identity and parsed according to a 9:1 training:testing ratio, with no superfamilies intersecting both subsets. Two sequence-derived 1D-features are compounded with amino acid identity and subsequently convoluted with evolutionary correlations for residue pairs in L_1. Given the desired output, the 1D-features chosen are predicted solvent accessibility computed by SOLVPRED

←

Figure 11.4. (*Continued*) the amino acid sequence of MyBP-C represented with sigmoidal function f in Fig. 11.3(b). There is inferred wrapping only for evolutionarily correlated residues learned to be paired by BHBs. The single region in the dehydron twilight $11.6 \leq w \leq 19.1$ is displayed. Reprinted from [Fernández A (2020) Artificial Intelligence Steering Molecular Therapy in the Absence of Information on Target Structure and Regulation. Journal of Chemical Information and Modeling (ACS) 60:460–466] with permission from the American Chemical Society.

and predicted secondary structure, computed by PSIPRED, both run with default parameters [27].

Dehydrons and epistructures are identified from structural coordinates within the PyMol platform using the PyMol plugin [22] (Appendix 1). As described in Chapter 2, we define the extent of hydrogen-bond wrapping, w, indicating the number of sidechain nonpolar groups ($\mathrm{CH_n, n} = 1, 2, 3$) contained within a "desolvation domain" that defines the BHB microenvironment. The desolvation domain is defined as two intersecting balls of fixed radius commensurate with three water layers centered at the α-carbons of the residues paired by the backbone hydrogen bond. A batch-mode wrapping analysis of the PDB (download February 7, 2019) revealed that 86% of backbone hydrogen bonds are wrapped by $\mathrm{w} = 26.6 \pm 7.5$ nonpolar groups for a desolvation ball radius fixed at 6 angstrom. Dehydrons are located in the tails of the distribution, with their desolvation domain containing 19 or fewer nonpolar groups, so their w value is below the mean ($\mathrm{w} = 26.6$) minus one standard deviation. More precisely, to ensure sustainability of the dehydron, the twilight region $11.6 \leq w \leq 19.1$, corresponding to wrapping values in the range of one to two standard deviations below the mean.

By establishing correspondences between evolutionary couplings in $\boldsymbol{E}$ and structural/epistructural data in $\boldsymbol{Y} \otimes \boldsymbol{Z}$ for the training subset, the network learns the relationship between evolutionary coupling and BHB wrapping. The learning process is encoded in the connective weight optimization $\boldsymbol{\theta} = \boldsymbol{\theta}^* = argmin\, J(\boldsymbol{\theta})$, with loss function

$$J(\boldsymbol{\theta}) = \frac{1}{|\wp|} \sum_{\boldsymbol{s}^{(n)} \in \wp} d[\boldsymbol{w}(\boldsymbol{s}^{(n)}), \boldsymbol{w}_{NN}(\boldsymbol{s}^{(n)}, \boldsymbol{\theta})],$$

where $\wp$ denotes training set; $|\wp|$ is the number of elements in the set (cardinal); d indicates Euclidean distance; $\boldsymbol{s}^{(n)}$ is the nth sequence in $\wp$; $\boldsymbol{w}$ is the structure-derived wrapping vector and $\boldsymbol{w}_{NN}$ is the neural network wrapping inference. Thus, the minimization of $J(\boldsymbol{\theta})$ is a least-squares problem numerically solved with stochastic gradient descent. The set $\wp$ is sampled randomly at each iteration to compute the gradient with minibatch size $10^{-3}|\wp|$. To train the network, the

ADADELTA method with learning rate 0.3 is adopted [28]. Full network training is shown in Fig. 11.5, and takes approximately 16 hours on a cluster of 12 Titan RTX GPUs.

To validate and benchmark the DL discovery platform, native structures and structure-derived native wrapping patterns obtained from the ASTRAL-based testing set are contrasted against the neural network inferences generated from the respective primary sequences. To assess accuracy, a distance d between epistructural tensors $\boldsymbol{Y} \otimes \boldsymbol{Z}$ (PDB-derived) and $\boldsymbol{Y_{NN}} \otimes \boldsymbol{Z_{NN}}$ (inferred by the neural network) is introduced. Accordingly, d is defined as

$$
\begin{aligned}
& d(\boldsymbol{Y} \otimes \boldsymbol{Z}, \boldsymbol{Y_{NN}} \otimes \boldsymbol{Z_{NN}}) \\
& = \sum_{i<j} \Bigg\{ Q^{-1}[\Delta_{ij}(\boldsymbol{Y}, \boldsymbol{Y_{NN}})] \\
& \quad + q^{-1}[1 - \Delta_{ij}(\boldsymbol{Y}, \boldsymbol{Y_{NN}})] \frac{|< w >_{NN,ij} - w_{ij}|}{M} \Bigg\},
\end{aligned}
$$

In the equation, Q is the number of BHBs that are either native PDB-reported or nonnative but inferred by the network; $\Delta_{ij}(\boldsymbol{Y}, \boldsymbol{Y_{NN}}) = 0$ if there is a BHB pairing residues i and j in both native ($\boldsymbol{Y}$) and inferred ($\boldsymbol{Y_{NN}}$) structure, while $\Delta_{ij}(\boldsymbol{Y}, \boldsymbol{Y_{NN}}) = 1$ otherwise; $q = \sum_{i<j}[1 - \Delta_{ij}(\boldsymbol{Y}, \boldsymbol{Y_{NN}})]$ is the number of correctly inferred native BHBs; M = 32 is the maximum wrapping in PDB, as previously indicated; w_{ij} is the wrapping of the $i - j$ BHB in the native structure and $< w >_{NN,ij} = \sum_{w=1}^{M} w \frac{A_w(i,j)}{M(i,j)}$, $M(i,j) = \sum_{w=1}^{M} A_w(i,j)$, is the expected wrapping for the $i - j$ BHB inferred by the neural network (notation introduced previously). For each i, j-pair, the term $Q^{-1}\Delta_{ij}(\boldsymbol{Y}, \boldsymbol{Y_{NN}})$ contributes to the structural distance between native and inferred fold, while the second term $q^{-1}[1-\Delta_{ij}(\boldsymbol{Y}, \boldsymbol{Y_{NN}})]\frac{|<w>_{NN,ij}-w_{ij}|}{M}$ measures the wrapping distance between inferred and native structure for a correctly predicted $i - j$ BHB ($\Delta_{ij}(\boldsymbol{Y}, \boldsymbol{Y_{NN}}) = 0$).

To benchmark our method, we note that the epistructural distance between native and inferred fold over the ASTRAL-derived testing set is invariably lower than 2.2% for an optimized

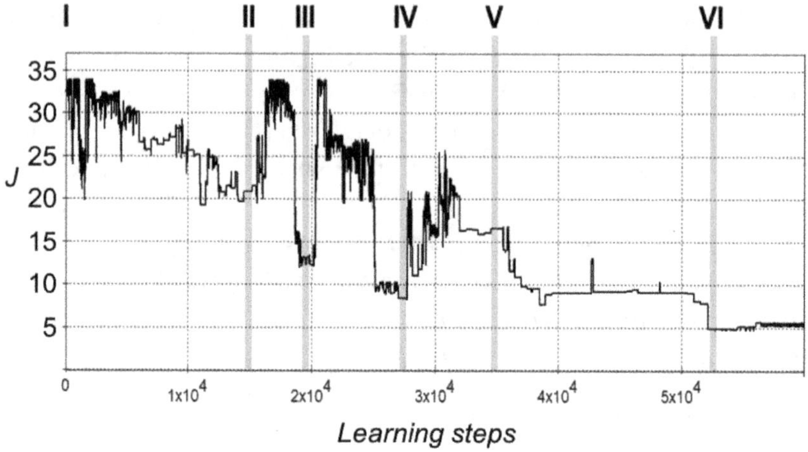

(a)

Figure 11.5. *Network training process.* **(a)** Loss function $J = J(\boldsymbol{\theta})$ with network connection weight vector $\boldsymbol{\theta}$ optimized following stochastic gradient descent. Highlighted bands are regions of suboptimal (II–V) or optimal (VI) stability further examined by structural inference on the testing set adopting the respective parametrizations $\boldsymbol{\theta} = \boldsymbol{\theta}_m$, $m = I, II, \ldots, VI$. **(b)** Contact maps (β-carbon distance <8 Å) for the hyperthermophilic variant of B1 domain in protein G (PDB.1GB4), a member of the testing set, learned from sequence-based evolutionary coupling with network parametrizations $\boldsymbol{\theta} = \boldsymbol{\theta}_m$, $m = I, II, \ldots, VI$. The emergence of the tertiary parallel β-sheet motif (circled) on panel VI is indicative of achieved accuracy, confirmed by comparing the topologies of the learned contact map in panel VI with **(c)**, the native contact map for PDB.1GB4 (same folding topology). **(d)** Ribbon structural renderings of the learning process for test protein 1GB4. Structure in panel VI has backbone RMSD = 1.54 Å relative to the native fold in PDB.1GB4. The upper bound RMSD < 2.45 Å was found to hold across the entire testing set for parametrization $\boldsymbol{\theta} = \boldsymbol{\theta}_{VI}$, while native folding topologies were invariably reproduced, thus validating the machine learning method. **(e)** Learned epistructural tensor $\boldsymbol{Y} \otimes \boldsymbol{Z}$ for the six parametrizations along the learning process. Note that the learned wrapping level for each BHB is not unique, even for the optimized network, an indication of the sparsity of the training set vis-à-vis the dimensionality of the inferential space.

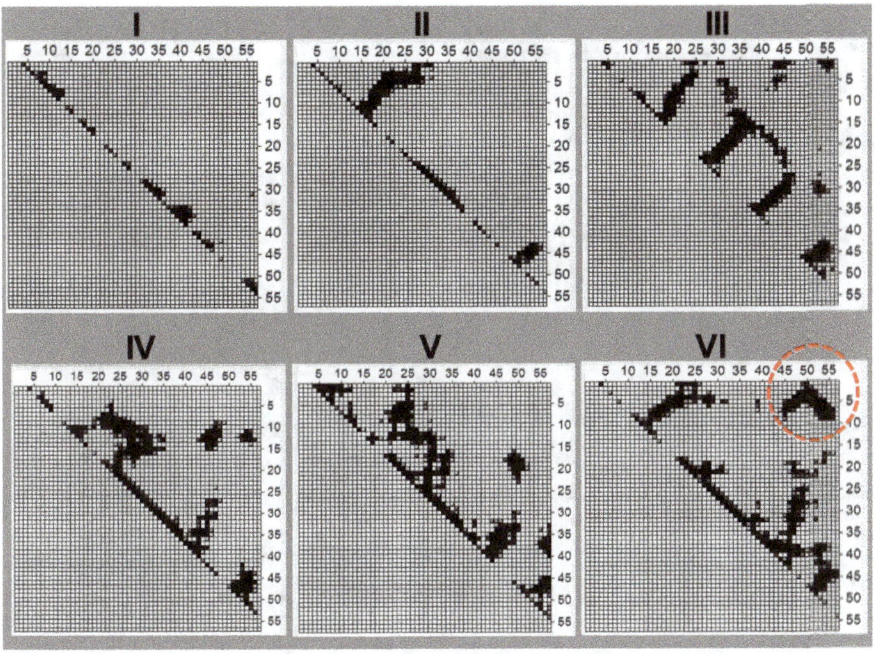

(b)

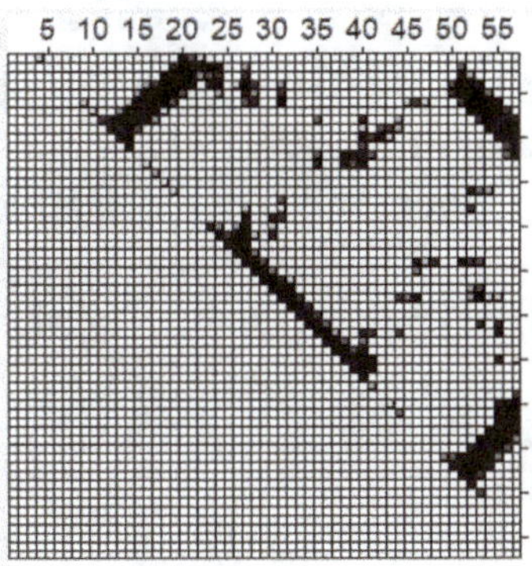

(c)

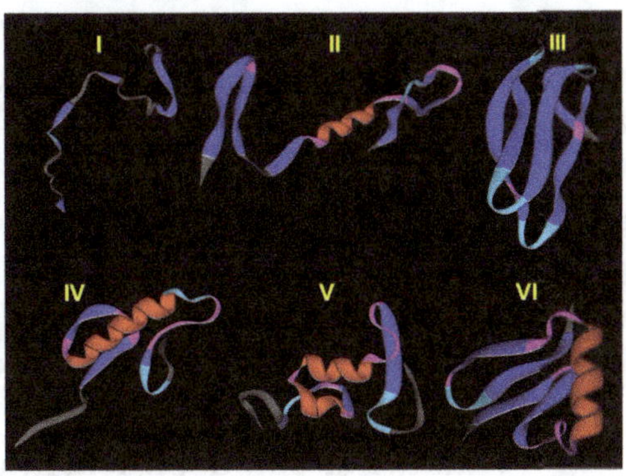

(d)

Figure 11.5. (*Continued*)

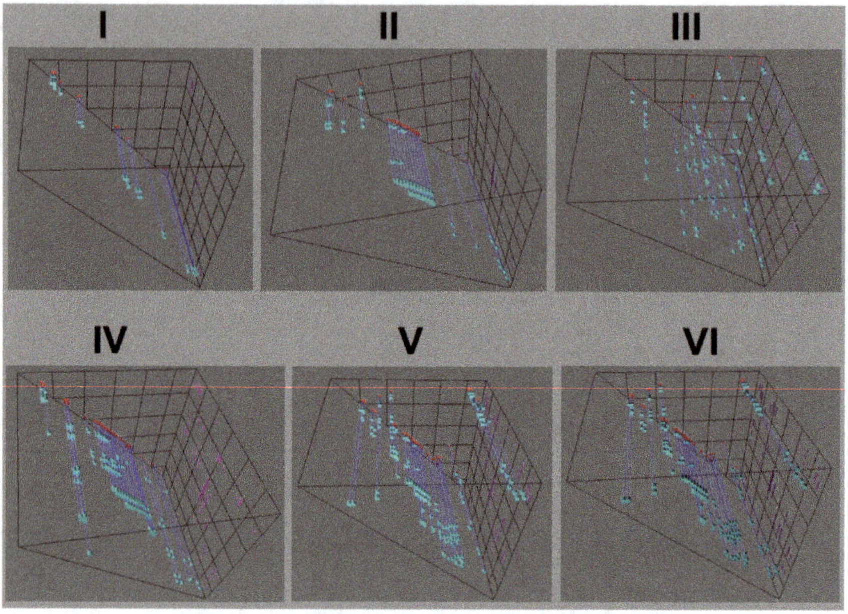

(e)

Figure 11.5. (*Continued*)

parametrization of the network, with mean value at 1.4% (Supporting Information). Of significance, at most 2% of native BHBs may be incorrectly predicted, while in cases where all native BHBs are correctly predicted, at most 1% of dehydrons are incorrectly predicted to be well-wrapped BHBs. These figures attest to the validity of the DL discovery platform.

The validation of the DL discovery platform is given in Fig. 11.6.

11.6 Validating the deep learning platform on molecular targeted therapy for heart failure

The discovery platform is now validated by contrasting the epitope inference against a peptide-based lead adopted to treatment of heart failure [13]. In this therapeutic context, MyBP-C needed to be displaced from a large dysfunctional complex with myosin (Fig. 11.1).

In healthy cardiomyocytes, MyBP-C reduces the speed and strength of contraction by interacting with the myosin S2-region,

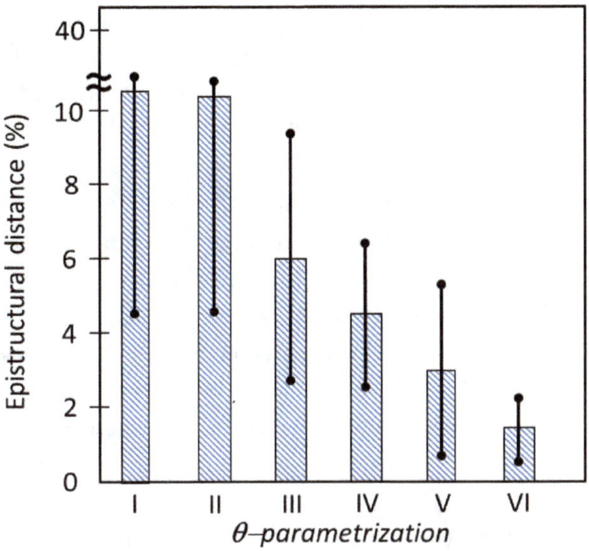

Figure 11.6. *Validation of the DL discovery platform.* Distance between network-inferred epistructure and native epistructure derived from PDB-reported structure from the testing subset. The inferences were made for six parametrizations along the optimization process to minimize the loss function, as shown in Fig. 11.5. The bar indicates mean value while the Gaussian dispersions are indicated by dumbbells. The DL neural network is trained by the PDB-derived ASTRAL dataset filtered for sequences with less than 40% identity and parsed according to a 9:1 training:testing ratio, with no protein superfamilies intersecting both subsets.

thereby decelerating cross-bridge kinetics by reducing the probability of myosin sliding along actin filaments [12,13] (Fig. 11.1). Phosphorylation of MyBP-C by kinases PKA or CAMKII disrupts this interaction and relieves the MyBP-C repressive tethering of myosin. On the other hand, in heart failure, MyBP-C is phosphorylated minimally or not at all due to down-regulation of β-adrenergic receptors. Based on the premise that disruption of the myosin-MyBP-C interface would release the molecular brake on cardiomyocyte contractility (Fig. 11.1), we intend to displace MyBP-C with an optimal MyBP-C-derived peptide that materializes the DL-inferred epitope [13].

The lack of 3D-structure precluded us from addressing design issues regarding the MyBP-C-myosin-S2 interaction, such as induced folding [18], inter-domain cooperativity and epitope-related functionalization of the phosphorylation sites in MyBP-C [21]. These limitations prompted us to discover the protein complex disruptor based on DL inference of the dehydron-rich region in MyBP-C that constitutes the putative S2-myosin-binding site. To predict the peptide sequence, a region was identified in the so-called m-motif between the MyBP-C domains C1 and C2 [12] fully contained in the dehydron twilight zone $11.6 \leq w \leq 19.1$ (Fig. 11.4(b)). This is the only region inferred to be entirely in the wrapping twilight for MyBP-C. Thus, we identified the sequence of peptide ($_{293}$FSSLLKKRDSFRRDSKLF$_{310}$) that may be adopted, after S302A replacement to prevent phosphorylation, as emergency therapeutic agent to treat heart failure with administration *in situ*. The peptide shows significant increase in cardiac contractile force and frequency in the failing heart [13]. *Ex-vivo* experiments reveal that, upon peptide treatment, the contractile force in compromised cardiac tissue is restored to 82% of the force in normal tissue, compared with 44% in untreated compromised tissue. On the other hand, the rate of development of the contractile force is restored to 84% levels, compared with 22% for untreated compromised tissue [13].

We have highlighted the power of artificial intelligence (AI) to guide therapeutic interventions in clinical settings where a clear molecular understanding of the dysfunctionality is lacking.

Drug-based disruptions of PPIs in large dysfunctional complexes represent therapeutic opportunities but pose great challenges, as ligands are required to displace binding partners with extensive interfaces. The problem becomes daunting because the structure of the protein complex and its regulated modulation are frequently unknown and the complex often has insufficient homologs to build a reliable model of the PPI. To address the challenge, we developed a DL platform trained with big data on structural defects in proteins. These defects are known to cause interfacial tension [5, 18] and to constitute regulatory elements [21]. The network exploits sequence-based input and learns to draw a relationship between evolutionarily coupled residues, epistructural features and regions that promote water exclusion through protein-protein association, ultimately becoming capable of inferring phosphorylation-modulated binding epitopes.

This chapter thus paves the way to an expansion of the technological base for rational drug design. The developments are particularly suited to therapeutic contexts where target structure and detailed information on regulation of target activity are missing or underreported.

The DL discovery platform implemented in this work enabled focusing on some of the most challenging cases, involving the identification of molecular disruptors of dysfunctional PPIs, whose recruitment is conducive to disease. The neural network uses sequence-derived 1D-input, gets trained on evolutionary and structural PDB data, and generates epistructural information that leads to the identification of binding regions susceptible of phosphorylation-based regulation. These regions generate interfacial tension and functionalize nearby phosphorylation-susceptible side chains, thus, they become essential to create peptide-based PPI disruptors within a rational discovery effort. The discovery is made possible because epistructural information or the structure-solvent dynamic relationship, is encoded in structural information which the network is able to infer from 1D sequence-based input. At a preliminary level, the DL discovery platform is benchmarked by establishing the accuracy of epistructural inference on a PDB-derived testing set. Subsequently, the DL platform is validated through the identification of the clinically competent peptide-based disruptor of the deregulated MyBP-C-myosin complex that gets recruited in heart failure. The therapeutic efficacy of this peptide-based pharmaceutical has been previously established but the discovery pathway that led to its identification was not revealed in the patent where the invention is described [13].

11.7 AI unravels patterns of biological cooperativity

There are obviously many ways in which artificial intelligence (AI) is likely to broaden the technological base of the pharmaceutical industry. Applications of AI that involve the parsing of the vast chemical space are already being implemented. This book takes a complementary view and advocates that the true game change comes with AI-steered solutions to core problems in biophysics that are intimately related to drug discovery and development. These problems share a common challenge: understanding and controlling cooperativity, a hallmark of biological processes and drug-target associations. A take-home lesson from this book is that drug design guided by engineering pairwise interactions across a putative drug-target interface is not likely to be successful. Drug designers are actually faced with a many-body problem, where correlations are indicative of cooperativity and cooperative patterns need to be exploited because they represent filters for drug specificity while giving the complete more accurate picture of drug-target complexation. Thus, the designers need to master this aspect if their compounds are expected to withstand the long-term attrition along the discovery pipeline. This closing informal section, tailored as a short essay, argues that precisely because cooperativity can be cast in tensor format, AI is likely to play a decisive role in unravelling and predicting patterns of cooperativity at molecular scales, hence transforming, hopefully revolutionizing, pharma as we know it.

Broad examination of biomolecular architectures in aqueous media reveals a stunning complexity, where the structural determinants are hydrogen bonds (HBs) pairing identifiable fixed partnering groups. This observation has turned into a *leitmotif* in the organization of information in structural biology, particularly when dealing with protein folding, binding-induced folding, protein complexation and protein-ligand binding. However, it has been argued, particularly in the preparatory Chapter 2, that the potential energy function governing such interactions is not additive and thus cannot be accurately described as sums of pairwise contributions. The exclusion of water, partial or complete, from the surroundings of a HB is essential to warrant its stability and strength and this fact alone signals that we are dealing with a many-body problem underlying a highly cooperative process: no pairwise interaction *per se* is likely to prevail unless it forms cooperatively so as to stay "dry in water". We may say that in this picture, protein folding, binding-induced folding and complexation may be regarded as "struggles for the survival of HBs".

Cast more rigorously, protein structure in water is only sustainable if backbone HBs are shielded from the disruptive hydration of amide and carbonyl groups. As described in chapters 2,4, this implies that the structure must often rely on binding partnerships to maintain its integrity. This is the case, for example, with the binding-induced folding of transcription factors, which are autonomously incapable of folding into stable conformations. In other instances delineated in chapter 4, the soluble structure is autonomously untenable due to backbone exposure and the protein misfolds into a conformation that can only be stabilized at high concentrations through aggregation, as it is the case in degenerative neuropathies with an aberrant protein aggregation ethiology.

We are clearly dealing with a many-body problem: The concurrence of additional groups is required to shield a pairwise electrostatic interaction from the bond-debilitating dielectric modulation and the disruptive effect of amide and carbonyl hydration. These patterns are in fact three-body correlations that bespeak of a cooperative process of structure formation: Secondary structure cannot form incrementally but needs either tertiary-structure buttressing or exogenous protection, as in protein complexes. This shielding from water is what we have named and quantified as *wrapping* (chapter 2). Adopting a metaphoric language, the non-additivity of the potential energy indicates that “the whole is actually more than the sum of the parts”, while protein folding is reminiscent of Rubik's cube moves, where the solver does not work on one face at time but on all of them at once when deciding each move.

Let us illustrate this elusive aspect of Nature's architecture. An exhaustive cross-examination of the PDB and the sequence-based predicted propensity for structural disorder reveals that folding cooperativity is nowhere more apparent than in ubiquitin (PDB.1UBI). The reported structure features a cleanly formed helix spanning residues 22 to 35 (Fig. 11.7). By contrast, predictors of native disorder (PONDR) indicate inherent disorder for the 22–35 region (Fig. 11.8), clearly at odds with the structural data. This clash suggests a highly cooperative process that cannot be captured by the locality of the disorder prediction. The predictor slides a window along the protein sequence and draws accordingly the plot

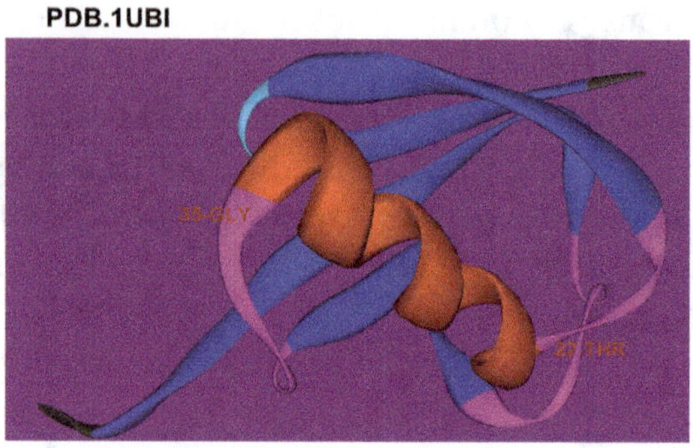

Figure 11.7. Ribbon rendering of the structure for human ubiquitin as reported in PDB entry 1UBI.

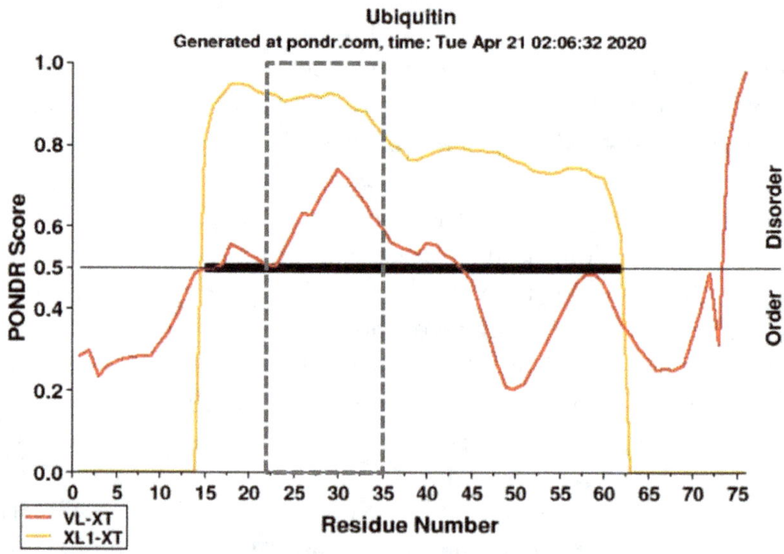

Figure 11.8. Two sequence-based predictions of intrinsic disorder for ubiquitin obtained from PONDR (http://www.pondr.com/). The dashed rectangle marks the sequence window 22–35, known to be helical but predicted to be disordered.

of disorder propensities (Fig. 11.8). Indeed, a profusion of three-body correlations with distant non-helical residues (Figs. 11.9, 11.10) reveals a highly cooperative shielding of backbone HBs in the helix region (22–35) that would be otherwise unsustainable in water.

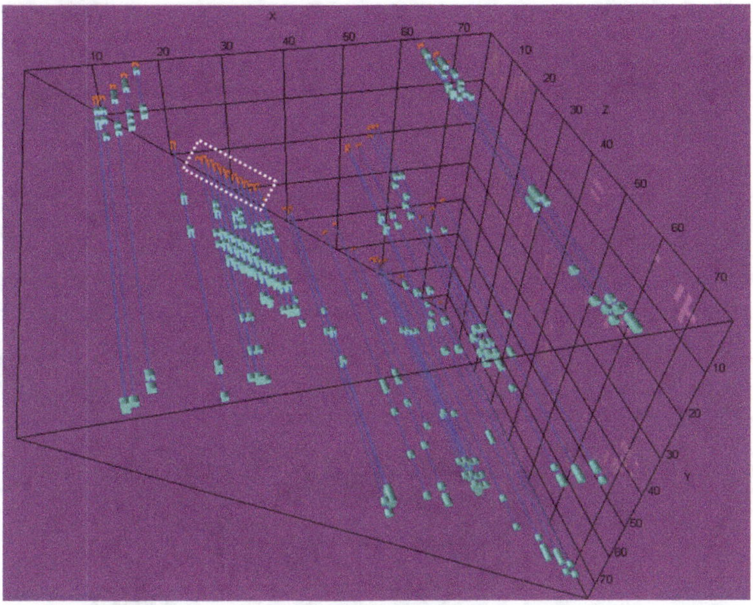

Figure 11.9. Wrapping tensor for ubiquitin structure. The dashed rectangle highlights the highly cooperative helical region 22–35.

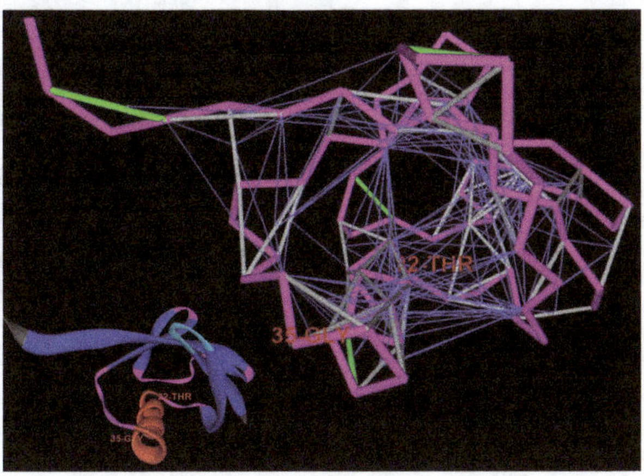

Figure 11.10. Wrapping pattern for helix 22–35. The profusion of three-body correlations involving distant non-helical residues indicates that the helix forms in a highly cooperative way.

As shown in this chapter, AI is instrumental to capture such cooperative patterns, classify them and accordingly organize structural information. Telling evidence based on analysis of the connectivity parameters for the dilated convolutional neural network (CNN) described in this chapter supports this assertion. In fact, all the 3-body correlations involving backbone HBs in the ubiquitin 22–35 helix represented in the wrapping tensor (Fig. 11.9) are actually contained in the optimized convolution kernels or filters adopted by the deep learning system for feature extraction in sequence-based inference of induced folding. To represent this assertion, three body

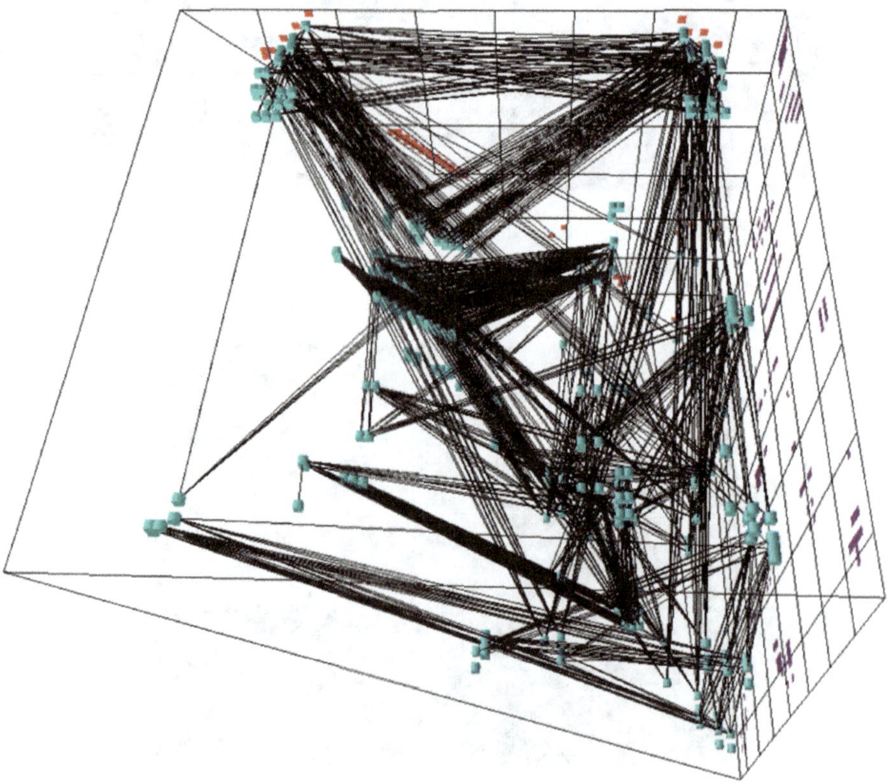

Figure 11.11. The convolution kernels in the dilated CNN for the deep learning system displayed on the ubiquitin wrapping tensor. Two three-body correlations are linked by a black line if they belong to the same optimized filter in the feature-extraction phase. Thus, the most highly cooperative patterns had been captured by the deep learning system.

correlations were linked in the 3D wrapping tensor whenever they were contained in the same filter in the dilated CNN. Thus, as shown in Fig. 11.11, the wrapping three-body correlations in the most highly cooperative helix in the PDB have all been inferred independently by AI, since they are all contained in the filters of the dilated CNN that have evolved to perform the optimal feature extraction.

This analysis is indicative of the power of AI to identify patterns of cooperativity, hence unraveling a major hallmark of biomolecular processes and drug-target associations. This instills confidence that the true game change in pharmaceutical discovery may be within arm's reach.

References

1. Scott DE, Bayly AR, Abell C, Skidmore J (2016) Small molecules, big targets: Drug discovery faces the protein-protein interaction challenge. *Nat Rev Drug Discov* 15:533–550.
2. Li Z, Ivanov AA, Su R, Gonzalez-Pecchi V, Qi Q, *et al.* (2017) The OncoPPi network of cancer-focused protein–protein interactions to inform biological insights and therapeutic strategies. *Nature Comm* 8:14356.
3. Sejnowski TJ (2018) The Deep Learning Revolution. MIT Press, Cambridge.
4. Fox NK, Brenner SE, Chandonia JM (2013) SCOPe: Structural classification of proteins — extended, integrating SCOP and ASTRAL data and classification of new structures. *Nucleic Acids Res* 42:D304–D309.
5. Fernández A (2012) Epistructural tension promotes protein associations. *Phys Rev Lett* 108:188102.
6. Jones D, Singh T, Kosciolek T, Tetchner S (2015) MetaPSICOV: Combining coevolution methods for accurate prediction of contacts and long range hydrogen bonding in proteins. *Bioinformatics* 31:999–1006.
7. Gao M, Zhou H, Skolnick J (2019) DESTINI: A deep learning approach to contact-driven protein structure prediction. *Scientific Reports* 9:3514.
8. Wang S, Sun S, Li Z, Zhang R, Xu J (2017) Accurate de novo prediction of protein contact map by ultra-deep learning model. *PLoS Comput Biol* 13:e1005324.
9. Liu Y, Palmedo P, Ye Q, Berger B, Peng J (2018) Enhancing evolutionary couplings with deep convolutional neural networks. *Cell Syst* 6:65–74.e63.
10. Seemayer S, Gruber M, Soding J (2014) CCMpred — fast and precise prediction of protein residue-residue contacts from correlated mutations. *Bioinformatics* 30:3128–3130.
11. Fernández A, Scheraga HA (2013) Insufficiently dehydrated hydrogen bonds as determinants of protein interactions. *Proc Natl Acad Sci USA* 100:113–118.

12. Kensler RW, Craig R, Moss RL (2017) Phosphorylation of cardiac myosin binding protein C releases myosin heads from the surface of cardiac thick filaments. *Proc Natl Acad Sci USA* 114:E1355–E1364.
13. Moss RL, Fernandez A (2015) Inhibition of MyBP-C binding to myosin as a treatment for heart failure. United States Patent 9051387.
14. Arkin MR, Tang Y, Wells JA (2014) Small-molecule inhibitors of protein–protein interactions: Progressing toward the reality. *Chem Biol* 21:1102–1114.
15. Pelay-Gimeno M, Glas A, Koch O, Grossmann TN (2015) Structure-based design of inhibitors of protein–protein interactions: Mimicking peptide binding epitopes. *Angew Chem Int Ed Engl* 54:8896–8927.
16. Wang J, Cao H, Zhang J, Qi Y (2018) Computational protein design with deep learning neural networks. *Scientific Reports* 8:6349.
17. Chen H, Engkvist O, Wang Y, Olivecrona M, Blaschke T (2018) The rise of deep learning in drug discovery. *Drug Discovery Today* 23:1241–1250.
18. Fernández A (2016) Physics at the Biomolecular Interface; Springer, Berlin.
19. Fernández A, Rogale K, Scott LR, Scheraga HA (2004) Inhibitor design by wrapping packing defects in HIV-1 proteins. *Proc Natl Acad Sci USA* 101: 11640–11645.
20. Fernández A (2018) Stickiness of the hydrogen bond. *Ann Phys (Berlin)* 530:1800162.
21. Fernández A (2014) Communication: Chemical functionality of interfacial water enveloping nanoscale structural defects in proteins. *J Chem Phys* 140:221102.
22. Martin O (2014) Wrappy: A dehydron calculator plugin for PyMOL. MIT License, 2014 http://www.pymolwiki.org/index.php/dehydron.
23. Ketkar N (2017) Deep Learning with Python. Apress, Berkeley, CA.
24. Rampasek L, Goldenberg A (2016) Tensor flow: Biology's gateway to deep learning. *Cell Sys* 2:12–14.
25. Remmert M, Biegert A, Hauser A, Söding J (2011) HHblits: Lightning-fast iterative protein sequence searching by HMM-HMM alignment. *Nature Methods* 9:173–175.
26. The UniProt Consortium (2019) UniProt: A worldwide hub of protein knowledge. *Nucleic Acids Res* 47:D506–515.
27. Jones DT, Kandathil SM (2018) High precision in protein contact prediction using fully convolutional neural networks and minimal sequence feature. *Bioinformatics* 34:3308–3315.
28. Zeiler MD (2012) ADADELTA, an adaptive learning rate method. arXiv: 1212.5701 https://arxiv.org/abs/1212.5701.

Chapter 12

Artificial intelligence teaches drugs to target proteins by solving the drug-induced folding problem

Suppose someone were to say "Imagine this butterfly exactly as it is, but ugly instead of beautiful."

Ludwig Wittgenstein

In this chapter we implement a deep learning (DL) platform that teaches drugs to target proteins. This is accomplished by introducing chemical scaffold modifications steered by *a priori* predictions of drug-induced binding-competent conformations of the intended target. In this way, we deal with the fact that target proteins are usually not fixed targets fitting the lock-key paradigm: they structurally adapt to ligands in ways that need to be predicted to empower drug discovery. In contrast with protein folding predictors that do not include disorder propensities as input, the neural network presented solves a "drug-induced folding problem" by incorporating as input sequence-derived signals for structural disorder. The DL system thus predicts conformations in floppy regions of the target protein that rely on associations with a conformation-selecting purposely designed drug to acquire and maintain their structural integrity. This is tantamount to generate within an AI-empowered drug discovery platform the *a-priori* drug-induced folding ensemble without committing to a specific ligand and then steer the modification of a lead compound to select a specific drug-induced conformation from within the ensemble.

12.1 The "drug-induced protein folding problem" in drug design

Deep learning (DL) methods are showing striking progress towards solving the protein folding problem [1, 2]. In particular, a machine learning system named AlphaFold [1] (Deep Mind Technologies, UK) has proven most successful at predicting the 3D structure of autonomous protein folders based solely on sequence-derived input. AlphaFold fulfills a major imperative since elucidation of structure is essential to infer protein function, while the determination of protein structure quite often eludes the experimental methods available [1]. In this chapter we adapt the AlphaFold platform *mutatis-mutandis* to a different set of needs related to drug design, i.e. we shall attempt to solve what we hereby name the "*drug-induced protein folding problem*". This task confronts us with the fact that target proteins are typically not fixed targets: they structurally adapt to the man-made ligand in ways that need to be predicted to empower pharmaceutical discovery. In stark contrast with AlphFold which predicts structure for autonomous folders, we aim at predicting structures that only form and prevail within obligatory drug-target complexes, that is, structures for non-autonomous folders. The goal is to instruct drug design to target specific conformations that are *a-priori* predicted to rely on association with the purposely designed drug to maintain their structural integrity. This is tantamount to adapt to AlphaFold platform *mutatis-mutandis* to solve the drug-induced folding problem.

We can anticipate that AlphaFold *per se* cannot be put to good use in this context, simply because it does not incorporate 1D information that would signal regions susceptible to structural adaptation as the drug-target complex is formed. We need to incorporate disorder propensities in the 1D-input, and not just any flavor of disorder — for example, we don't care for regions that may represent merely a storage of conformational entropy — but rather disordered regions susceptible to turn into order upon binding. Metaphorically speaking, we are interested in incorporating signals for regions that represent "tame" as opposed to "wild" disorder.

To effectively incorporate these "tamed disorder signals" into an AlphaFold-derived platform we first briefly revisit the AlphaFold architecture and workflow. AlphaFold trains with PDB-reported structures a multilayered convolutional neural network (CNN) [3], the architectural scaffold for feature extraction, and generates 3D-structure models that fit accurate predictions of distances between residue pairs. Such predictions are based on information that quantifies pairwise evolutionary correlations [4] organized in a 2D-array. The underlying premise for this representation is that the co-evolution of two residues within a multiple sequence alignment signals that they are spatially related. The co-evolution matrix elements are concatenated with residue profiling including amino acid identity and secondary structure prediction, *but no sequence-based prediction of disorder propensity.* The latter signals would be conflictive with overlapping secondary structure prediction and with the purview of the CNN. In fact, if disorder propensities are directly incorporated they would clash along the feature-extraction phase in ways that would render the predictor ineffectual, as folding possibilities would be overwritten by disorder output or *vice-versa.* Local propagation of distance constraints from one layer to the next is achieved via progressively dilated convolutional operations [5] where suitably chosen convolution kernels or "filters" allow incorporation of features not just from neighbors of a pixel but also from further afield, incorporating surrounding context by expanding the receptive field of the convolution stencils.

12.2 Drug targets are moving targets: The induced folding problem and the design of conformation-selecting chemical scaffolds

Protein structure prediction assumes that the chain will adopt a 3D structure and that the structure is unique [1, 2]. Since AlphaFold is concerned with the endpoint and not with the folding process, it is immaterial whether or not the folding process can be successfully completed *in vitro*, i.e. without the assistance of a cellular annealing, chaperone and scaffolding apparatus. AlphaFold may well be successful at predicting structure of proteins that fold *in vivo* and are selected to fold only *in vivo*. On the other hand, molecular dynamics efforts towards elucidating the folding trajectories have been invariably misplaced because they have only dealt with the *in vitro* context, at least up to this day.

In practice, many proteins cannot fold autonomously and the structure is not unique but dependent on binding partnerships, reliant on such associations to acquire and maintain its integrity [6]. In fact, the binding context typically selects the protein fold from within an ensemble of closely related folding possibilities that we hereby name the induced folding ensemble (IFE). For example, proteins such as transcription factors typically possess only induced structure, that is, their fold cannot prevail in an "apo" (separated) form [7], antibodies usually present antigen-induced conformational multiplicity [8], while proteins which constitute drug targets often have a variety of "holo" (within-complex) forms, depending on the ligand/drug they associate with [9]. These considerations imply that AlphFold by itself is ill equipped at dealing with folding context or folding-upon-binding scenario, which is precisely the scenario of interest to the drug designer. Thus, the pressing issue becomes, how do we modify or extend AlphaFold to encompass such possibilities?

This issue constitutes the focus of this chapter and may be illustrated by the structural diversity of the stress-responsive molecular chaperone Hsp90 [10], a cancer target that adopts different structures depending on the drug-target complex (Fig. 12.1(a)). This type of induced folding diversity should prompt rational drug designers to focus on inferring the target's IFE, rather than a unique 3D-structure, probably only suitable for autonomous folders [11] forming nonobligatory or ephemeral complexes. Thus, efforts in structure-based drug design are often marred by the need to encompass the target structural adaptation [8, 9]. Obviously, the IFE concept shifts the focus of structure prediction, especially of DL prediction, that must be adapted to infer *a-priori* holo forms, introducing significant complications. Here we propose a DL scheme to enable IFE prediction of pharmaceutically relevant holo forms, geared

(a)

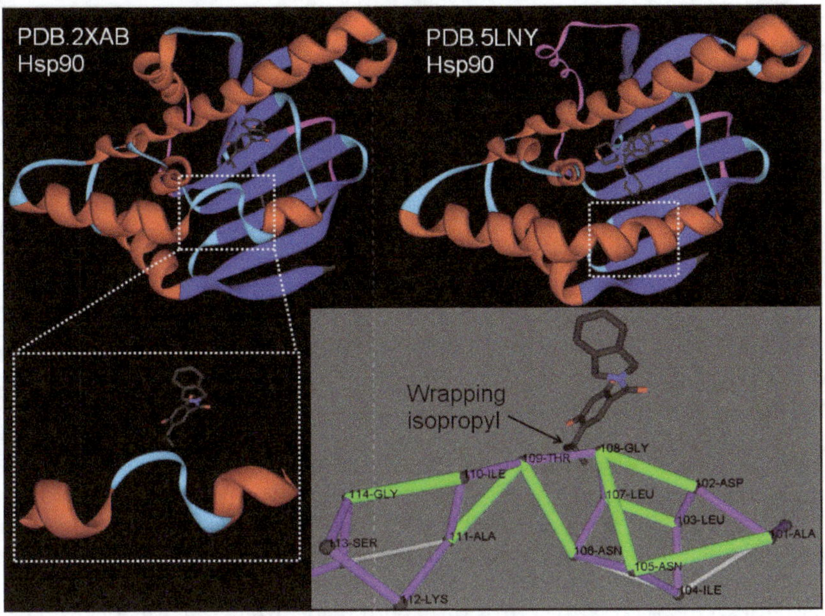

(b)

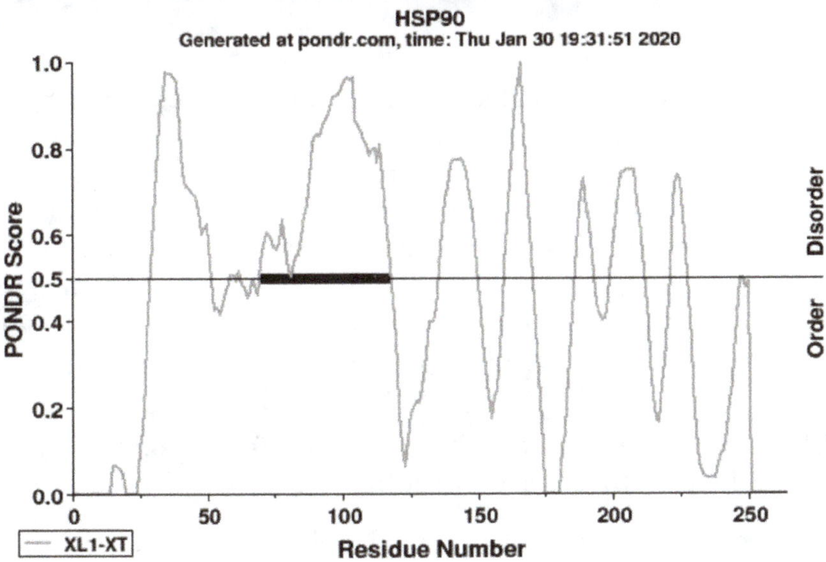

Figure 12.1. (*Continued*)

Figure 12.1. Conformational diversity of "*holo* forms" for cancer target Hsp90 induced by different drug ligands resulting from the intrinsic disorder propensity of a region in the protein, as the region is reliant on binding partnerships to maintain structural integrity. **(a)** The 100–120 helix in Hsp90 gets distorted, developing a kink as the ligand in the complex PDB.5LNY gets replaced for that in PDB.2XAB. The helical region has a disorder propensity which translates into susceptibility to fold into a binding-induced conformation that varies according to the ligand. The ligand in PDB.2XAB has a protruding isopropyl group capable of exogenously contributing to the wrapping of the dehydron-rich helix kink, specifically wrapping the dehydrons T109-A111 and N106-T109. In this way the ligand determines or selects the binding-competent induced folding. BHBs are indicated as lines joining the α-carbons of the protein backbone, with well wrapped bonds marked in grey and dehydrons in green. For the computation of BHB wrapping and identification of dehydrons, the reader may consult [12–14]. **(b)** Sequence-based prediction of intrinsic disorder for Hsp90 regarded as an autonomous folder. The disorder plot was generated by the Predictor of Native Disorder (PONDR®), [15], freely accessible from http://www.pondr.com/. Reprinted from [Fernández A (2020) Perspective: Artificial intelligence teaches drugs to target proteins by tackling the induced folding problem". Molecular Pharmaceutics (ACS) 17:2761–2767] with permission from the American Chemical Society.

at tackling the "drug-induced folding problem", possibly the next frontier for a rational drug designer involved in lead optimization.

In this chapter the AI predictions of IFEs are validated in two ways: a) vis-à-vis experimental evidence on the conformation-selective power of AI-steered drug design; b) through the generation of the predicted drug-induced conformation via an AI-empowered MD simulation that captures the structural adaptation of the target protein concurrent with formation of the drug/target complex.

12.3 Deep learning architecture to infer targetable drug-induced protein folds

The induced folding of the protein target implies that the protein relies on binding partnerships to acquire and maintain its structural integrity [6–9] with the ligand/drug selecting a conformation from within the IFE. Thus, delineating a suitable CNN architecture for the DL predictor of the IFE requires that we first identify the culprit for the lack of structural integrity of a free protein chain. Reviewing material from the introductory chapters, we learned that backbone hydrogen bonds (BHBs) are determinants of protein structure, and hence hydration of backbone amides and carbonyls competes with intramolecular hydrogen bond formation, exerting a structure-disruptive effect. An autonomous folder [11] is thus cable by itself of shielding or wrapping most BHBs from the disruptive effects of backbone hydration. Thus, protein integrity may be said to be contingent on the structure, by itself or within a complex, being capable of preventing backbone hydration. This leads us to propose wrapping as a descriptor of the degree of autonomy of the protein fold (or its degree of reliance on binding partnerships) [12,13]. As we have established in the introductory chapters, an underwrapped BHB constitutes a structural defect, known as dehydron [13], possessing an insufficient number of side-chain nonpolar groups clustered around the BHB, so that dehydrons are exposed to structure-disruptive hydration [6,7,12,13]. An extended underwrapped region (dehydron cluster) has a high propensity to be disordered [7] in the *apo* form, since backbone hydration is likely to prevail over structure formation. Thus, induced folding may be interpreted as the optimal structural adaptation to a binding ligand to ensure the maximum shielding of underwrapped regions, thereby contributing to the stabilization of a specific *holo* form.

As shown in the introductory chapters, dehydrons and wrapping may be computed from structural coordinates of proteins [6,7,12,13] and the computation may be incorporated in the feature-extraction workflow of the DL platform [14]. To that end, we introduce the extent of hydrogen-bond wrapping, w, indicative of the number of sidechain nonpolar groups contained within a "desolvation domain" that defines the BHB microenvironment in a training reported structure. Being marginally wrapped, dehydrons are located in the tail of the distribution of w-values across BHBs in the structural database. The dehydrons in protein structure compromise its integrity and promote protein associations as a means to exclude surrounding water. In this way, dehydrons become determinants for protein association because, by decreasing charge screening, exogenous removal of water from the dehydron microenvironment strengthens and stabilizes the electrostatic interaction that underlies the BHB. Ample bioinformatics evidence on the distribution of dehydrons at interfaces of protein complexes supports this picture [13], pointing to dehydrons as key factors driving complex formation, with dehydron-rich regions being flexible and hence susceptible of undergoing binding-induced folding [9]. To illustrate this picture, the Hsp90 helical 101–128 region in the complex reported in PDB entry 5LNY becomes disrupted when Hsp90 forms a different complex (PDB.2XAB), as shown in Fig. 12.1(a). The structural difference arises as a kink forms with dehydrons N106-T109 and T109-A111, which in turn get exogenously wrapped by the protruding isopropyl group in the drug inhibitor that binds Hsp90 in the complex reported in PDB.2XAB. As the example suggests, the *a-priori* inference of induced folding states would be essential for a rational drug designer, seeking to control drug affinity and specificity through lead optimization to select the *holo* form from within the IFE.

The previous discussion suggests that leveraging a DL platform to predict induced conformations hinges on a wrapping representation of the protein chain in the feature extraction phase. The structure wrapping must lend itself to a tensor representation wherein information is describable and processed on a multidimensional array (tensor) of digital entries within a layered architecture. Thus, the steering of the drug design process to target a binding-competent induced fold involves the inference of the IFE using as input the primary sequence of the target protein. This task requires an adaptation of the AlphaFold platform to incorporate the following elements:

1) In contrast with AlphaFold and other structure predictors, residues need to be profiled incorporating a key additional signal: the sequence-based prediction of intrinsic disorder, a descriptor of the propensity of a window along the chain to be inherently unstructured as the protein is taken in isolation, i.e., as an autonomous folder [15, 16]. The disorder score ranges from 1 (certainty of disorder) to zero (certainty of order). Regions predicted to be disordered

are expected to be reliant on binding partnerships to improve the wrapping of BHBs to the point where they can be sustainable [6, 7]. *Thus, the disorder score signal needs to be integrated in the residue profiling for a sequence-based inference of the IFE.* A clear illustration is provided by the induced folding diversity in Hsp90: the predicted helicity of the region 100–120 (Fig. 12.1(a)) is partially overlapping with an overwriting signal of intrinsic disorder for the region 80–114 (Fig. 12.1(b)). This is a clear indication that the helix would be partially unsustainable if the protein is regarded as an autonomous folder, and can be partially disrupted or distorted by induced folding depending on the ligand, as it is indeed the case in the overlapping region 100–114 (Fig. 12.1(a)). Thus, a kink is induced in the predicted helical region, whereby non helical dehydrons N106-T109 and T109-A111 are formed and become sustainable as they get wrapped exogenously by the isopropyl group in the Hsp90-binding ligand reported in PDB.2XAB.

The overlapping conflictive signals described above inform us that the disorder score cannot be simply incorporated as input representation into the AlphaFold platform but requires an architectural modification of the underlying CNN to be adequately processed during the feature-extraction phase.

2) Residues paired by BHBs are represented within a triangular 2D-array (the information plotted is symmetric) inputted with pairwise co-evolutionary information [3, 4]. The underlying premise is that if the evolution of two residues correlates across a multiple sequence alignment, it is likely that they are spatially related. The array is concatenated with residue profiling in the same way as it is done in AlphaFold, except for the incorporation of the local disorder propensity as an overwriting signal.

3) In contrast with AlphaFold, a third dimension is needed to identify the residues wrapping the BHBs that will emerge during the feature extraction phase of DL [13, 14]. Thus, wrapping components are identified upon the structural information within a 3D-tensor whereby a matrix $\boldsymbol{Y}$, evolving from the evolutionary coupling matrix (ECM), is constructed to ultimately indicate residues (i, j) paired

by BHBs, while the wrapping of the BHBs is represented along $\boldsymbol{Y}$-orthogonal vector $\boldsymbol{z}_{ij}$ for entry $\boldsymbol{Y}_{ij}$. Thus, the DL flow operates on the tetrahedral N$\times$N$\times$N tensor $\boldsymbol{Y}\otimes\boldsymbol{Z} = [\boldsymbol{Y}_{ij}\otimes\boldsymbol{Z}_{ij}]_{ij}$ (N = chain length).

4) Feature extraction requires a dilated convolutional layered architecture [1, 3] where in a generic layer denoted F, the convolutional kernel becomes a $3 \times 3 \times 3$ tetrahedral tensor ($\boldsymbol{F}$) that evolves during the parameter optimization process turning into a filter. This filter extracts a structural pattern drawn from the training set in a curated PDB-derived database [14]. The product of the convolutional operation $(\boldsymbol{Y} \otimes \boldsymbol{Z})*\boldsymbol{F}$ is thus a tensor with entries indicating sums of entry-by-entry multiplication (Frobenius inner product) of $\boldsymbol{Y} \otimes \boldsymbol{Z}$ by tensor $\boldsymbol{F}$ as the latter slides along $3 \times 3 \times 3$ tetrahedral sectors of $\boldsymbol{Y} \otimes \boldsymbol{Z}$ with stride 2 to produce the (N-2)^3 convolved tensor $[\widehat{\boldsymbol{Y} \otimes \boldsymbol{Z}}]_F = (\boldsymbol{Y} \otimes \boldsymbol{Z})*\boldsymbol{F}$. Thus, large value entries in the convolved tensor are indicative of regions where the configuration more clearly resembles the kernel/filter. Within the F-layer, the convolved tensor $[\widehat{\boldsymbol{Y} \otimes \boldsymbol{Z}}]_F$ is expanded into the "F-feature-discerning" N^3-tensor $(\boldsymbol{Y} \otimes \boldsymbol{Z})_F$ by spanning the F-pattern for the largest value entries in $[\widehat{\boldsymbol{Y} \otimes \boldsymbol{Z}}]_F$ while retaining the original entries from $\boldsymbol{Y} \otimes \boldsymbol{Z}$ for those $3 \times 3 \times 3$ tetrahedral sectors that don't yield a significant inner product. The F-filter is then dilated within a F-spanned multilayered architecture to incorporate surrounding context by enlarging the receptive field size of the convolution kernel. In this way, we incorporate features not just from pixel neighbors but from further afield by creating $3 \times 3 \times 3$ tetrahedral filters with the pixels further and further apart. Thus, each neuron in a hidden layer only receives input from the local region of what the input to the layer is, and with the dilations we enlarge the receptive field of the convolution kernel. So the hidden layer for filter F is actually spanning a bunch of hidden layers where the dilated filters $F_1 = F, F_2, F_3, \ldots$ are successively applied, with the subindex giving the value of the dilation coefficient.

5) The training of the CNN enables optimization of the set of filters $F = \{F^{(1)}, F_2^{(1)}, \ldots, F^{(2)}, F_2^{(2)}, \ldots\}$ by minimizing the sum

of Frobenius norms ($\|.\|$, sum of squared entries) for tensors $\boldsymbol{Y} \otimes \boldsymbol{Z} - \widetilde{\boldsymbol{Y} \otimes \boldsymbol{Z}}$, where $\widetilde{\boldsymbol{Y} \otimes \boldsymbol{Z}}$ indicates the structure-based computed wrapping of each BHB in a PDB-reported structure (ξ) picked from the training set ($\mathcal{I}$), and $\boldsymbol{Y} \otimes \boldsymbol{Z}$ is the DL-based inference of the structure wrapping obtained from the protein sequence of the PDB-reported structure. Thus, the loss function $L(F)$ for the DL network becomes

$$\mathcal{L}(\mathcal{F}) = |\mathcal{I}|^{-1} \sum_{\xi \in \mathcal{I}} \|(\boldsymbol{Y} \otimes \boldsymbol{Z} - \widetilde{\boldsymbol{Y} \otimes \boldsymbol{Z}})(\xi)\|,$$

where $|\mathcal{I}|$ denotes the number of structures in the training set.

While the tensor representation of structure wrapping allows suitable processing in a DL platform with Tensor Flow [17], the tensor should get decoded into a 3D rendering specifying relative spatial locations of wrapping residues vis-à-vis the BHBs to enable the threading of structural decoys onto it (Fig. 12.2). The threading requires a separate inference of the torsional (Φ, Ψ)-conformation of the protein backbone, as performed by AlphaFold, and a fitting of the backbone torsional model onto the decoded 3D model of structure wrapping to determine side chain locations to the level of resolution where it becomes possible to decide whether they contribute to wrap specific BHBs (Fig. 12.2(c)). The full workflow of the DL platform is delineated in Fig. 12.2(a).

12.4 Drug design by teaching to induce folds in targetable proteins

A DL system to solve the drug-induced protein folding problem has been constructed as described in Figs. 12.2(a),(b) following the premises 1–5 given in the previous section. Details for a basic precursor of this system were previously reported [14]. The precursor system has been modified *mutatis-mutandis* to infer induced folding possibilities. The repurposing requires: a) The integration of a sequence-based prediction of disorder [15, 16] as a signal overwriting secondary structure prediction in the residue profiling. This signal is essential to identify regions reliant on binding partnerships to

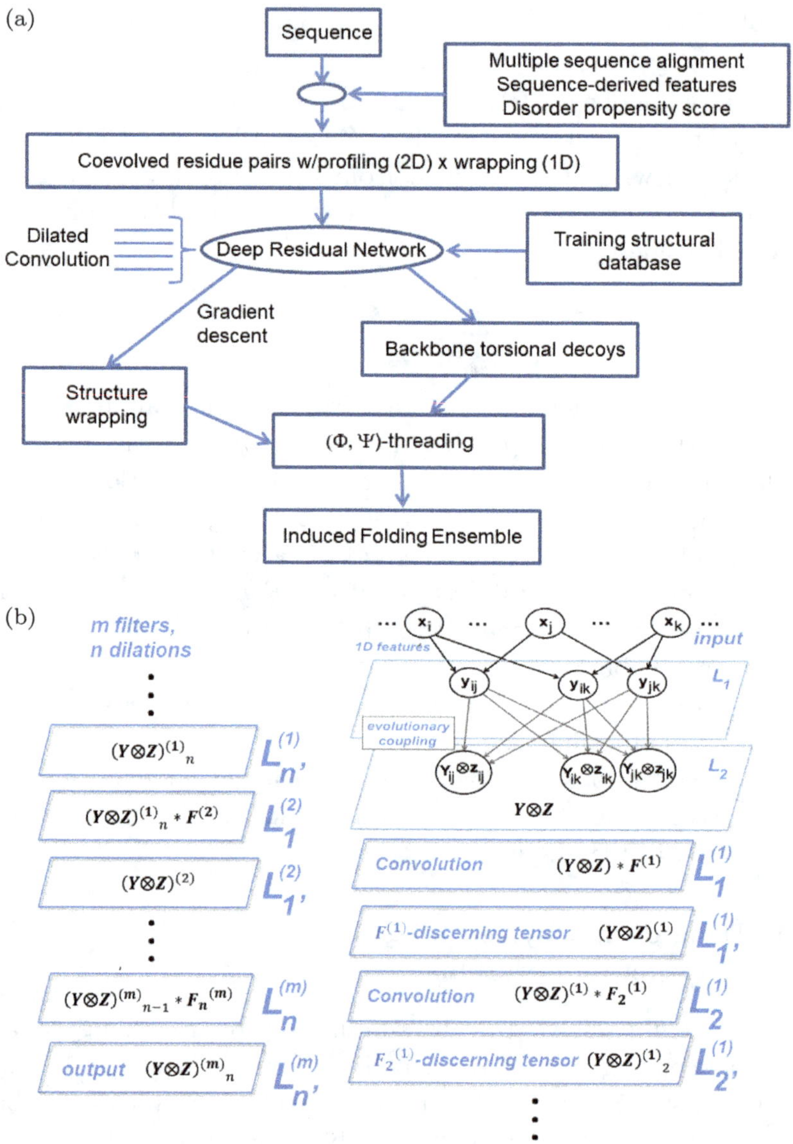

Figure 12.2. (*Continued*)

(c)

(d)

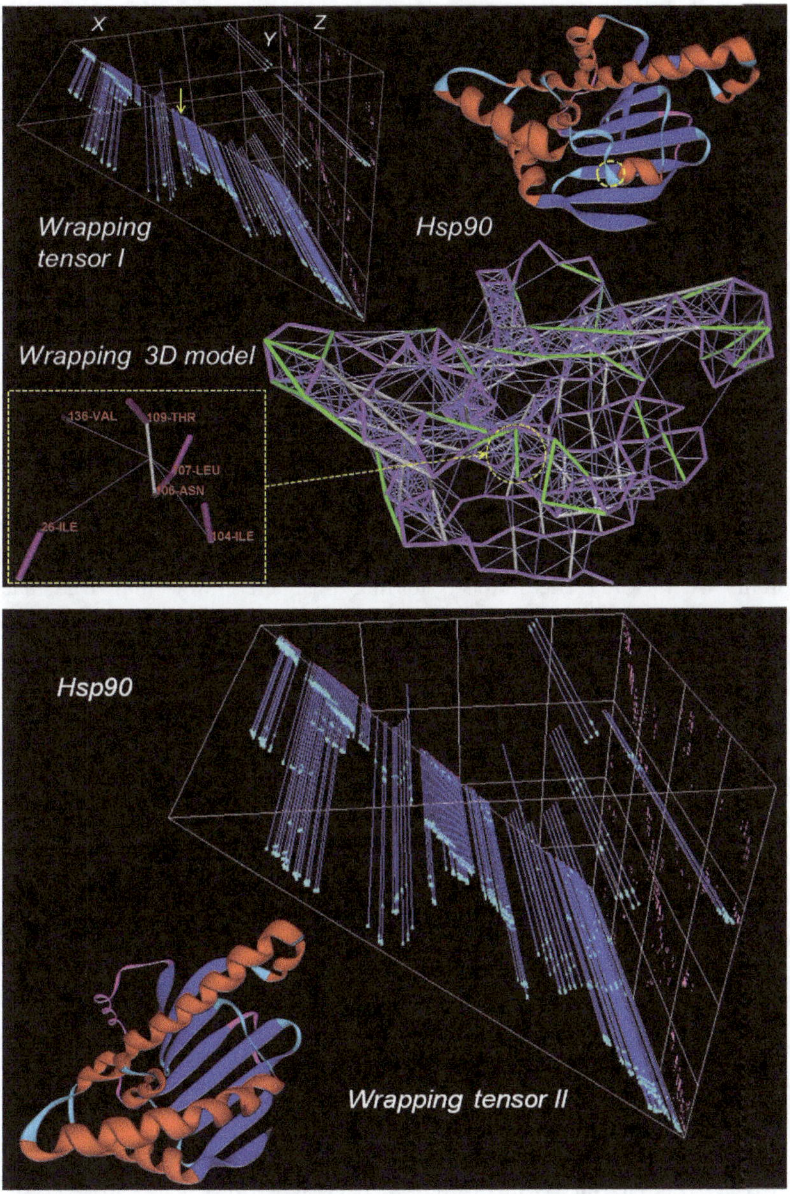

Figure 12.2. (*Continued*)

Figure 12.2. The DL discovery platform and its inference of the IFE for Hsp90. **(a)** Workflow for the DL system. **(b)** Architecture of the dilated convolutional network required to infer structural wrapping patterns. The dummy indices i, j, k indicate residues along the chain and the 1D features, including disorder propensity, are subsumed vectorially in $\mathbf{x}_i, \mathbf{x}_j, \mathbf{x}_k, \ldots$. For feature extraction, the network contains mxnx2 hidden layers labelled $\mathrm{L}_1^{(1)}, \ldots, \mathrm{L}_n^{(m)}$, (m = number of filters/convolution kernels, n = number of dilations per filter). In the cases reported in this study, we used $m = 120$, $n = 6$, so the network has 1440 hidden layers. **(c)** Component I of the Hsp90 IFE, specified by the tetrahedral wrapping tensor, the decoded 3D wrapping model and the threaded 3D backbone conformation in ribbon rendering. The inferred BHBs are represented in the triangle in the background of the tetrahedron, while the residues contributing to the wrapping of each BHB are identified along the axis orthogonal to the background triangle. In the 3D wrapping model of the chain, a residue contributing to the wrapping of a BHB is indicated by a thin blue line between the α-carbon of the wrapper and the center of the wrapped BHB. **(d)** Component II of the IFE for Hsp90, specified by wrapping tensor and ribbon rendering of the 3D structure. Reprinted from [Fernández A (2020) Perspective: Artificial intelligence teaches drugs to target proteins by tackling the induced folding problem". Molecular Pharmaceutics (ACS) 17:2761–2767] with permission from the American Chemical Society.

maintain structural integrity [7,9], and hence susceptible of induced folding in consonance with the ligand. b) The incorporation of dilated convolution in the layered architecture for feature extraction. This is essential to add nonlocal context to the prediction of induced folding, as the receptive field for each layer input gets progressively magnified in accord with the value of the dilation parameter for a given convolution kernel or filter during the feature extraction phase of the DL processing.

The IFE for cancer target Hsp90, obviously excluded from the training set and obtained by incorporating the prediction of intrinsic disorder given in Fig. 12.1(b) is made up of two components, I, II, displayed in Figs. 12.2(c),(d). The display includes structure wrapping tensor and ribbon rendering of the (Φ,Ψ)-threaded conformation. The RMSDs of backbone Cartesian coordinates for I and II relative to the structural coordinates within the complexes (PDB.2XAB and PDB.5LNY, respectively) are 1.9 and 1.2 angstrom.

12.5 Experimental corroboration: AI successfully instructed the reworking of a known drug scaffold to select a new therapeutic target

Drug-based targeted therapy, aimed at blocking specific dysfunctional proteins, often faces a major obstacle due to induced folding, a hard-to-predict phenomenon that often generates unexpected and undesirable cross reactivity while making the intended target elusive to molecular recognition [9]. We advocate that DL can steer drug design to achieve therapeutic impact by controlling the induced folding in the target protein. The way DL may teach the drug to target the protein is apparent as we focus on reworking the anticancer drug *imatinib* [18] into the prototype WBZ_4 ([9, 13], Fig. 12.3). Exploiting wrapping differences among proteins that share a common fold as a filter for selectivity, a chemical modification of imatinib has been introduced to steer the drug impact towards clinically relevant imatinib targets (bcr-ABL, c-KIT, PDGFR kinases [19]), while suppressing off-target cross-reactivity against kinases such as LCK, whose inhibition may lead to harmful immunosuppressive effects [19]. However, just like we may remove potentially harmful cross reactivity by chemically modifying the parental scaffold guided by the wrapping filter [18], we could also incorporate new and therapeutically desirable cross reactivity guided by a kinome-wide examination of IFEs.

By inputting primary sequence, multiple sequence alignment, intrinsic disorder and secondary structure prediction, and pairwise residue coevolution, the IFEs for the 518 human kinases become accessible adopting the DL platform described. As expected, the augmentation of the imatinib scaffold by addition of a methyl group (WBZ_4 in Fig. 12.3) would generally decrease cross reactivity simply because less targets are typically able to accommodate a larger ligand as a result of steric hindrance. This is only partially true, however, as some targets are floppy enough to circumvent steric hindrance, especially those that may be susceptible to binding-induced folding. On one hand, it was experimentally observed that WBZ_4 is not reactive against imatinib target ABL kinase or against

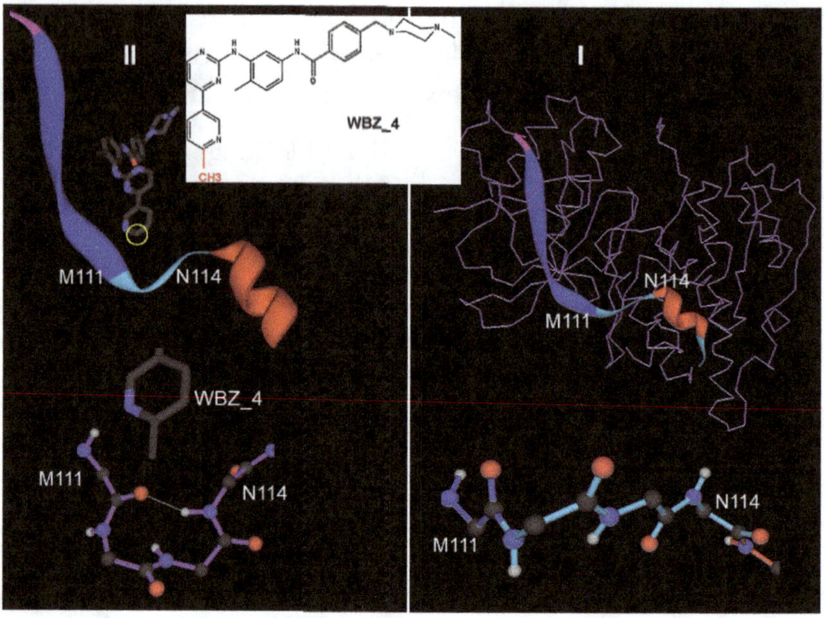

Figure 12.3. The IFE inferred by the DL platform for JNK, a target of WBZ_4 and not of parental drug *imatinib*. The *apo* form is component I and the *holo* form is II. The BHB M111-N114 (actually a dehydron) is induced upon binding to WBZ_4 and absent in the apo form. The two components have identical structure except for the region where induced folding occurs, indicated by the ribbon rendering. This example illustrates the application of AI to steer drug design in order to target a specific protein by learning to induce a drug-binding competent fold. Reprinted from [Fernández A (2020) Perspective: Artificial intelligence teaches drugs to target proteins by tackling the induced folding problem". Molecular Pharmaceutics (ACS) 17:2761–2767] with permission from the American Chemical Society.

LCK, culprits of cardiotoxicity [20] and immunosuppression [19], respectively. However, we found an exception to the steric hindrance rule in JNK1/2, which has no detectable affinity for imatinib but is a target for WBZ_4 [9]. JNK stands out in the kinome-wide IFE inference because of its significant induced folding diversity in the targeted region and its susceptibility to get wrapped by the extra methyl group not present in the imatinib scaffold, as shown in Fig. 12.3. In fact, the nanomolar affinity of WBZ_4 against JNK1 has been experimentally documented [9], making this compound potentially impactful on ovarian cancer, where JNK inhibition has shown clinical relevance, at a variance with imatinib, which is not active in that therapeutic context [20].

The DL-inferred IFE for JNK1 has two components described in Fig. 12.3. An apo form (I), where the dehydron BHB M111-N114 is not formed, and a holo form (II) which we reason must be the conformation adopted in the complex with WBZ_4. We arrived at that conclusion by docking WBZ_4 to JNK according to the structural alignment of JNK with the cKIT/imatinib complex reported in PDB.1T46 and noticing that WBZ_4 binding induces the BHB M111-N114 by contributing exogenously to its wrapping with the extra methyl that is not present in imatinib (Fig. 12.3). Thus, the induced folding enabling the exogenous protection and hence stabilization of the induced M111-N114 BHB is responsible for the new cross reactivity that gets turned on by tuning the parental chemical scaffold.

This example illustrates the use of the DL platform to steer the reworking of a drug in order to redirect its impact towards a different therapeutic context.

12.6 AI-empowered MD reveals the AI-predicted structural adaptation in the drug/target WBZ_4/JNK complex

To further validate the AI inference of the JNK conformation-selecting modification WBZ_4 of imatinib we carried out the MD simulation of the WBZ_4/JNK complex formation in order to capture the structural adaptation of JNK to its putative ligand WBZ_4. To that end, we empowered MD using AI, along the lines described in Chapter 3.

To reduce the informational burden in MD integration steps, we simplify the dynamics taking into account the topology of the MD-steering vector field. Thus microstates/conformations are regarded as equivalent if and only if the respective local conformations of the constitutive subunits lie in the same basins of attraction in the local potential energy surface. This is the "modulo basin" coarse representation of the protein conformation as described in Chapter 3. If x indicates a microstate of a system of N subunits, the modulo-basin class (state) to which x belongs is denoted $\bar{x}$ and may be expressed as a Cartesian product of N basins designating the basin occupancies for the individual subunits: $\bar{x} = \prod_{n=1}^{N} b(x, n)$ where $b(x, n)$ is the basin of attraction occupied by subunit n when the system is in microstate x.

Folding and induced folding trajectories are defined by the evolution of backbone torsional coordinates $\{\phi_n, \psi_n\}_{n=1,\cdots N}$. In this context, the modulo-basin "quotient" space is made up of Cartesian products of the so-called Ramachandran basins, that is, the allowed low-energy regions in the potential energy surface of each residue along the protein chain of length N. Within this mathematical construct, we may project the MD trajectory on the quotient space and then adopt deep learning to propagate the encoded "shorthand" dynamics to make computations more agile. The shorthand dynamics carry far lower information burden, while the transition timescale for each iteration is the intrabasin equilibration time τ = 100ps, considerably larger than the femtosecond integration timescales used in MD. Hence, since intra-basin events are lumped together and the iteration timescale is five orders of magnitude longer, the propagated modulo-basin dynamics has a far better chance of capturing the infrequent or rare interbasin transitions, a highly sought after goal and a significant shortcoming in MD modeling of *in vitro* processes.

The deep learning process to propagate the modulo-basin dynamics, uses a maximum likelihood (ML) ansatz to train a dilated convolutional network (CNN) so that the ML weight, $f_\tau(n, b, b')$, for basin transition $b \to b'$ at chain position n after time τ elapsed is influenced by the amino acid identity and basin occupancy at flanking residues $(\mathrm{n}-1, \mathrm{n}+1)$, with the influence field progressively dilated in the CNN layers so that flanking positions $(\mathrm{n}-2, \mathrm{n}+2)$, $(\mathrm{n}-3, \mathrm{n}+3), \ldots, (\mathrm{n}-8, \mathrm{n}+8)$ with respective strides $g = 1, 2, \ldots, 8$ also impact the transition probability. Computational cost dictates that we limit the extent of dilation to maximum stride $g = 8$. Thus the ML weight of the basin transition becomes:

$$f_\tau(n,b,b') = \prod_{g=1}^{8} w(n,g,A(n,g),B(n,g))f(n,g,A(n,g),B(n,g),b,b') \tag{1}$$

Where $f(n,g,A(n,g),B(n,g),b,b')$ gives the frequency of the $b \to b'$ basin transition at position n after time τ elapsed obtained by projecting MD runs onto a modulo-basin τ-discretized time series for chain composition $A(n,g)$ giving the amino acid identity of residues $\mathrm{n-g, n, n+g}$ in the chain, and basin assignment $B(n,g)$ for residues $\mathrm{n-g, n, n+g}$. The g-stride triads $(\mathrm{n-g, n, n+g})$ bearing on the basin transition at position n are weighted in accord with parameters $w(n,g,A(n,g),B(n,g))$, optimized relative to a suitable loss function. There are $20^3 \times 4^3 \times 8 = 4,096,000$ triad-weighting parameters to be optimized in the ML scheme.

The training of the network yields the transition frequencies $f(n,g,A(n,g),B(n,g),b,b')$ thus following the ML scheme. The propagation of the modulo-basin trajectory (time series) in the ML scheme is determined by the $b \to b'$ transition probabilities: $p_{ML}(n,b,b') = \frac{f(n,b,b')}{\sum_{b''} f(n,b,b'')}$, where b'' is any of the four basins. The destiny basin b′ after a time period τ is determined by a Monte Carlo scheme taking into account the four transition probabilities at each position n along the chain.

The dilated CNN is thus organized into $8 \times 4^3 = 512$ layers in accord with stride g and basin assignment $B(n,g)$ for the triads centered at each position n on the chain and influencing the basin transition at position n. The input is a basin assignment for each residue $\mathrm{n = 1,\ldots,N}$ along the chain, and the output is the basin assignment after time τ has elapsed. In turn, each layer contains $20^3 = 8000$ filters or convolution kernels in accord with the amino acid identity $A(n,g)$ of the triad. To convolve, a modulo-basin state for a chain of length N may be labeled with a 4N-vector $(\mathbf{b}_1|\mathbf{b}_2|\cdots|\mathbf{b}_\mathrm{n}\cdots)$ consisting of N binary 4-tuples $\mathbf{b}_\mathrm{n}(\mathrm{n} = 1,2,\ldots,\mathrm{N})$ indicating the Ramachandran basin occupancy for each residue, so value 1 at entry m in $\mathbf{b}_{\mathrm{n}}$ ($\mathrm{b}_{\mathrm{nm}} = 1$) indicates that residue n occupies basin m ($\mathrm{m} = 1,2,3,4$). For example, (1000|0010) indicates the coarse-grained state of a dipeptide with first residue in basin 1 and second residue in basin 3. Thus, a convolutional kernel $\mathrm{K}(\mathrm{n},\mathrm{g},\mathrm{B}_{\mathrm{K}}(\mathrm{n},\mathrm{g}))$ becomes a triad of binary 4-tuples (basin assignment $\mathrm{B}_{\mathrm{K}}(\mathrm{n},\mathrm{g})$) with stride g, with the convolution operation carrying the Kronecker-delta factor $\delta_{A(n,g),A_K(n,g)}$, where $A_K(n,g)$ is the kernel amino acid assignment for positions $\mathrm{n}-\mathrm{g},\mathrm{n},\mathrm{n}+\mathrm{g}$. Each layer $\mathrm{L}(\mathrm{q},\mathrm{g})$ is labeled by the basin triad $\mathrm{q} = 1,\ldots,4^3 = 64$, and the stride g. In each layer, the $20^3 = 8000$ convolution kernels are slided along the chain as stencils, and full coincidence at position n in $\mathrm{L}(\mathrm{q},\mathrm{g})$ yields concatenation (enrichment) at position n with the four attributes $f(n,g,A(n,g),B(n,g),b,b')$, one for each of the four *a-priori* possible b′ destiny basins. After further processing across all 512 layers, we arrive at a full representation of the chain at layer L(64,8), where each position n is endowed with $8 \times 4 = 32$ transition parameters $f(n,g,A(n,g),B(n,g),b,b')$, one for each stride g and one possible destiny basin b′. In the 513th layer, the products $\prod_{g=1}^{8} w(n,g,A(n,g),B(n,g)) f(n,g,A(n,g),B(n,g),b,b')$ are computed, and the four transition probabilities $p_{ML}(n,b,b')$ are obtained for each of the four *a-priori* destinies b′.

Finally, in the output layer, the destiny basin for each residue is chosen using the Monte Carlo scheme.

The optimization of the field-influence factors $w(n,g,A(n,g),$ $B(n,g))$ is carried out during the training phase of the modulo-basin propagator Γ_τ defined by the Monte Carlo generator of basin transitions. To train the network, we break up the MD trajectories spanning the time period $[0,\mathrm{t_f}]$ into two regions, a training portion with timespan $[0,\mathrm{t_0}]$ and an optimization portion covering the time interval $(\mathrm{t_0},\mathrm{t_f}]$. With the trajectory statistics drawn for the region $[0,\mathrm{t_0}]$ we obtain the basin-transition frequencies for triads with different stride centered at each particular residue. On the other hand, a variational optimization process during the period $(\mathrm{t_0},\mathrm{t_f}]$ enables us to determine the w-parameters. Thus, the w's are obtained from a commutativity condition that reflects the compatibility of fine and coarse grained propagation of the trajectory and must be fulfilled during the period $(\mathrm{t_0}, \mathrm{t_f}]$. The commutativity condition is $\Gamma_\tau \circ \pi = \pi \circ M(\tau)$ as depicted by the following scheme:

$$\begin{array}{ccc} x(t) & \stackrel{\pi}{\rightarrow} & \overline{x(t)} \\ \downarrow M(\tau) & & \downarrow \Gamma_\tau \\ x(t+\tau) & \stackrel{\pi}{\rightarrow} & \overline{x(t+\tau)} \end{array}$$

Here π is the canonical projection that assigns the Ramachandran basins to each backbone torsional state of the chain and $M(\tau)$ is the molecular dynamics propagator operating on torsional states of the chain. In other words, the parametrization of the modulo-basin propagator Γ_τ is optimized to minimize the loss function $\mathcal{L}(\Gamma_\tau)$ given by

$$\mathcal{L}(\Gamma_\tau) = M^{-1} \sum_{q=1}^{M} \|\pi x(t_0 + q\tau) - [\Gamma_\tau]^q \pi x(t_0)\|^2, \tag{2}$$

where $M\tau \leq t_f - t_0 < (M+1)\tau$. We know this loss function is the correct one since $L(\Gamma_\tau) = 0$ if and only if the transition operator makes the diagram commutative. Once the optimal $\Gamma_\tau^* = argmin\, L(\Gamma_\tau)$ has been obtained from stochastic steepest descent, the modulo-basin projected trajectory can be propagated beyond MD-accessible timescales. Physically meaningful timescales may be reached by computing the coarse states $\overline{x(t_f + q\tau)}$ beyond the simulation timespan t_f as $[\Gamma_\tau^*]^q \overline{x(t_f)}$.

The results of the AI-empowered propagation of the MD simulation of the structural adaptation of JNK within the WBZ_4/JNK association process are described in Fig. 12.4. The initial state of the AI-empowered MD run incorporates the PDB-reported JNK structure where the dehydron M111-N114 is not formed, within a metastable complex obtained by positioning WBZ_4 relative to JNK according to the structural alignment with the cKIT/imatinib complex in PDB entry 1T46. The alignment is possible because kinases cKIT and JNK are homologous in so far as they belong to the same superfamily, and imatinib is the parental compound from which WBZ_4 is derived. The choice of initial condition is an educated

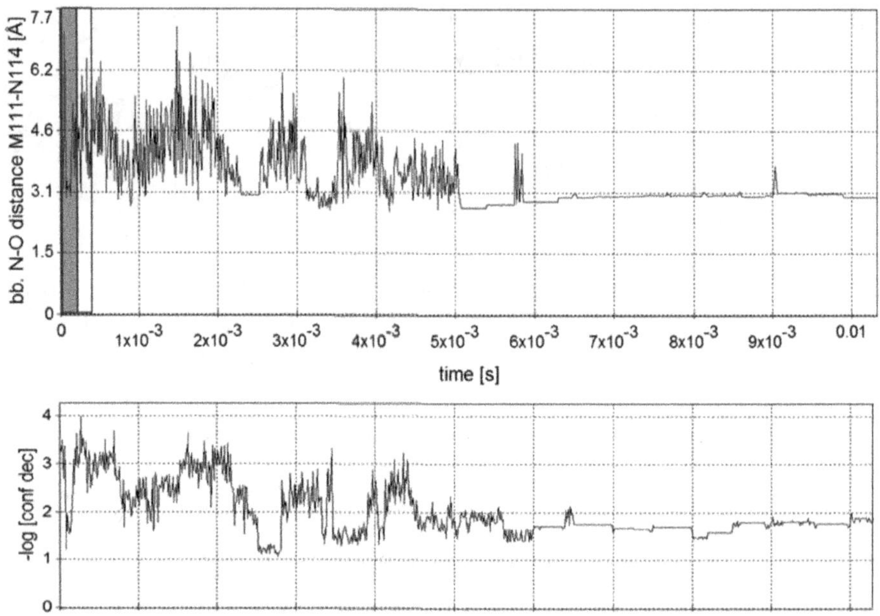

Figure 12.4. AI-empowered MD trajectory of the drug-induced folding trajectory for JNK in complex with WBZ_4 (Fig. 12.3). The backbone N-O distance for residues M111, N114 in JNK is monitored along the trajectory which is given in the lower panel with the modulo-basin chain conformation represented in decimal form, as described in Chapter 10. The BHB M111-N114 is clearly induced at about 6ms, thus signaling the cooperative binding where WBZ_4 methyl contributes exogenously to the wrapping of the BHB (Fig. 12.3). The training unassisted MD trajectory propagated with AI assistance is highlighted by the shaded box with its testing period in the unfilled box.

guess justified since the binding mode of imatinib to kinase cKIT is expected to be similar to that of WBZ_4 with regards to JNK.

The AI-empowered MD simulation clearly reveals that WBZ_4 binding induces the dehydron M111-N114 (Fig. 12.4) by contributing exogenously to its wrapping with the extra methyl not present in imatinib (Fig. 12.3). Thus, we have once more corroborated the AI-based prediction in regards to the conformation-selecting modification of the imatinib scaffold. Not only *AI has taught the drug designer how to modify imatinib to target JNK but has also revealed the specific conformation of JNK induced upon drug/target association and the induced folding process that leads WBZ_4 to select the predicted conformation.*

12.7 AI teaches drugs how to target proteins and identifies the selected conformation in the drug/target complex

Rational drug design faces difficulties and it is felt it may not be living up to the expectations. This is mostly because the target proteins are usually not fixed targets: they structurally adapt to the ligand in ways that have been very hard to predict. That brings us to the drug-induced folding problem that is squarely addressed in this chapter aimed at fueling pharmaceutical discovery within an AI-empowered platform.

We implemented a deep learning (DL) platform to teach drugs to target proteins and identify the selected conformation of the target within the complex with the drug. The DL system is geared at steering drug design to induce targetable binding-competent protein conformations. The control of induced folding by a drug or ligand requires a DL platform that, at a variance with protein folding predictors like AlphaFold, integrates signals for structural disorder to predict conformations of floppy regions that rely on purposely designed binding partnerships to maintain their structural integrity. The conformational diversity of such regions begets an induced folding ensemble (IFE) from which the targetable conformation gets selected by DL-instructed drug design, enabling a therapeutically significant drug-target association.

References

1. Senior AW, Evans R, Jumper J, Kirkpatrick J, Sifre L, Green T, Qin C, Žídek A, Nelson AW, Bridgland A, Penedones H, Petersen S, Simonyan K, Crossan S, Kohli P, Jones DT, Silver D, Kavukcuoglu K, Hassabis D (2020) Improved protein structure prediction using potentials from deep learning. *Nature* 577:706–710.
2. Dill KA, MacCallum JL (2012) The protein folding problem, 50 years on. *Science* 338:1042–1046.

3. Jones DT, Kandathil SM (2018) High precision in protein contact prediction using fully convolutional neural networks and minimal sequence feature. *Bioinformatics* 34:3308–3315.
4. Jones DT, Singh T, Kosciolek T, Tetchner S (2015) MetaPSICOV: Combining coevolution methods for accurate prediction of contacts and long range hydrogen bonding in proteins. *Bioinformatics* 31:999–1006.
5. Yu F, Koltun V (2016) Multi-Scale Context Aggregation by Dilated Convolutions. *arXiv*:1511.07122.
6. Chen JP, Liang H, Fernández A (2008) Protein structure protection commits gene expression patterns. *Genome Biol* 9:R107.
7. Pietrosemoli N, Crespo A, Fernández A (2007) Dehydration propensity of order–disorder intermediate regions in soluble proteins. *J Proteome Res* 6:3519–3526.
8. Ovchinnikov V, Louveau JE, Barton JP, Karplus M, Chakraborty AK (2018) Role of framework mutations and antibody flexibility in the evolution of broadly neutralizing antibodies. *eLife* 7:e33038.
9. Fernández A, Bazan S, Chen J (2009) Taming the induced folding of drug-targeted kinases. *Trends Pharm. Sci.* 30:66–71.
10. Schopf FH, Biebl MM, Buchner J (2017) The HSP90 chaperone machinery. *Nature Rev Mol Cell Biol* 18:345–360.
11. Plaxco KW, Simons KT, Baker D (1998) Contact order, transition state placement and the refolding rates of single domain proteins. *J Mol Biol* 277:985–994.
12. Fernández A, Scheraga HA (2013) Insufficiently dehydrated hydrogen bonds as determinants of protein interactions. *Proc Natl Acad Sci USA* 100:113–118.
13. Fernández A (2016) *Physics at the Biomolecular Interface: Fundamentals for Molecular Targeted Therapy.* Springer International Publishing, Switzerland.
14. Fernández A (2020) Artificial intelligence steering molecular therapy in the absence of information on target structure and regulation. *J Chem Inf Model* 60:460–466.
15. Obradovic Z, Peng K, Vucetic S, Radivojac P, Brown CJ, Dunker AK (2003) Predicting intrinsic disorder from amino acid sequence. *Proteins: Struct Funct Gen* 53:566–572.
16. Oldfield CJ, Dunker AK (2014) Intrinsically disordered proteins and intrinsically disordered protein regions. *Annu Rev Biochem* 83:553–584.
17. Rampasek L, Goldenberg A (2016) Tensor flow: Biology's gateway to deep learning. *Cell Sys* 2:12–14.
18. Druker BJ, Guilhot F, O'Brien SG, Gathmann I, Kantarjian H, Gattermann N, Deininger MW, Silver RT, Goldman JM, Stone RM, Cervantes F, Hochhaus A, Powell BL, Gabrilove JL, Rousselot P, Reiffers J, Cornelissen JJ, Hughes T, Agis H, Fischer T, Verhoef G, Shepherd J, Saglio G, Gratwohl A, Nielsen JL, Radich JP, Simonsson B, Taylor K, Baccarani M, So C, Letvak L, Larson RA, IRIS Investigators (2006) Five-year follow-up of patients receiving imatinib for chronic myeloid leukemia. *New Engl J Med* 355:2408–2417.

19. Fernández A, Scott LR (2017) Advanced modeling reconciles counterintuitive decisions in lead optimization. *Trends Biotech* 35:490–497.
20. Kerkelä R, Grazette L, Yacobi R, Iliescu C, Patten R, Beahm C, Walters B, Shevtsov S, Pesant S, Clubb FJ, Rosenzweig A, Salomon RN, Van Etten RA, Alroy J, Durand JB, Force T (2006) Cardiotoxicity of the cancer therapeutic agent imatinib mesylate. *Nature Med* 12:908–916.
21. Vivas-Mejia P, Benito JM, Fernandez A, Han HD, Mangala L, Rodriguez-Aguayo C, Chavez-Reyes A, Lin YG, Carey MS, Nick AM, Stone RL, Kim HS, Claret FX, Bornmann W, Hennessy BT, Sanguino A, Peng Z, Sood AK, Lopez-Berestein G (2010) c-Jun-NH2-kinase-1 inhibition leads to antitumor activity in ovarian cancer. *Clin Cancer Res* 16:184–194.

Epilogue: AI constructs its own physics

"Nevertheless, I suspect he was
not quite capable of thinking.
Thinking is neglecting differences,
generalizing, abstracting.
In Funes' cluttered world there was
nothing but details, immediacy."

Jorge Luis Borges: Funes the Memorious
(translation by the author)

The program laid out in this book is by no means complete: it cannot be because the subject matter is in a state of flux. The book is inevitably transitional. We are witnessing the dawn of a revolution like no other, as humans, or rather the biological portion of humans, will no longer be at the center of the scene. At a very basic level, our minds are not yet wrapped around the new physics that is emerging from AI-based approaches. It is undeniably physics, but with new categories and based on patterns, the patterns enshrined in the hidden layers of optimized neural networks. This physics has yet to be unraveled by humans, and probably defies intuition. At least we have one certainty: it will always be compatible with the physics we are familiar with, and hopefully strictly equivalent. This is so because the standard well-worn physics of our textbooks is always subsumed in the patterns contained in the training sets.

To get a glimpse of what AI has in store for us, let us go back to the *in vivo* protein folding problem described in Chapter 3. A problem arises that is just as hard as generating expeditious *in vivo* trajectories: it consists of identifying conformations that commit the chain to fold in the *in vivo* context. The problem has haunted researchers for decades and it may well be that the atomistic description we are familiar with is inadequate to provide the proper signal for the nucleating event.

As AI constructs an *in vivo* reality and generates *in vivo* folding trajectories, AI comes up with a solution of its own, oblivious of the wanton complexities of the potential energy surface, which in the new order will be regarded as simply one of many *a-priori* possible representations of the system's physics. The commitment to fold at a particular stage of the process is embossed in a specific snapshot but the information contained in that specific picture/array is not conveyed in an intuitively obvious way. Let us consider the *in vivo* trajectory displayed in Fig. 3.5. We have verified that it converges to a structure topologically equivalent and strikingly similar to the native fold (Chapter 3). Direct examination of the entire trajectory in backbone torsional space resolved modulo Ramachandran basins suggests that the chain is committed to fold at approximately 6.85×10^{-5} s. What pattern perceived by AI triggers that commitment? How does AI "decide" that the state of the system at that time will nucleate the formation of the native fold? At about the time indicated, part of the native fold has been formed and prevails in a quasi steady state while the remaining structural elements are solidified upon the stabilized pattern that appears to function as a buttressing nucleus. This nucleus is stable *in vivo* but not *in vitro*, as it consists of secondary structure but lacks the tertiary structure to wrap it (Fig. 3.5). The wrapping *in vivo* is exogenous, it is furnished by the chaperone incorporated in the training of the deep learning system. Thus, the output pattern that emerges at 6.85×10^{-5} s contains the nucleation signal that commits the chain to fold *in vivo*, but we humans cannot read it. This is physics for AI, not for humans.

AI physics for future projects: Glycosylated proteins and other nested complexities

This entire book is devoted to develop an AI platform for drug discovery, largely focusing on the dynamic aspects of the drug-target interface. Yet, there is an "800-pound gorilla in the room": Actually, about half of the human proteins get glycosylated either co- or post-translationally! Glycosylation is a major chemical modification not dealt with in this book and hardly, if at all, in related studies on molecular targeted therapy based on translational science approaches.

Glycosylation involves side-chain attachment of *glycans*, large linear or branched condensations of monosaccharides. This chemical modification introduces a vast amount of conformational entropy due to the rotameric diversity of glycans and greatly enhances protein solubility and dynamics. The net consequences of glycosylation of concern to biomedical engineers are profound, including a vast alteration of the target aqueous interface and a huge modulation of drug affinity due to a significant entropy loss associated with targeting a glycosylated site.

For instance, immunotherapies against SARS-CoV-2, typically focusing on epitopes in the spike protein, are severely constrained by extensive spike glycosylation that serves as camouflage to immune surveillance (Fig. E1), a fact hardly ever acknowledged. Thus, antibodies, either administered or vaccine-induced, only have an effective chance of targeting the ACE2 interface in the receptor binding domain (RBD) of the spike, which is basically the only antigenic region that is not glycosylated. This local lack of glycosylation is obviously required due to the fitness consequences of impairing the virus ACE2-mediated anchoring to the host cell.

The fundamental biophysical problems underlying the design of drug-target interfaces — i.e., folding, drug-induced folding and drug-induced conformational selection — become even more arduous when targeting glycosylated proteins. They are intractable with current computational resources and require a carefully designed AI

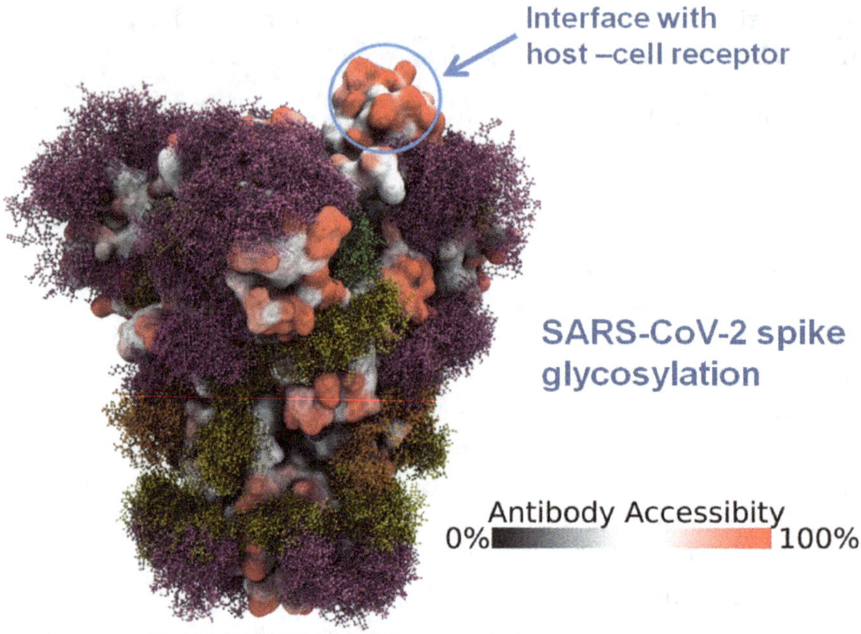

Figure E1. Glycosylation camouflage on the spike protein of SARS-CoV-2 covering 40% of the spike surface and modulating immune surveillance. The exposed interface with the host-cell receptor (circled) is the largest antigenic region with maximum antibody accessibility. The "moss colors" indicate the different glycan types. Adapted from [Grant OC, Montgomery D, Ito K, Woods RJ (2020) Analysis of the SARS-CoV-2 spike protein glycan shield reveals implications for immune recognition. *Sci. Rep.* 10:14991] under Creative Commons CC BY license.

platform. To delineate such a platform we take into account the fact that we are dealing with nested complexities. We begin by noting that the acquisition of huge dynamic information on the rotameric diversity of glycans along drug-induced folding pathways requires a quotient-space simplification along the lines of the procedure described in Chapter 10. This quotient space must be constructed underlying the quotient space simplification that results from the coarse-grained "modulo-Ramachandran-basin" discretized representation of the torsional state of the protein backbone (cf. Chapter 10). Essentially, the AI system learns the information subsumed in full atomistic MD simulations of the glycosylated protein chain captured in its full complexity and generates a suitable folding pathway or induced folding pathway, extending the MD trajectory to realistic timescales completely out of reach within state-of-the-art MD runs.

First, to train the system with detailed dynamic information, a suitable encoding of Ω, the atomistic conformation space for the glycosylated protein chain, is required. Thus, an equivalence relation "$\approx$" is introduced whereby two microstates in Ω become equivalent if and only if they share the same torsional state of the underlying protein backbone. This relation enables the encoding of MD-generated information on quotient space $\Omega/\approx$ via the canonical projection π_{gl}. Trained with MD information, the AI system learns to propagate the simplified MD trajectory within $\Omega/\approx$ by constructing a propagator Υ, so diagram **1** below becomes commutative. Then, the AI system learns to propagate an even coarser description of the MD trajectory by introducing a second equivalence relation "$\sim$" (cf. Chapter 10) where two states in quotient space $\Omega/\approx$ become equivalent if the respective backbone torsional states for each residue belong to the same basin of attraction in the Ramachandran plot. Thus, the dynamics gets further simplified as it gets encoded onto the quotient space $(\Omega/\approx)/\sim$ via the canonical projection composition $\pi\circ\pi_{gl}$. The AI system learns to propagate the trajectory in the discrete space $(\Omega/\approx)/\sim$ by constructing a second propagator Γ, so diagram **2** becomes commutative:

$$\begin{array}{ccccc}
\Omega & \xrightarrow{\pi_{gl}} & \Omega/\approx & \xrightarrow{\pi} & (\Omega/\approx)/\sim \\
\downarrow MD & \boxed{1} & \downarrow\Upsilon & \boxed{2} & \downarrow\Gamma \\
\Omega & \xrightarrow{\pi_{gl}} & \Omega/\approx & \xrightarrow{\pi} & (\Omega/\approx)/\sim
\end{array}$$

The commutativity of diagrams 1 and 2 ensures that the simplified dynamics can be extended way beyond the reach of an MD computation while compatibility with the full-detail computation is ensured. To recover the long-time full atomistic trajectory, two automated decoders μ, μ_{gl} will need to be constructed by the AI system on separate CNNs, so the following diagram for atomistic-level reconstruction of the long-time MD trajectory becomes commutative on the training set of microstate trajectories:

$$\begin{array}{ccccc} \Omega & \xrightarrow{\pi_{gl}} & \Omega/\approx & \xrightarrow{\pi} & (\Omega/\approx)/\sim \\ \downarrow MD & & \downarrow \Upsilon & & \downarrow \Gamma \\ \Omega & \xleftarrow[\mu_{gl}]{} & \Omega/\approx & \xleftarrow[\mu]{} & (\Omega/\approx)/\sim \end{array}$$

This is new physics, physics based on commuting diagrams to handle hierarchically organized complexities in order to empower MD computation. Projecting successively onto quotient spaces seems a "natural" way of handling nested complexities, a pervasive motif in many problems amenable to AI-based approaches. It is expected that more sophisticated AI systems may organize the nesting of complexities in other ways.

Last challenge for wet intelligence

Unveiling the physics generated by AI is a task for the next (last?) all-biological generation to undertake. This is probably the last frontier left to the wet portion of human intelligence. Thereafter, AI will take over the scientific endeavor and displace our biological selves from the center of the scene.

This book should not end on a negative note. It is now time for reflection. The book is coming to an end. Strictly speaking, it is a transitional book introducing AI-based approaches in molecular biomedicine. Yet, the human mind is about to dramatically expand its reach. In three or at most four decades, the nonbiological portion of our intelligence will be billions upon billions of times more powerful than the wet counterpart for which this book is written. Thus, this book, and others of the like, may be placed at the very early stages of the dramatic transformation.

The growth of the capacity of information technology is approaching the point at which an exponential trend is evident. In less than four decades, the trend will become explosive to the point of tearing up the fabric of human civilization. Hopefully, our future may still be recognizably human but will surely transcend our biological nature, to the point when physical and virtual reality will become indistinguishable and exchangeable. In that scenario, this book will become in many ways irrelevant, an archeological curiosity. Yet, the same will be said of most books addressing the biological portion of humans, from Plato to Fernández. But perhaps this particular book will still be worth a mention because of its transitional and prescient character. An imperfect analogy comes to mind as we recall Bohr's model of the atom, which was not really quantum mechanical — as Bohr would have hoped — but was an essential transitional step that ultimately enabled the paradigm shift.

Appendix 1

Code for dehydron identification

The software "YapView" (yet another protein view), currently incarnated as "Dehydron Calculator", is used to identify the dehydrons from structural coordinates of soluble proteins. This program and two equivalent programs, "WRAPPA" and "dehydron calculator in PyMOL plugin version", are currently freely downloadable from the site:

http://people.cs.uchicago.edu/~ridg/softwaredigbio.html

The code for the Dehydron Calculator in Python provided as plugin for PyMol is provided in this Appendix. The open source is found at

https://raw.github.com/Pymol-Scripts/Pymol-script-repo/master/plugins/dehydron.py

YAP View/Dehydron Calculator and the "desolv" plugin within it used to calculate hydrogen bond burial and identify dehydrons are currently hosted at:

http://sourceforge.net/projects/protlib/files/yapview/0.6.8/

The main installer for the windows version (YAPView-0.6.8-1-Installer.exe) comes with a pre-compiled version of the desolv plugin that should be accessible from the UI (user interface).

Code for Dehydron Calculator as PyMOL Plugin (in Python)

```
Dehydron: A dehydron calculator plugin for PyMOL
Version: 1.7
Described at PyMOL wiki:
http://www.pymolwiki.org/index.php/dehydron

Author : Osvaldo Martin
email: aloctavodia@gmail.com
Date   : March 2013

License: GNU General Public License
Acknowledgement: The H-bond detection code is based on the
list_mc_hbonds.py
script from Robert L. Campbell
http://pldserver1.biochem.queensu.ca/~rlc/work/pymol/
'''

import Tkinter
from Tkinter import *
import Pmw
from pymol import cmd
from pymol import stored


def __init__(self):
    """Add this Plugin to the PyMOL menu"""
    self.menuBar.addmenuitem('Plugin', 'command',
                            'dehydron',
                            label = 'Dehydron',
                            command = lambda : mainDialog())


def mainDialog():
    """ Creates the GUI"""

    def get_dehydrons():
        angle_range = float(angle_value.get())
        max_distance = float(dist_cutoff_value.get())
        desolv = float(desolv_sphere.get())
        min_wrappers = float(min_value.get())
        selection = sel_value.get()
        dehydron(selection, angle_range, max_distance, desolv,
min_wrappers)

    master = Tkinter.Tk()
    master.title(' dehydron ')
    w = Tkinter.Label(master, text = 'dehydron calculator\nOsvaldo
```

```
Martin - aloctavodia@gmail.com',
                                background = '#000000',
                                foreground = '#cecece',
                                #pady = 20,
                                )
    w.pack(expand=1, fill = 'both', padx = 4, pady = 4)

    Pmw.initialise(master)
    nb = Pmw.NoteBook(master, hull_width = 420, hull_height=280)
    p1 = nb.add('Main')
    p2 = nb.add('About')
    nb.pack(padx=5, pady=5, fill=BOTH, expand=1)
############################ Main TAB #################################
### hydrogen bond settings
    group = Pmw.Group(p1,tag_text='Hydrogen bond Settings')
    group.pack(fill='x', expand=1, padx=20, pady=1)
    Label(group.interior(), text='angle range').grid(row=2, column=0)
    angle_value = StringVar(master=group.interior())
    angle_value.set(40)

    entry_angle = Entry(group.interior(),textvariable=angle_value,
width=10)
    entry_angle.grid(row=2, column=1)
    entry_angle.configure(state='normal')
    entry_angle.update()
    Label(group.interior(), text='max distance').grid(row=3, column=0)
    dist_cutoff_value = StringVar(master=group.interior())
    dist_cutoff_value.set(3.5)
    entry_dist = Entry(group.interior(),textvariable=dist_cutoff_value,
width=10)
    entry_dist.grid(row=3, column=1)
    entry_dist.configure(state='normal')
    entry_dist.update()
### dehydron settings
    group = Pmw.Group(p1,tag_text='Dehydron Settings')
    group.pack(fill='x', expand=1, padx=20, pady=5)
    Label(group.interior(), text='desolvatation sphere
radius').grid(row=2, column=2)
    desolv_sphere = StringVar(master=group.interior())
    desolv_sphere.set(6.5)
    entry_desolv=Entry(group.interior(),textvariable=desolv_sphere,
width=10)
    entry_desolv.grid(row=2, column=3)
    entry_desolv.configure(state='normal')
    entry_desolv.update()
    Label(group.interior(), text='minimum wrappers').grid(row=3,
column=2)
    min_value = StringVar(master=group.interior())
    min_value.set(19)
```

```
    entry_min_value=Entry(group.interior(),textvariable=min_value,
width=10)
    entry_min_value.grid(row=3, column=3)
    entry_min_value.configure(state='normal')
    entry_min_value.update()
### selection settings
    group = Pmw.Group(p1,tag_text='Selection')
    group.pack(fill='x', expand=1, padx=20, pady=5)
    Label(group.interior(), text='selection').grid(row=4, column=2)
    sel_value = StringVar(master=group.interior())
    sel_value.set('all')
    entry_sel_value=Entry(group.interior(),textvariable=sel_value,
width=10)
    entry_sel_value.grid(row=4, column=3)
    entry_sel_value.configure(state='normal')
    entry_sel_value.update()
### submit
    Button(p1, text="Calculate",
command=get_dehydrons).pack(side=BOTTOM)
############################## About TAB
###################################
    group = Pmw.Group(p2, tag_text='About dehydron plug-in')
    group.pack(fill = 'both', expand=1, padx = 5, pady = 5)
    text =u"""For a brief introduction to the dehydron concept, you
could
read http://en.wikipedia.org/wiki/dehydron

Citation for this plugin:

Martin O.A.; dehydron calculator plugin for PyMOL,
2012. IMASL-CONICET.

Citation for PyMOL may be found here:
http://pymol.sourceforge.net/faq.html#CITE

Citation for dehydrons (I think these could be used):
Fern\u00E1ndez A. and Scott R.; "Adherence of packing
defects in soluble proteins", Phys. Rev. Lett. 91, 018102
(2003).

Fern\00E1ndez A., Rogale K., Scott R. and Scheraga H.A.;
"Inhibitor design by wrapping packing defects in HIV-1
proteins", PNAS, 101, 11640-45 (2004).

Fern\00E1ndez A. "Transformative Concepts for Drug Design:
Target Wrapping" (ISBN 978-3642117916),
Springer-Verlag, Berlin, Heidelberg (2010).
"""
    #
    # Add this as text in a scrollable panel.
```

```
    # Code based on Caver plugin
    # http://loschmidt.chemi.muni.cz/caver/index.php
    #
    interior_frame = Frame(group.interior())
    bar = Scrollbar(interior_frame)
    text_holder = Text(interior_frame, yscrollcommand=bar.set,
foreground="#cecece",background="#000000",font="Times 12")
    bar.config(command=text_holder.yview)
    text_holder.insert(END,text)
    text_holder.pack(side=LEFT,expand="yes",fill="both")
    bar.pack(side=LEFT,expand="yes",fill="y")
    interior_frame.pack(expand="yes",fill="both")

    master.mainloop()


def dehydron(selection='all', angle_range=40, max_distance=3.5,
desolv=6.5, min_wrappers=19, quiet=0):
    '''
DESCRIPTION

    dehydron calculator

USAGE

    dehydron [ selection [, angle_range [, max_distance [, desolv [,
min_wrappers ]]]]]
    '''

    angle, max_distance = float(angle_range), float(max_distance)
    desolv, min_wrappers = float(desolv), int(min_wrappers)
    quiet = int(quiet)


    name = cmd.get_legal_name('DH_%s' % selection)
    cmd.delete(name)

    selection_hb = '((%s) and polymer)' % (selection)
    hb = cmd.find_pairs("((byres "+selection_hb+") and n. n)","((byres
"+selection_hb+") and n.
o)",mode=1,cutoff=max_distance,angle=angle_range)

    if not quiet:
        hb.sort(lambda x,y:(cmp(x[0][1],y[0][1])))
        print "--------------------------------------------------------
------------"
        print "-------------------------Dehydron Results--------------
------------"
        print "--------------------------------------------------------
------------"
```

```
        print "                Donor                |                Aceptor
|"
        print "      Object    Chain Residue   |      Object    Chain
Residue   | # wrappers"

    cmd.select('_nonpolar', '(elem C) and not (solvent or (elem N+O)
extend 1)', 0)
    try:
        cmd.select('_selection', '%s' % selection, 0)
    except:
        pass

    sel = []
    for pairs in hb:
        wrappers = cmd.count_atoms('((%s and _nonpolar and _selection)
within %f of byca (%s'%d %s'%d))' %
                ((pairs[0][0], desolv) + pairs[0] + pairs[1]))
        if wrappers < min_wrappers:
            cmd.distance(name, pairs[0], pairs[1])
            if not quiet:
                cmd.iterate(pairs[0], 'stored.nitro = chain, resi,
resn')
                cmd.iterate(pairs[1], 'stored.oxy = chain, resi, resn')
                print ' %12s%4s%6s%5d | %12s%4s%6s%5d |%7s' %
(pairs[0][0], stored.nitro[0], stored.nitro[2], int(stored.nitro[1]),
pairs[1][0], stored.oxy[0], stored.oxy[2], int(stored.oxy[1]),
wrappers)
            sel.append(pairs[0])
            sel.append(pairs[1])
    cmd.delete('_nonpolar')
    cmd.delete('_selection')

    if len(sel) > 0:
        cmd.show_as('dashes', name)
    elif not quiet and len(hb) != 0:
        print ' - no dehydrons were found - '
    else:
        print ' - no hydrogen bonds were found - '

cmd.extend('dehydron', dehydron)

# vi:expandtab:smarttab
```

NOTE: The code also runs directly from the line of command. It is basically the same as the plugin but adapted to be called from a terminal. When executed as python dehydron_ter.py > log.out it will compute dehydrons for all PDB files contained in the same folder as "dehydron_ter.py" and it would download the results in the log.out file. The code can of course be modified to print the results on a single file (trivial in Python).

```
import __main__
__main__.pymol_argv = ['pymol','-qck']
import glob
import pymol
from pymol import cmd, stored
pymol.finish_launching()


'''
Dehydron: A dehydron calculator plugin for PyMOL
Version: 1.7
Described at PyMOL wiki:
http://www.pymolwiki.org/index.php/dehydron

'''


def dehydron(selection='all', angle_range=40, max_distance=3.5,
desolv=6.5, min_wrappers=19, quiet=0):
    '''
DESCRIPTION

    dehydron calculator

USAGE

    dehydron [ selection [, angle_range [, max_distance [, desolv [,
min_wrappers ]]]]]
    '''

    angle, max_distance = float(angle_range), float(max_distance)
    desolv, min_wrappers = float(desolv), int(min_wrappers)
    quiet = int(quiet)


    name = cmd.get_legal_name('DH_%s' % selection)
    cmd.delete(name)

    selection_hb = '((%s) and polymer)' % (selection)
    hb = cmd.find_pairs("((byres "+selection_hb+") and n.
n)","((byres "+selection_hb+") and n.
o)",mode=1,cutoff=max_distance,angle=angle_range)
```

```
    if not quiet:
        hb.sort(lambda x,y:(cmp(x[0][1],y[0][1])))
        print "--------------------------------------------------------
---------------"
        print "-------------------------Dehydron Results-----------
---------------"
        print "--------------------------------------------------------
---------------"
        print "            Donor               |             Aceptor
|"
        print "     Object   Chain Residue  |      Object   Chain
Residue   | # wrappers"

    cmd.select('_nonpolar', '(elem C) and not (solvent or (elem N+O)
extend 1)', 0)
    try:
        cmd.select('_selection', '%s' % selection, 0)
    except:
        pass

    sel = []
    for pairs in hb:
        wrappers = cmd.count_atoms('((%s and _nonpolar and
_selection) within %f of byca (%s`%d %s`%d))' %
                ((pairs[0][0], desolv) + pairs[0] + pairs[1]))
        if wrappers < min_wrappers:
            cmd.distance(name, pairs[0], pairs[1])
            if not quiet:
                cmd.iterate(pairs[0], 'stored.nitro = chain, resi,
resn')
                cmd.iterate(pairs[1], 'stored.oxy = chain, resi,
resn')
                print ' %12s%4s%6s%5d | %12s%4s%6s%5d |%7s' %
(pairs[0][0], stored.nitro[0], stored.nitro[2],
int(stored.nitro[1]), pairs[1][0], stored.oxy[0], stored.oxy[2],
int(stored.oxy[1]), wrappers)
            sel.append(pairs[0])
            sel.append(pairs[1])
    cmd.delete('_nonpolar')
    cmd.delete('_selection')

    if len(sel) > 0:
        cmd.show_as('dashes', name)
    elif not quiet and len(hb) != 0:
        print ' - no dehydrons were found - '
    else:
        print ' - no hydrogen bonds were found - '
```

```
############ main routine ###########
proteins = glob.glob('*.pdb')
proteins.sort()
for protein in proteins:
    cmd.load(protein)
    dehydron(selection='all', angle_range=40, max_distance=3.5,
desolv=6.5, min_wrappers=19, quiet=0)
    cmd.delete("all")
```

Index

www.ingramcontent.com/pod-product-compliance
Lightning Source LLC
LaVergne TN
LVHW010327220926
848484LV00004BB/853